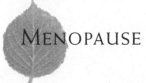

MENOPAUSE

Bridging the Gap Between
Natural and Conventional Medicine

MENOPAUSE

Bridging the Gap Between Natural and Conventional Medicine

LORILEE SCHOENBECK, N.D.,
with CHERYL GIBSON, M.D.,
and M. BROOKE BARSS, M.D.

Foreword by Tori Hudson, N.D.

TWIN STREAMS
Kensington Publishing Corp.
http://www.kensingtonbooks.com

TWIN STREAM BOOKS are published by

Kensington Publishing Corp.
850 Third Avenue
New York, NY 10022

To our patients

Contents

ACKNOWLEDGMENTS

This book was conceived and created in a spirit of collaboration. Many diverse voices have lent their support and expertise, and made this work possible.

First of all, we would like to thank our patients, who have challenged us to bridge the gaps between our (often oppositional) fields of health care, and forge a path that honors their choices to use the best of all their options. This book exists because of you.

Next, we'd like to offer a very special thanks to our illustrator, Donna Harley, who combined menopausal wisdom and incredible talent to produce the images that have brought this book to life. Thank you, Donna, for adding much joy to the project. Thanks also to Amy Dinitz for her work on graphics and patience with endless revisions.

To Elaine Will Sparber, our editor at Kensington; thank you for your expert guidance, patience, and always personable nature in shepherding this book. Many thanks also go out to our literary agent, Nancy Love, who initiated and persevered with this project through its various permutations.

We have received support from many colleagues, and are grateful for the richness of their expertise and their generosity in sharing it. Edward Leib, M.D., Director of the Osteoporosis Center at the University of Vermont, went way beyond the call of duty in editing and contributing to our chapter on bone health. To Cate Nicholas, M.S., P.A., for her continued support, to pioneering researcher Eric Poehlman, M.D., for his contributions to our sections on metabolism, to Jeanne Watson Driscoll, M.S., R.N., C.S., for her groundbreaking work in mental health with Deborah Sichel, M.D., and generosity in sharing it; to author Susun Weed, for the inspiration to stress the importance of "breast health," and to Tori Hudson, N.D., for her immense contribution to the field of women's health and for teaching many of the principles embraced in this book, thank you.

Lorilee would also like to thank the naturopathic medical community, for championing and daily applying the principles of holistic healthcare. Thank you to Bart for his lasting friendship and "on call" I.T. support. Special thanks go to Beverly Jacobson and carolyn V. Brown, M.D., for all their work on this book while it was still in proposal form. To Phillip J. Schoenbeck, M.D. (aka Dad), for his unending support and to Lynn Bliss, R.N. (aka Mom), for always believing in this path, thank you. And finally, to Robin, for his love, patience and understanding and for modeling what's possible in being a human being, thank you.

FOREWORD

In the last few years, many books have been written in the attempt to meet the many needs of perimenopausal and menopausal women. Women are seeking reliable sources of information for relief of their varied symptoms, prevention strategies for osteoporosis and heart disease, information to allay their fears of breast cancer, and answers to their many questions related to hormone replacement therapy. Women are also eager to learn more about herbal, nutritional, and natural hormone alternatives for menopause.

Women want safe, effective, affordable medicine. Women want to be educated about their bodies and their health. Women want to make choices in their health care that they have determined are right for them. Women increasingly choose a more collaborative and cooperative approach to their health care, sorting, sifting, and integrating alternative therapies with conventional medicine options. By philosophy, design, and commitment, this approach to one's health care can give women what they want: cooperation with their health care provider, and collaboration amongst their health care providers. This new concept is called integrative medicine. I believe it is the menopausal woman who is the greatest force behind this new medical framework. It is the menopausal woman who is most responsible for her varied health care practitioners working together, and who most questions the status quo, demands information, asks questions, and wants to make informed decisions.

When Dr. Schoenbeck asked me if I would be willing to write the foreword for the book she was writing with a gynecologist and a psychiatrist, I was very happy to oblige. I have been acquainted with Dr. Schoenbeck since she was a medical student and I have known her to be a committed proponent of this new practice of integrative medicine. In collaborating on such a project, Dr. Schoenbeck, Dr. Cheryl Gibson, and Dr. Brooke Barss have accomplished the task of providing everything a woman needs to know to find solutions to her own menopausal issues.

Many of the naturopathic approaches discussed in this book can stand alone as viable, safe, and effective treatment options. Others can be used in an integrative approach along with conventional treatments. Some women and situations will require conventional medical treatments and it may be the purpose of the natural therapies to minimize the side effects of those treatments. This book, *Menopause: Bridging the Gap Between Natural and Conventional Medicine*, will help to sort through the many decisions to be made. I found it thorough, reliable, and an extremely valuable guide for all women facing perimenopause and menopause.

The authors of *Menopause: Bridging the Gap Between Natural and Conventional Medicine* have astutely recognized the need for an integrative approach by listening to their patients. They have been willing to communicate with each other, across medical perspectives, and build bridges on behalf of their patients. They are helping to create this new medicine because they recognize its value and they recognize that while both conventional and alternative medicine are inadequate alone, they are here to stay. The strengths of each are magnified in the presence of the other. The weaknesses of each are minimized in the presence of the other. Women and their health care needs in menopause will be much better met, and women will be empowered and healthier, by following the principles and practice of *Menopause: Bridging the Gap Between Natural and Conventional Medicine*. I will be pleased to recommend this book to my patients, knowing that the choices they make will be based on accurate information and principles they can trust.

—Tori Hudson, N.D., author of
Women's Encyclopedia of Natural Medicine

PREFACE

Because of our patients, we have evolved as doctors. Women's demands for better health care have forced us to break down the invisible barriers that existed between us and build bridges instead. Because of our patients, we—a naturopathic physician, a gynecologist, and a psychiatrist—have found ourselves collaborating on patient care. In response to those who want the best of both natural *and* conventional medicine, we have written this book.

It is largely pioneering, *female* patients, with their instinctive knowledge of the mind-body connection, who are opening the lines of communication between practitioners historically at odds with one another, and are thereby fueling *integrative medicine*. In our case, patients of Cheryl's gynecology practice would ask her for a natural treatment for hot flashes. Cheryl would send them to Lorilee, a naturopathic physician. Lorilee or Brooke (a psychiatrist) would refer one of their patients to Cheryl for an important gynecological problem. As the patients traveled between practitioners, so did the communication. Women requested that we talk to one another about their concerns. It wasn't such an odd request—after all, isn't that what doctors should do? When we collaborated, our patients were relieved and often thrilled that experts from such different worlds were working together on their behalf. No longer forced into the middle between "dueling practitioners," they were able to concentrate on finding the right solutions for their problems—using the best of natural and conventional medicine *together.*

Building bridges between the worlds of gynecology, naturopathic medicine, and mental health has certainly caused evolution for we three as practitioners. Each of us remains firmly grounded in our own respective field, yet has come to recognize when another view might work better. We are interested in providing accurate information to our patients, which means also making appropriate referrals to those with more knowledge in certain areas. We are also committed to recognizing and challenging our *own* biases. We prioritize our patient's well-being and are willing to challenge personal and professional beliefs, if appropriate.

One of the greatest gifts of our collaboration has been the discovery that our similarities greatly outweigh our differences. Our commitment to empowering women through active participation in their own health care forms, perhaps, the basis of our connection. More important, we are adamantly opposed to any "one size fits all" definition of a woman's experience of menopause, and firmly support women in finding their unique path.

This book brings together what we feel are the most viable, successful approaches to maintaining wellness during the menopausal transition and beyond, from the fields of natural and conventional medicine and mental health. We have integrated our treatments within each chapter because we believe it is time to erase the divisions between natural and conventional medicine, and between mind and body health. By bridging the gap between natural and conventional medicine, we have created a continuum of health care options that supports a comprehensive, whole-woman approach to well-being. With it, hundreds of our patients have found unique combinations of lifestyle, dietary, psychological, herbal, pharmaceutical, and even sometimes surgical supports on their menopausal journeys. We hope to help you find the right combination of these, too.

Through our collaboration, we also hope to provide a model for *practitioners* to reach across professional barriers, and work together in the best interests of patients. (To encourage the process, buy a copy of this book for your practitioner!) It's you, the woman going through menopause, who has changed everything else you've touched so far in this lifetime. It's you again who will challenge your practitioners to collaborate, thereby changing the face of medicine. We owe this to future generations, and we owe this to ourselves.

INTRODUCTION

Women of the baby-boom generation have changed everything. They've completely altered the face of the workplace, transformed woman's role in society and redefined family life. Baby boomers are a powerful economic and political force, and their persistent questioning of authority has brought about evolution in every part of their collective experience. As they encounter menopause, it's no surprise that this generation is changing everything about that, too.

Women today are demanding more *choices* and more accurate *information* regarding their health care. More than ever, women are taking charge of their medical decisions. In sharp contrast to their mothers' generation, they do not sit quietly in the doctor's office and nod with complacency. Instead, they show up with a list of questions, an article, or a bag of supplements, requesting guidance amid a barrage of new information about menopause. Sometimes they get their questions answered. Too frequently, however, they don't.

Today's health consumers are catching their health care practitioners off guard. First of all, most practitioners weren't trained to expect patients to assume such an active role in their health care. Secondly, clinicians and consumers alike are finding themselves inundated with new and constantly changing information about women's healthcare. This has a great deal to do with the onslaught of results from research initiated in the 1980s and 1990s, when women successfully got medicine to stop ignoring their unique health issues. Now, while tons of new information is pouring in every day, we have precious little time to sift through it all. And the young research has yet to gain consensus on some issues. Many questions remain unanswered.

The volumes of rapidly changing, conflicting reports can take only part of the blame for the difficulty facing women who need to make important health care decisions. *Enter natural medicine*—a vast field that has rapidly expanded women's options. It was hard enough to make a decision about hormones. Now, we have to think about herbs, vitamins, and all the rest!

Women have instinctively known for a long time that neither natural nor conventional medicine has all the answers. That's why we've been using herbs, supplements, chiropractic, and other modalities along with regular gynecological health care for years. Yet it wasn't until Harvard researchers discovered that 42 percent of the population uses alternative medicine—and spends more out of pocket on it than they do on conventional medicine—that many *practitioners* started to take this force seriously. A few opened their minds to the alternatives. Those who felt threatened when patients looked to alternatives continued to reinforce the gap between these two medical worlds.

Today, we desperately need collaboration between practitioners from all sides of health care. The alternative—lack of interest or frank disdain toward practices on "the other side"—has left patients in the middle of a turf war, trying to sort out the mass of conflicting information about therapies. "Take hormones or you'll get osteoporosis," says one source. "No, don't take hormones—they cause cancer. Herbs are safer," retorts another. "Herbs haven't been studied. They could be dangerous," counters another source. "Natural is best—I'm eating soy." And on it goes . . . When all the various sources are in such disagreement, it is no wonder that confusion arises. How do you know who is right?

One thing is certain: anyone claiming to have all the answers doesn't. A dogmatic proponent of *any* health care method who categorically dismisses or attacks another approach does health consumers a disservice. Both natural and conventional practitioners are guilty of stubbornly trying to sell their approach when a patient could benefit more from a different one.

Health care practitioners aren't the only ones to blame when it comes to confusing the public about whether to use natural or conventional medicine. The very nature of our competitive, market-driven culture sets us up for a war between advertisers. With nearly 5,000 women in the United States entering menopause *each day*[1] perimenopausal and menopausal women have become the largest target of commercial campaigns for natural products. Since every pill or supplement maker wants a piece of your wallet, they all are going to promote their wares as if they're "the answer" for everyone.

Whole industries, in fact, have capitalized on the huge baby-boomer menopausal market. Vitamins and supplements have become big business almost overnight. New manufacturers and distributors for these items have grown up spontaneously. Once-conventional pharmacies now carry full lines of herbal, homeopathic, and nutritional products. Clinics and hospitals have added alternative medicine to their offerings. Books on alternative medicine have mushroomed on the shelves of bookstores, and it seems like every magazine cover boasts a "new" natural medicine cure.

Importantly, *the demand for alternative medicine has outstripped the access to reliable, accurate information about its use.* As a result, some practitioners, pharmacies, and distributors are promoting therapies in which they have little or no training, or are selling products that have shown little evidence of effectiveness.

So what are we to do?

As part of our collaborative approach, the authors of this book have created a basic strategy that can transform an often overwhelming process of navigating through menopausal options into an empowering one. It consists of three basic components: *individual assessment, accurate information,* and *supportive practitioners.* We believe that if all three components are in place, a woman has an excellent chance of being able to use the health care system to support her well-being in her menopausal years. These components are important enough to spell out.

Individual Assessment

Product advertisements and even many well-intentioned books and articles are aimed at a mass audience. The writers have no idea who *you* are, what kind of family medical history you have, and what your experience of menopause is. In an attempt to sell you on a particular product or idea, some information sources may be delivering a message that has nothing to do with you. Understanding the notion that *each woman's menopause is a unique experience* is the first step in simplifying the process. Our book will guide you in assessing what's unique about your situation.

A comprehensive clinical assessment by a qualified health practitioner can help you know both what to focus on and what to ignore. It should include not only attention to current symptoms, but also an evaluation of health issues likely to crop up for you in the coming decades. Because most of us will survive to age 85 or beyond,[2] with one-third to one-half of our lifetime lived after menopause, we need to factor in issues like bone and heart health when making lifestyle, medication, and other health-related choices at menopause. In this book, we'll help you ascertain which areas are most important for *you.*

In addition to getting a good clinical assessment, it's also important to access your own inner knowing. Throughout this book, we will guide you in integrating your intuition into an overall assessment. We're getting older, and we're getting wiser. It's time to put that wisdom to good use.

Accurate Information

Just as no single profession has all the answers regarding health, no one type of practitioner has all the information we want at menopause, especially if we intend to explore both natural and conventional options. No matter how highly qualified health professionals may be in their own area, they cannot be proficient at therapies for which they have no training. This applies to all fields of health care. Many practitioners in fields of alternative medicine have deficiencies in clinical experience with pathology, pharmaceutical drugs, and diagnosis. It's unwise to ask a homeopath to assess a broken leg or a nutritionist to recommend medications. Likewise, if you ask your pharmacist, a health-food store worker, or even your gynecologist about herbs for menopause, you may be looking for information where it is not available.

Learning *who* to consult for *what* information is the first step to getting expert guidance. This usually means meeting with two different types of practitioners, if you really want accurate advice about two very different approaches.

Supportive Practitioners

Finally, there is likely to be bias inherent in any advice you receive. Historically, the institutions of conventional and natural medicine have been at odds with one another. Each side lacks knowledge about other approaches and comes armed with its own agenda. Practitioner bias, whether toward natural or conventional approaches, often colors the advice that is given. Although this dynamic is changing, particularly among the younger generation of practitioners, it still slips out insidiously whenever a practitioner warns her patient against a therapy that the practitioner knows little or nothing about.

It's important to choose practitioners who respect your questions, support you if you choose to explore another option and are committed to helping you find the best choices for *you*—whether they be natural or conventional options. A practitioner from any field who discourages or frankly dismisses other options out of hand is probably more committed to his or her own dogma than to your health.

We think women today deserve the best that both natural and conventional medicine has to offer for their menopause. They deserve accurate and thoughtful advice, respectful dialogue, and plenty of options when approaching this transition. Our offering to you, *Menopause: Bridging the Gap Between Natural and Conventional Medicine*, models the change that women everywhere are demanding and are partners in creating. We hope it touches you, and helps you find radiant health in these, your "crowning" years.

Menopause and Perimenopause

1

Menopause is a natural transition in a woman's life. Derived from the Greek words "men" (month) and "pausis" (cessation), menopause signals an end to monthly menstruation and to the reproductive years. *Perimenopause* is the time before the actual menopause, when cycles may change and symptoms appear. Perimenopause can last only a few months or up to several years, and is different for every woman. Some women sail through the perimenopause with no symptoms except changes in their monthly cycles, while others experience hot flashes, mood swings, erratic bleeding, and other discomforts.

Your Reproductive Years

Let's go back to the beginning. Way back. Your reproductive history actually starts before your actual birthday. As you grow inside your mother's uterus, your tiny ovaries are developing. By the time you are born, your ovaries will have made and stored all of the potential eggs that you will use throughout your cycling years. These eggs, some 1–2 million in number at birth,[1] rest in wait during childhood. They await their chance to gain center stage during your reproductive years, when about 400 will have the chance to mature into follicles (maturing eggs) and ovulate.

Your first ovulation marks puberty. This means that one pioneer follicle leaves home (the ovary) and travels down the fallopian tube to the inside of the uterus. (See Figure 1.1.) If not fertilized by a sperm on its journey, this follicle disintegrates and washes away in a couple of weeks along with tissue that lined the inside of your uterus (called the *endometrium*)—and this is your first menstrual period.

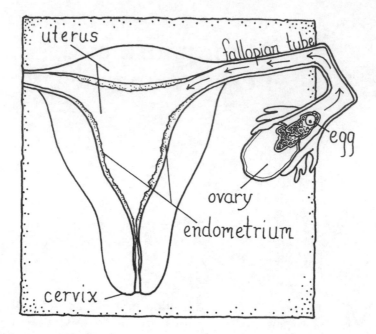

Figure 1.1.   An egg leaves the ovary and travels down the fallopian tube to the inside of the uterus.

By knowing what happens during a complete menstrual cycle, you will then easily understand what can happen around menopause. Let's look at Figure 1.2.

Figure 1.2 is read from left to right, the numbers corresponding with the days of the menstrual cycle. Most women's cycles vary somewhat between 25 and 32 days. We've chosen 28 days as an average, even though only about 15% of women hit this number right on the dot.[2]

Look what's happening to the levels of your female sex hormones, estrogen and progesterone, throughout a normal reproductive cycle. Notice that they do not remain constant. Their up-and-down fluctuations, in fact, cause (or caused) you to cycle.

Both estrogen and progesterone are at their lowest points beginning on the first day of your menses, which we call "Day One" of your cycle. The cycling process begins with the pituitary gland in the brain secreting follicle stimulating hormone (FSH) in response to the low levels of estrogen. Accordingly, estrogen levels begin to climb in the beginning of your cycle.

Days 1–14 are known as the "follicular phase," because one of your eggs is maturing into a follicle and preparing to exit—or ovulate. In fact, it is actually this growing follicle, along with a support group of sorts—some of

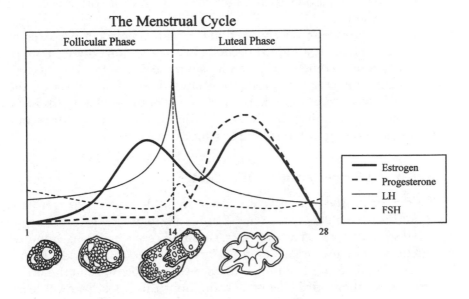

Figure 1.2. *Hormone levels and development of follicle during one menstrual cycle.*

its neighboring follicles—that produce the estrogen you see rising on the chart.

Ovulation

Lots of interesting things happen in the middle of the cycle, at ovulation. Around Day 14, after a sustained rise in estrogen, the pituitary gland releases surges of leuteinizing hormone (LH). The LH surge causes ovulation. The egg is shot out of the ovary, and begins its descent down the fallopian tube toward the uterus.

One possible fate for this egg is to encounter a sperm and become fertilized as it travels toward the uterus (pregnancy). During the follicular phase, the uterus was actually preparing itself for just such a possibility. (Just imagine—this happens every month!) Those high estrogen levels caused the endometrium to grow, so that just in case a fertilized egg came down the fallopian tube this month, it would have a nice, cushy, nutrient-rich bed to burrow into, and there, a fetus would develop.

Progesterone plays its part too. Notice how it rises on the right half of our graph. Produced during the second half of the cycle, the "luteal phase," progesterone stabilizes the endometrium. It does this by encouraging the growth of blood vessels, which bring oxygen and other nutrients to the uterine lining.

This entire production occurs so that the body is perfectly prepared to support a pregnancy, if it indeed occurs. Most of the time, however, we're just running a dress rehearsal. When no sperm arrive to fertilize the egg, progesterone and estrogen production shut down. It is primarily the decline of progesterone (and therefore the loss of those blood vessels stabilizing the uterine lining) at the end of the cycle that makes the endometrium die and shed off, resulting in a menstrual period.

Estrogen and Progesterone's Other Roles

Besides being the key players in your monthly cycles, estrogen and progesterone have many other roles. Estrogen initiates the growth of your so-called secondary sex characteristics, causing breasts, pubic hair, and reproductive tissues and organs to grow. Progesterone usually adds the finishing touches, like contributing to the growth of milk ducts in the breast and preparing them for lactation. Throughout this book, you will learn many other important ways that these female sex hormones affect not only reproductive organs, but almost every area of the body: from the brain to the bones to the heart, and many places in between.

> *The moon's choreography*
> *is less reliable now.*
> *Unlike the obedient tides*
> *my body chooses its own tempo,*
> *sways out of rhythm*
> *then drifts in step again*
> *for a measure or two . . .*
>   (from "Cross Currents," by Noelle Sickels)

Changes in Bleeding Patterns

Changes in bleeding patterns occur for every woman during the perimenopause. For about 10% of women, periods simply end, without any fanfare whatsoever. For others, periods may lighten and come less frequently. Yet other women experience erratic cycles and heavy bleeding. The adage "The only thing certain is *change* itself" definitely applies to menstruation at perimenopause.

Many women notice that their periods take on different characteristics—whether lighter or heavier, longer or shorter—as early as their late 30s. However, true perimenopausal cycle irregularities begin, on average,

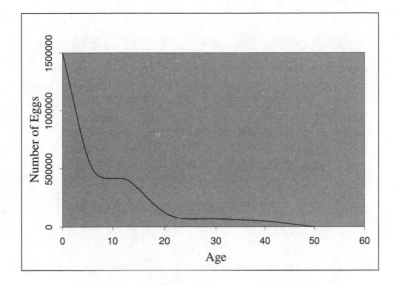

Figure 1.3.   Number of viable eggs a woman has during her lifetime.

between ages 45 and 47½.[3,4] We see a huge variability in how long these bleeding changes persist. Studies show the average length of this time to be 4 years.[5] After the variability stops, generally so do the periods.

Let's look at why changes in our cycles happen. Remember that you were born with all the eggs you will ever have. After 30 35 or so years of ovulating, you begin to actually run out of viable eggs. (See Figure 1.3.)

As we mentioned, some women just stop cycling all of a sudden, and go from having regular periods to none at all. Most women, however, experience some type of cycle irregularities.

Figure 1.4 shows the expected estrogen levels throughout a woman's lifetime—perhaps yours. You will notice that during childhood, as expected, you produced almost no estrogen until puberty. Estrogen levels shot up suddenly at that time, and for a few years, may have fluctuated quite a bit. No doubt, you remember the effects that estrogen had on your body, as well as your emotions, at puberty.

Peak cycling estrogen levels remain relatively constant throughout your reproductive years, until the perimenopause begins. At this time, fluctuations in estrogen levels mirror those you may have experienced in puberty. Beginning 2 to 8 years before menopause, most (but definitely not all) women experience longer cycles.[6] Periods may become a little lighter.

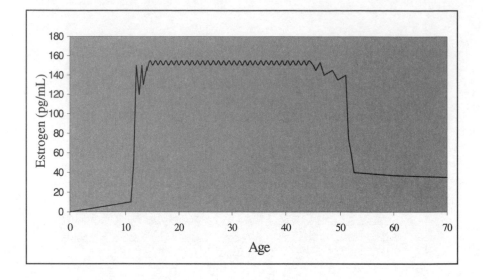

Figure 1.4.   Average estrogen levels throughout a woman's lifetime.

Many women in their 40s, who are still a long way from the actual cessation of their periods, report that instead of having several days of moderate or heavy bleeding during their periods, they'll have only one or two days of moderate bleeding, followed by two to four days of very light bleeding or spotting.

Although the above pattern is common, many variations exist. It is also common for women to report heavier periods as they go through their 40s. Depending on factors such as weight fluctuations, diet, exercise, medications, supplements, stress levels, thyroid function and metabolism, your cycles may be different compared to how they were in the past. These changes are usually perfectly normal.

It is important to note, however, that conditions other than menopausal hormone changes can cause unpredictable bleeding. These include uterine fibroids, polyps and overgrowth, or even cancer of the endometrium. If you are concerned about bleeding irregularities, particularly in the absence of other signs of perimenopause, it's a good idea to speak with your practitioner about what could be causing your symptoms.

When Ovulation Doesn't Happen

By the time of perimenopause, the number of estrogen-producing follicles has dwindled significantly. Some months, the ovaries are able to produce enough estrogen to stimulate endometrial growth, but not enough to trigger the LH surge that causes ovulation. A woman might then skip a period altogether. If she ovulates the next month, the period may be heavier than usual, as the endometrium was growing for a longer time.

Prolonged and/or heavy bleeding can also result from an anovulatory cycle. This occurs because without ovulation, there will be no second half of the cycle or luteal phase, and hence, little or no progesterone production. (Remember that progesterone stabilizes the endometrium after estrogen initiates its growth.) A relative excess of estrogen and deficiency of progesterone means this tissue grows, but is very unstable. "Flooding," or excessive bleeding can result. Heavy or prolonged periods can sometimes cause anemia, so if you experience either, you should contact your health care practitioner.

On the other hand, if the tissue does not shed, or doesn't shed completely, a buildup of tissue, known as endometrial hyperplasia, can occur. This is a condition that needs to be managed by a health care provider experienced in managing gynecological problems, and usually calls for a temporary prescription of progesterone.

Although sometimes uncomfortable, bleeding irregularities are usually normal—and treatable. Only very rarely does heavy bleeding during the time of perimenopause signal a serious problem, such as abnormal endometrial growth or cancer. If you have prolonged heavy bleeding, periods that just won't quit, or are otherwise concerned, please consult with a health care practitioner who can recommend an ultrasound or a biopsy if she or he feels it is warranted. Much of the time, however, you are more likely to be reassured that perimenopausal hormonal changes are the culprits.

Is There a Test for Perimenopause?

Menstrual irregularities, hot flashes, and other fairly obvious signs make testing for perimenopause seldom necessary. If there's any question about what's causing symptoms you may have, your health care practitioner can order a blood test known as an FSH level. Recall that FSH rises in the beginning of the cycle during your reproductive years in response to low levels of estrogen. *In perimenopause, FSH keeps rising*, as fewer and fewer follicles are capable of making estrogen.

Because FSH levels tend to fluctuate from month to month in perimenopause, you could have a normal FSH level even if you are definitely in this phase. A high FSH level, on the other hand, can be information that supports the diagnosis of perimenopause, and sometimes reassures a woman who would like an explanation for her symptoms.

When you're really out of follicles (menopausal), your FSH will remain steadily high. *You are technically in menopause if your FSH level remains consistently over 30 to 40 milli international units per milliliter (mIU/mL)*, depending on the laboratory used, *or if you have completed a full year without a period or spotting*. Important note: You can still become pregnant until then.

Women often ask if testing estrogen or progesterone levels can help diagnose menopause. If you recall how widely these hormones fluctuate during a normal cycle, you can understand how different your hormone levels would be depending upon what day you obtained them. Today estrogen could be high, and a week later it could be low. Because of this, we don't recommend blood testing for estrogen and progesterone as reliable indicators of menopausal status. For *post*menopausal women, whose estrogen levels remain constant, a clinician may get some good information by checking estrogen levels, say—to monitor someone's course of hormone replacement therapy (HRT), for example.

Growing interest as well as controversy surround the emerging technique of salivary hormone testing. Proponents of these tests state that hormone levels in the saliva more closely resemble the levels found in the organs that respond to them (such as the breasts or uterus) than do blood levels. In addition, the relative ease and absence of needles in this testing method make it attractive to many people.

Furthermore, proponents argue, salivary testing measures the "unbound" or active form of hormones, whereas blood tests largely measure "bound" or inactive hormones. Hormones, like estrogen, travel around the bloodstream attached to proteins, much like you or I would travel down a highway in a car. Only when we actually get out of the car—or in this case, when the hormone actually detaches from the carrier protein, is it active. Salivary hormone testing measures "free" or active hormone.

The accuracy of salivary hormone testing depends on the hormone being tested. For instance, testing of cortisol (a nonsex hormone produced by the adrenal glands) levels via saliva has gained acceptance in medical research, because salivary and blood levels correlate well. Likewise, testosterone levels in blood and saliva demonstrate a predictable relationship, and may be equally accurate.

On the other hand, data concerning the accuracy of testing estrogen in the saliva varies from good to poor. Research into salivary progesterone is mostly limited to fertility studies at this time, with little information available yet about menopausal or perimenopausal women. One study which compared salivary progesterone levels with that in the bloodstream for 23 normally-cycling, 10 pregnant, and 5 postmenopausal women on HRT did find salivary progesterone measurements to accurately correlate with levels in the bloodstream.[7]

Besides the lack of consistent correlation between blood and saliva hormone levels, there is a significant technical difficulty with this method. Saliva itself flows more or less abundantly at different times,[8] leading to fluctuating salivary hormone levels throughout the day. In other words, an 8 A.M. "deficiency" could turn "normal" by 3 P.M. Additionally, collection of saliva with cotton-based materials can lead to artificially high results for estrogen, progesterone, testosterone, and DHEA.[9]

Perhaps in the future we will have information and experience with salivary testing to make it an affordable and largely accepted guide for women in perimenopause. It is possible that today, a clinician experienced with these testing methods may glean some information helpful to understanding your situation. But you need to know that these testing methods are still considered experimental and are not proven to be accurate measures of perimenopausal estrogen and progesterone status.

Our collective experience as clinicians tells us that following a woman's symptom picture closely is usually a more reliable way to manage the perimenopausal symptoms than either blood or salivary hormone testing. Given the changeable nature of perimenopausal hormones, you're likely to find different values from one month to the next anyway, no matter what form of testing is used. In other words, you can usually save time, energy, and money by foregoing the added tests. There's an old doctor's saying that goes like this: "Treat the *patient,* not the lab work." Nowhere is this more true than during perimenopause.

Factors Affecting Menopause

Many women find their mother, or older sister's experience of menopause somewhat predictive of their own. If you do a little research into your family history, you can use the information you learn to your advantage. For example, knowing when your mother entered menopause gives you an indication of when yours may begin. Likewise, if you begin having symptoms reminiscent of Mom's or older sister's perimenopause, you might recognize them, and be better equipped to handle them.

Not every woman's perimenopause will be like that of her female relatives, however. Significant differences in lifestyle, medication use, and surgery history are some of the things that can alter the ability to predict what might happen at this time. For example, current smokers stop menstruating on average 1.5 years before nonsmokers. Even a past history of smoking can lead to earlier menopause, and the more cigarettes and longer you have smoked, the earlier menopause begins.[10,11] Thin women as well as undernourished women experience earlier menopause,[12,13,14] because body fat produces estrogen. Vegetarians have a slightly earlier menopause,[15] probably because they are overall thinner than nonvegetarians. Alcohol consumption is associated with later menopause,[16] probably because it interferes with the metabolism of estrogen.

A Family History Checklist

Fill in the following information about your mother or an older sister:
1. Age she stopped having periods _____
(If she had a hysterectomy, what age and for what reason? Were her ovaries removed?)
2. Age when perimenopausal symptoms first appeared, if any _____
3. Types and severity of perimenopausal discomforts _____
_____
4. Did she take hormones? Dates, type, effectiveness, and side effects
_____
_____
5. General lifestyle habits affecting health (Did/does she smoke? Eat a healthy or unhealthy diet? Exercise?) _____
_____

If you begin experiencing bleeding changes or what seems like perimenopausal symptoms and are concerned about them, fill out the "Family History Checklist" above and bring it to your clinician. It will help you both assess whether or not your symptoms are perimenopausal in nature, and help you more quickly find relief. It can also help you both gauge how strong your tendency might be toward this symptom, and therefore choose a therapy of the appropriate strength. For example, if your mother and older sister had intolerable and incessant hot flashes, and you begin to have them as well, you may opt to begin on a relatively strong therapy, for faster and more complete relief. In Chapter 3, we will discuss the whole range of remedies for hot flashes.

Perimenopausal Symptoms

Aside from changes in—and an eventual end to—menstrual periods, some women experience absolutely no perimenopausal discomforts at all. While we discuss symptoms, please keep in mind that you are not obligated to have any! Just know that in case any of these discomforts do show up, they are likely to be normal, related to hormones, and often quite treatable, should you desire help.

Night Sweat

You wake, holding nothing in your arms
but your arms, and try to call back your dream. . . .
You don't move, waiting for the night to wipe off your forehead,
dry your neck, your arms, your legs now free
of covers, your side slick against the sheet,
the moon behind the dark leaves of the magnolia
a clock's face over your shoulder . . .

(from *Wanting to Know the End* by Judy Goldman)

Hot Flashes and Night Sweats

Women talk about flashes more than any other perimenopausal or menopausal experience.[17] Ten to 25% of perimenopausal women have them at any given time.[18] According to the National Institute on Aging, more than 60 percent of women in the United States experience hot flashes at menopause.[19]

Hot flashes are affected by changes in the temperature of our environment, stress, diet, exercise, and other factors. In Chapter 2, we will discuss how incidence of hot flashes and night sweats varies in women living under different conditions, and in different countries.

Hot flashes and night sweats are known to health practitioners as *vasomotor changes*. "Vaso" refers to blood flow and "motor" means movement. Vasomotor changes occur, therefore, when blood flow suddenly shifts from one part of the body to another. Hot flashes decrease without treatment, for most women, after one or two years. For some women, however, hot flashes and night sweats can last up to five years or more. We'll talk more about vasomotor changes in Chapter 4.

Insomnia

Nighttime waking at perimenopause usually results from vasomotor fluctuations. Research shows that perimenopausal insomnia results from the same fluctuations in blood flow and temperature that cause hot flashes and night sweats.[20, 21, 22] In many cases, it is an actual night sweat that wakes a woman up. In other cases, although temperature elevations aren't high enough to cause noticeable heat or sweating, the fluctuation itself is enough to disturb sleep.

Many women notice a particular pattern to their insomnia at this time. They usually get to sleep without difficulty, but wake in the middle of the night. In Chapter 4, we will further discuss patterns of insomnia, other contributing causes, and what to do about them.

Mood Changes

Some people are surprised to learn that the majority of women report an improvement in their psychological health at menopause. In Chapter 6, we will explore this issue more deeply, and shed light on the myth that menopause is a time of emotional turmoil and depression.

That said, we all know women (perhaps family members, friends, or even ourselves) who experience mood swings, irritability or depression around the time of menopause. In Chapter 6, we'll highlight fascinating new work which links hormones and moods, and outline an approach to mental wellness for any woman, regardless of her menopausal status.

Memory Changes

"Now why did I come into this room?" "Where are those keys?—I just had them." "Please hand me the . . . whatchamacallit . . . that thing over there!"

Do these phrases sound familiar? Many perimenopausal women are surprised to find themselves at a loss for words, literally, when referring to common objects or names of people—even people they know well. Within what seems like a relatively short period of time, a perfectly adequate brain can become fuzzy, easily distracted, or lose its train of thought. If making lists has become a survival tactic for you—you'll find help in Chapter 8. We'll also explore the role estrogen and some natural medicines might have in slowing the progression of Alzheimer's disease. Please note that changes in mental function do not occur for every woman. Some women, in fact, report that after an initial period of "fuzzy thinking," their concentration returns and becomes even sharper than before, and they later become more focused than ever.

Vaginal Issues

Vaginal tissue relies on estrogen in order to maintain strength and elasticity. While some women are not aware of any vaginal symptoms, others may experience itchiness, discomfort or even pain. This can become especially apparent during sexual activity.

Lower estrogen levels can also raise the acid-base balance, or pH, in the vagina, making some women more susceptible to vaginal infections. Fortunately, most vaginal problems at menopause respond quickly to therapy. In Chapter 8, "Sexuality and Bladder Health," we will point you toward the most effective natural and conventional treatments.

Urinary Issues

Like vaginal tissue, the lining of the bladder and urethra (the opening out of the bladder) also depend on estrogen for thickness and general health. Increased bladder "sensitivity" often accompanies dropping estrogen levels. A frequent urge to urinate is a common menopausal complaint.

Stress incontinence, or the loss of urine while sneezing, coughing or lifting can develop for some women at menopause. This is partially influenced by a decrease in bladder "tone" or integrity of tissues, which occurs when estrogen levels fall. Some women experience an increased susceptibility to bladder infections at menopause, again as a result of decreased estrogen levels and ensuing changes in tissues and pH. The good news again, is that all of these problems can usually be treated and prevented with natural and conventional means. In Chapter 8 we'll show you how.

Changes in Skin and Hair

Estrogen receptors are found on the skin and may be involved in proper function of collagen, which gives our skin elasticity and strength. The skin's elasticity and moisture decrease when we enter menopause, and this can show up as wrinkles and a general loosening of the skin. Also, scalp, underarm, and pubic hair may gradually thin, as we age. These issues can be some of the most challenging for women who live in our culture, where beauty is narrowly defined and arbitrarily promoted as being "young-looking." Likewise, hair cropping up in unwanted places, like on our chin or nipples, can challenge our feminine identity. In Chapter 2, we will explore more expansive cultural definitions of beauty and promote a necessary change in how we approach menopause psychologically. Then, in Chapter 5, we will describe available treatments and realistic outcomes in slowing the visible signs of aging.

Weight Gain

"It's occurring right in the middle," says 50-year-old Elizabeth, a bank teller and mother of three. "It is my belly, mainly. Nothing else is bigger— not my arms or legs or breasts. And no matter how many sit-ups I do, it doesn't seem to change."

Several factors can contribute to changes in weight around menopause. These include changes in thyroid function (and therefore changes in metabolism), activity levels, diet, and, indirectly, hormone levels. In Chapter 5, we'll learn what's happening at menopause, what can actually be healthy about some weight gain for thin women, how much is too much, and what to do about it.

"Perimenopausal PMS"

As the menopausal years approach, changes in cycles can sometimes include changes in our experience with premenstrual syndrome (PMS). Elizabeth also describes experiencing a longer time of premenstrual discomfort before her periods. "I used to have about three days of breast tenderness and bloating before my period—and I was able to predict when it was coming. Now I can get those changes for two weeks or longer. It feels like my period should be coming, but it might not come for weeks." Stories like Elizabeth's are common. Other premenstrual discomforts, such as "hormonal headaches," mood disturbances, and food cravings can stretch out for days, when they had previously been short-lived or rarely present.

Theories about the cause of PMS range from imbalance in brain chemicals, to imbalance in female hormones, to social and cultural feelings about menstruation. In Chapter 3, we will examine these potential causes more closely and offer several very effective approaches for what we call "perimenopausal PMS."

Heart Palpitations

Some women experience an increase in heart palpitations or "flutters" around the time of menopause. This can include a sense of rapid or irregular heart beat, and usually lasts for just a few seconds. Episodes may occur rarely or several times per day. Of course, if you are concerned about them, experience shortness of breath, fatigue or pains that accompany the palpitations, please see your practitioner to have them checked out. However, the vast majority of heart palpitations at perimenopause are benign. In Chapter 4, we'll offer treatments for these.

Loss of Sexual Desire

Sex is one of the most complex issues in the human experience. Factors as diverse as social structure, illness and medications, depression, relationship status, and hormones contribute to a woman's *libido*, or sexual desire. Researchers generally agree that testosterone, produced in small amounts in women by the ovaries, plays an important role.

Testosterone production can end abruptly if a woman's ovaries are removed. This is sometimes referred to as a "surgical menopause." In a nonsurgical or natural menopause, testosterone production may decline slightly at menopause. Although this varies from woman to woman, a decline in testosterone can sometimes be found prior to menopause.[23]

There is considerable debate about just how much estrogen itself contributes to sexual desire. Certainly estrogen effects the health of sexual tissues and affects how enjoyable sex can be. In Chapter 8, we will expand upon sexuality in menopause, and teach you about the herbal, hormonal, and other therapies that work best in promoting what *you* consider a healthy sex life well into the menopausal years.

Fatigue

Aside from changes in sexual energy, some women experience a drop in overall energy at perimenopause. It is important to rule out medical causes of fatigue, such as low thyroid function, anemia or depression. Low testosterone levels can contribute to fatigue in a minority of women at menopause. A decline in hormones produced by the adrenal glands can also contribute to fatigue. In our chapters on sexuality and HRT choices, we have included lengthy discussions about testosterone and adrenal hormones along with all the other hormones.

Most commonly, fatigue can be caused by several contributing factors at perimenopause—not the least of which is lack of sleep. An overly demanding life can tire us out too. If you and your practitioner have ruled out medical causes for fatigue, it may be time to ask yourself, "Am I doing too much?"

Aches and Pains

Forty-six-year-old Marian scheduled a visit to her massage therapist, hoping it would help with some minor aches and pains she had been experiencing lately. "I just feel 'creaky,' " she explained. Osteoarthritis, which is caused by normal wear and tear on the cartilage which cushions our joints, has been shown in some studies to accelerate at menopause. In Chapter 12, we'll discuss the emerging data on the relationship of hormones to arthritis, as well as excellent natural options for maintaining our joints.

Positively Menopause

If the list above seems worrisome, remember this: *you aren't obligated to experience any of these symptoms!* If you do find some of them to be interfering with your life, there is help. In this book, you will find natural and con-

ventional remedies for everything listed above, and will be guided in helping you work with your health care practitioners to decide which solutions
will work best for you.

For many women, menopause provides relief from long-time gynecological symptoms. Uterine fibroids, which can cause intense cramping and
excessive bleeding, will shrink as estrogen declines. The pain associated
with endometriosis usually vanishes at menopause. Fibrocystic breast tissue softens, making it easier for most women to perform breast examina-
tions. Women with severe PMS, who have been at the mercy of their
fluctuating hormones, can look forward one day soon to a smoother ride
from month to month. When cycling has finally ended, the breast tenderness, bloating, food cravings, mood swings, and other discomforts some
women experience as PMS will be history—or should we say *herstory*. And
important to note, once menopause has been firmly established, there's
no need to worry about birth control. Many women report feeling relieved and more at ease about their sex lives without that responsibility.

The menopausal years can have profoundly positive effects on our psychological health as well. Throughout this book, we will explore not only
the challenges, but perhaps as much or more important, some of the mental, emotional, and spiritual benefits available to us in menopause.

2 Menopause in Transition

The views her culture carries of menopause make an indelible impression on every woman within the culture and can color, if not define, her experience of "The Change." This is especially true if a woman is unaware of the cultural biases that grip her and likewise unaware that she can, to some extent, choose a different path. Knowing how beliefs and practices can influence the feel of this transition time for women in different cultures and different points in history can help us see that we are not obligated to have any one particular experience of menopause. Rather, this insight helps free us to make more conscious choices about what to expect, which will undoubtedly influence what's to come.

Menopause Across Cultures

The stories told by menopausal women across the globe, collected by pioneering female anthropologists, have advanced our understanding of how much culture affects the look and feel of menopause. In general, women in developing nations or traditional cultures have a much easier time in menopause than Western women. By studying what these women are doing and *thinking* that allows for a more graceful transition, we'll learn what we can do to influence our own transition.

Japan

During the 1980s, anthropologist Margaret Lock, Ph.D., of McGill University in Montreal, compared the menopausal experiences of over 10,000 women between 45 and 55 years of age in Japan, Canada, and the

United States. Lock also interviewed the physicians of these women. What she found advanced our understanding of how menopause looks and feels very different, depending on what culture in which a woman lives.[1]

At the start, Lock was astonished that there was no Japanese word for "hot flash," and more so when she found no word for *menopause!* She would later conclude that the Japanese had no word to signify the end of menstruation simply because it was not a significant event. Specifically, the Japanese women interviewed experienced no more symptoms at this time than at any other time.

Lock learned that the closest word in Japanese to "menopause" is the term *konenki.* Similar in meaning to the English "climacteric," *konenki* traditionally referred to "a long, gradual process, to which the end of menstruation is just one contributing factor."[2] Originally, the *konenki* was described as a time of life roughly between the ages of 40 and 60, rather than any particular medical event. In recent years, Western notions of menopause have rubbed off on the Japanese. Accordingly, the *konenki* has now popularly come to be associated with the cessation of a woman's menses—and a natural event has turned into a health issue to be singled out and concerned about.

Lock's next finding was that the actual symptoms experienced by Japanese women at this time were very different than those of the Western women. Some Japanese physicians involved in her study, in fact, did not even mention hot flashes as a menopausal symptom. Rather, these doctors indicated that *shoulder stiffness* was the most common symptom reported by Japanese women at the time of menopause. Likewise, "ringing in the ears" and "a heavy feeling in the head" were symptoms that the Japanese women and their doctors commonly associated with *konenki* but are not known to be menopausal symptoms in the West. Indeed, Japanese doctors today are looking for effective (even hormonal) treatments for the common menopausal symptom known as "AST," or abnormal sensation in the throat,[3] another symptom that you won't find on the list of Western women's experiences at menopause.

Lock found that vasomotor symptoms did exist for the Japanese, but that their incidence was much less than that for the North American women. When "hot flash" was translated as best as possible into Japanese, 14.7% of women reported experiencing this in the previous two weeks, compared to 38% and 36% in the United States and Canada, respectively. Night sweats were uncommon. Only 3.8% of the Japanese women had these, and the women did not associate them with menopause. By contrast, 11.4% of women in the United States and 19.8% of Canadians had hot flashes in the same time period. Additionally the Western women were three times as likely to have trouble sleeping than the Japanese women.

Lock found yet further differences in experience. Western women complained of depression two to three times more frequently than Japanese women. Lack of energy, a symptom in nearly 40% of the Western women, was present for only 6% of Japanese women. In fact, the Japanese women reported a less overall number of complaints when compared to Canadian and American women. Their most common problems were joint stiffness, diarrhea/constipation, and backaches.[4] Contrary to the North Americans, Japanese women did not have more complaints during menopause or perimenopause than they did at other times.

One can certainly argue that Japanese women may be less prone to mention their complaints than women in the West. Lock points out, however, that Japanese women are known to be keenly aware of subtle bodily sensations, and that their language has many more descriptive terms for physical sensation than does English—so any lack of words describing discomforts at menopause is probably not due to an economy of language or a lack of awareness. Most notably, the difference in *types* of complaints suggests a different overall experience with this phase of life across the cultures.

The now famous dietary influence of phytoestrogen-containing soy products in the traditional Japanese diet likely contributed to the lack of symptoms Lock found in Japanese women. In addition, cigarette, alcohol, fat, and coffee intake were extremely low in comparison to those of Western women at the time of Lock's study, and vegetable and fish consumption were high. Exercise and herbal medicines are popular among Japanese. All of these factors may have played a part in minimizing "menopausal" complaints for the Japanese.

Bone health seems to differ between Japanese and Western women too. Other researchers have described a historic lack of osteoporotic fractures in Japanese women,[5] and proposed phytoestrogens, as well as vitamin D-containing dietary fish as supporting bone health.[6] (We'll learn more about vitamin D for bones in Chapter 7.) These and other factors may be the reasons why Japanese women are the longest living women in the world despite the fact that only 2% of them take hormones.[7]

Another cultural influence on Japanese women's experience of *konenki* may be the historical practice of traditional Japanese medicine. Sino/Japanese medicine dominated this country's health care practices until the twentieth century, and persists to varying degrees in Japanese culture today. This system, akin to Chinese medicine, describes the end of menstruation as potentially causing symptoms of headaches, dizziness, palpitations, chilliness, and dry mouth.[8] These symptoms, the explanation goes, results from "stale blood," a condition not specific to the cessation of menses, nor specific to women.

Lock writes that modern, Western-trained gynecologists in Japan began to "medicalize" *konenki* at the end of the twentieth century after attending international meetings on the subject of menopause. Returning to their country, some began to write articles in prominent women's magazines in Japan, describing hot flashes as the "typical" menopausal symptom. In her conversations with Japanese gynecologists, she learned that some had newly focused their work on treating *konenki*. These doctors suggested that "economic pressures" had forced them into finding a new market for their practices.

By 1990, Japanese gynecologists began holding seminars to inform health care workers about menopause and Western treatments. Their work led to the formation of the Japan Menopause Society for practitioners, and spawned the founding of the Japan Amarant Society, an information and support group for menopausal Japanese women. To the women who join this society, these gynecologists are viewed as "modern specialists" and "heroic" whose intentions are to reform the Japanese health care system for women and improve access to therapies such as hormone replacement. An editorial in an international medical journal for menopause, written by the founder of the Japan Amarant Society, supported the doctors' efforts. The author, Lady Nobuko Albery, stated in 1999 that Japanese women today *do* suffer from hot flashes and more. She writes: "the menopause and all its symptoms and suffering are alive and unwell in Japan!" [9]

It is difficult to understand another culture through the lenses of one's own, and impossible to know exactly *why* Japanese women complain of more menopausal problems now than in the past. However, the rapid integration of Western health care ideas and practices seems a likely contributor. In fact, Japanese society is undergoing a rapid decline in *many* areas of health, including heart disease and colon cancer (which we'll talk about in upcoming chapters), as it Westernizes many areas of lifestyle. By witnessing certain declines in the health status of this traditional Eastern nation as it adopts our Western beliefs and practices, we have an unprecedented opportunity to see just how much *our* culture affects our health.

More Cultural Variations on Menopause

Over time, many additional researchers have found cultural variation in both the attitudes toward, and experience of menopause. Australian anthropologist Gabriella Berger surveyed the existing studies of menopause in other cultures, and included her own research in her book *Menopause and Culture*.[10] Like Lock, Berger has consistently found that both menopausal symptoms and mental outlook differ significantly across cultures. The differences, furthermore, are to some extent predictable.

Among Western or industrialized cultures, hot flashes and night sweats are particularly prominent. Western women generally report that they have

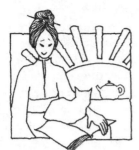

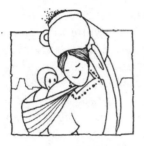

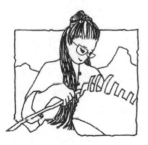

been told to expect these symptoms, and that menopause will be difficult and unpleasant. In her interviews with Australian women for example, Berger noted that several women felt abnormal if they had no symptoms. Also, fears about changes in appearance predominate in the West.

By contrast, women in Eastern or developing countries may not even recognize the "pause" in menstruation as a significant event. They experience fewer, but also different symptoms than Westerners, as evidenced by the lack of a word for "hot flash" in the traditional languages of China, Japan, Indonesia, and the Yucatan.[11,12] Finally, women in developing nations tend to regard this transition more positively than Western women. They look forward to release from childbearing, and to enjoying the position of respect that these cultures associate with age.

One study Berger refers to compared Indonesian and Greek women for menopausal symptoms. Indonesian women complained of fewer and also different types of menopausal symptoms compared to Greek women. Indonesian women complained most frequently of fatigue and weight gain. Greek women, on the other hand, had an overall larger number of complaints, and vasomotor symptoms predominated (with an astonishing 73% complaining of hot flashes).

Berger points out that Mayan women "welcomed [menopause] as a favorable transition to a new niche in the village lifestyle, characterized by relief from childbearing, acceptance as a respected elder, and a surrendering of many household chores to the wives of married sons."[13] Anthropologist Y. Beyene interviewed Mayan women who claimed to welcome menopause, using phrases such as "being happy," "free like a young girl again," "content and good health" to describe this time of life. "No Mayan woman reported having hot flashes or cold sweats," Beyene writes, theorizing that their habituation to a warmer climate may affect this. "Anxiety, negative attitudes, health concerns, and stress for Mayan women were associated with the childbearing years, not with menopause."[14]

Of note is the fact that despite the fact that the Mayan women lived 30 years into menopause, they have a very low incidence of osteoporosis. A study printed in the *American Journal of Obstetrics and Gynecology* by researchers at the University of California Medical School at San Francisco found that although bone density decreased with age in Mayan women from Mexico, height did not decrease and no clinical evidence of osteoporosis was detected. The reason for this is unclear. Genetics and bone structure may play a role. It is also probable that a lifetime of weight-bearing exercise, unprocessed foods, and absence of smoking and alcohol contributed to the Mayan women's health. Finally, it is also possible that their cultural outlook on the cessation of menses, which they associated with freedom, played a part as well. Mayan women simply expect to be better off at menopause.

The reports from Mayan women again illustrate that a variety of cultural differences, rather than just one factor, may contribute to women's different experience of menopause. Diet, environment, pregnancies and genes, in addition to attitudes, factor into the menopausal equation.[15] (Important—it isn't estrogen levels which account for the difference. Mayan women in menopause have been found to be just as "estrogen deprived" as any other menopausal women.[16]) Therefore, we might benefit from an overhaul of our Western thinking—in which we tend to separate out the pieces when seeking a cause, and look for a single "magic bullet" for a cure. These other cultures may be showing us the benefits of a holistic approach, where many interconnected parts affect a person's well-being.

The reports from Filipino women, both living in their native land and in the United States, further demonstrate that menopause feels different among women of different cultures. A study of Filipino women living in Manila found that headaches, irritability, and dizziness were more common experiences during perimenopause and menopause than hot flashes.[17] A second study of Filipino women, those living in the United States, found that the vast majority (86.1%) of these women reported that they "felt energetic," and 83.6% described a sense of "well-being" in menopause.[18] Only 17% of women experienced distress associated with estrogen-related symptoms. Filipino women, both living in Manila and the United States, regarded menopause in a positive light.

Cross-cultural differences in menopausal experiences persist even among women who live in the same nation. Interviews with over 16,000 Chinese, Japanese, Hispanic, African-American, and Caucasian women, all living in the United States, were tabulated in the Study of Women's Health Across the Nation.[19] Incidence of hot flashes, night sweats, sleep problems, urine leakage, and aches and pains differed significantly, depending on ethnicity. Financial strain also increased symptoms, which indicates that economics could also play a role in a woman's experience of menopause.[20]

A study in Thailand of 150 Thai women and 20 health professionals illustrates an example how even two distinct groups within one culture (presumably with different agendas) perceive menopause differently. While women described menopause as a "simple and natural biological event," health professionals described it as a "medical problem requiring treatment."[21]

Berger chronicles the "medicalization of menopause" in Australia, which parallels that of the United States. She pinpoints the adoption of the definition of "menopause as deficiency disease" by the medical community historically, and tracks its infusion into cultural belief. Even the word "symptom," she argues, implies that menopause is a "disease." She advances the notion that perimenopausal discomfort or ease could be self-fulfilling prophecies. She proposed that Western cultures, like Australia and the United States, contribute to women's menopausal symptoms via planting the expectation that each woman who goes into menopause will inevitably fall prey to the symptoms of this "deficiency disease."

The Changing Face of Menopause in the West

Even within the same culture, changes in attitudes and opinions about menopause over time can manifest in radically different experiences for women. Fortunately for us, Western society today supports a much more empowered version of menopause than it did for previous generations, though it may not always be a realistic one. When we can clearly see the ridiculous nature of arguments that support negative or unrealistic images of what's supposed to happen to women at menopause, we loosen their grip on us and become free to create our own experience.

Menopause Then

The image of the menopausal woman that the mothers and grandmothers of Western women had to contend with left them little encouragement for a positive "change." Prominent (and mostly male) artists, philosophers, and physicians painted a picture of a hysterical, hypochondriacal, and shriveled woman, depressed at her inevitable loss of femininity, and therefore, reason for being. Western culture adopted these erroneous images, and the menopause, which for many civilizations is recognized as a natural and welcome transition, was then culturally constructed in the West to be a dreaded and disempowering event.

Medical diagnoses reflected and promoted these cultural beliefs. Early editions of the Diagnostic and Statistics Manual (DSM—the standard manual still used by medical and mental health professionals to categorize mental illness) included menopause as a "depressive psychosis involutionary syndrome." Around 1900, the diagnosis of "involutionary melancholia" was applied to a unique form of depression that was believed to happen around menopause,[22] and electric shock therapy was promoted as a potential therapy.[23] These diagnoses were later to be dismissed and dropped from standard texts for lack of sufficient evidence.

In their book *The Curse*, authors Jane Delaney, Mary Jane Lupton, and Emily Toth traced the origins of cultural beliefs about menopause to highly influential Western thinkers like Freud and Shakespeare. They point out that Freud frequently commented on the menopause as a time of crisis, when women often "become quarrelsome and obstinate, petty and stingy."[24] In 1945, Freudian psychologist Helena Deutsch added her interpretation that the menopause is woman's last traumatic sexual experience. "The tragi-comic result is that the older and less attractive she becomes, the greater is her desire to be loved. Under the pressure of failure, the vagina gives up the struggle."[25] Deutsch taught that basically, women become depressed at menopause because they can no longer compensate for not having a penis by having a baby.

Philosopher Eric Erickson writes about the loss of menstruation leaving a "permanent scar" for the woman who can no longer bear children.[26] Even Shakespeare contributes to the belittlement of the menopausal woman, where, in *Hamlet*, his main character denies that an older woman can experience romance, or even her own sexuality. Hamlet, furious at his mother for marrying soon after his father's death, punishes her by denying that she could, at her age, experience new passion; rather she is supposed to just wait for her own death: "You cannot call it love, for at your age, the heyday in the blood is tame, it's humble, and waits upon the judgment."[27]

The notion of the defeminized, dispassionate, and depressed woman was picked up by Robert Wilson, M.D., one of the first and certainly the most vocal of physicians to have claimed to medically pinpoint the reason women were apparently so despondent in menopause. His universal explanation: estrogen deprivation.

Estrogen had actually been used by physicians since the 1920s. For several decades, it was primarily offered, however, to younger women who had undergone removal of the ovaries in conjunction with a hysterectomy, for temporary relief of severe discomforts. Wilson's writings would soon change all that. His book, *Feminine Forever*, which sold 100,000 copies in the first seven months, first painted the image of women who underwent a natural (meaning nonsurgical) menopause as shriveled, depressed, and useless. "Though the physical suffering can be truly dreadful, what impressed me most tragically is the destruction of personality," Wilson writes. "Some women, when they realize that they are no longer women, subside into a stupor of indifference."[28] He then promised women they could avoid becoming like the image he created, with the aid of a simple, natural, and universally safe remedy: estrogen.

Prominent endocrinologist Robert B. Greenblatt, M.D., wrote the foreword to Wilson's *Feminine Forever.* In it, Greenblatt states "The effects of estrogen deprivation are physically and emotionally devastating; for a fortunate few the damage is minimal, the scars only slightly visible." Greenblatt echoes Hamlet by warning women against "the threat of declining femininity, of waning romance." He proclaims that "Women will be emancipated only when the shackles of hormonal deprivation are loosed," and introduces Wilson as women's best hope of survival beyond menopause: "Like a gallant knight he has come to rescue his fair lady, not at the time of her bloom and flowering, but in her despairing years; at the time of her life when the preservation and prolongation of her femaleness are so paramount."[29]

While the public bought his books and consequently began to demand estrogen, Wilson was meanwhile carrying out his crusade within the medical profession. "Perimenopausal women suffer from a deficiency disease which requires treatment," he wrote in the *Journal of the American Geriatric Society* in October 1966. "Deprived of her ovaries, a woman is only a caricature of her former self—defeminized and a castrate."[30]

In 1972, Wilson "explained" to doctors that estrogen is "the essential fuel for all stages of life," literally from birth to "up to age 100." Estrogen, he implores physicians, gives a woman her beauty and allure. As evidence, he asserts that "ovarian failure in the twenties will preclude success in marriage, business and the arts," and advances the ideology that "administering natural estrogens plus an appropriate progestagen to middle-aged women will prevent the climacteric and menopause—a syndrome that seems unnecessary for most of the women in the civilized world."[31]

In her excellent historical account of menopause, *The Change,* feminist writer Germain Greer takes an in-depth look into the psyche of Wilson and others who were shaping our culture's views on menopause and inventing medical protocols around what they saw as pathology. Greer draws our attention to Wilson's own account of the menopause, as seen in his "gentle, almost angelic mother" when he was a young boy:

> Something terrible was obviously happening. I was appalled at the transformation of the vital, wonderful woman who had been the dynamic focal point of our family into a pain-racked, petulant invalid. I could feel the deep wounds her senseless rages inflicted in my father, myself, and the younger children. It was this frightful ex-

perience that later directed my interest as a physician to the problem of menopause.[32]

Wilson also thought of the postmenopausal uterus as merely a disease waiting to happen. "Fortunate indeed, is many an older woman who does not have a uterus," he writes to his colleagues. As history would unfortunately play out, this statement of Wilson's would come to be eerily prophetic—but not in the way he'd intended it.

Remember that the majority of women on estrogen during its first decades of use did not have a uterus. Wilson and other proponents of estrogen replacement therapy (ERT) did not realize the importance of this fact—an oversight that would later come back to haunt the medical profession a few years after a new generation of women were placed on ERT—that is, estrogen alone. As we learned in Chapter 1, estrogen acts to promote growth of the uterine lining while progesterone stabilizes this tissue. Unchecked by progesterone, a uterine lining constantly stimulated by estrogen can grow, thicken, and even produce abnormal cells. Uterine cancer developed in a significant percentage of women who were on ERT, or "unopposed estrogen."

Wilson's enduring contribution to the growing field of women's medicine was to change the medical view of menopause as a natural event to a pathological one. His treatises to the medical profession condemned a past in which doctors opted not to tamper with nature. "Today, however," he extols in 1966, "a revolution in thinking indicates that the menopause is both unnecessary and harmful . . ."[33]

Harvard-trained psychiatrist David Reubin further dramatized Wilson's vision of the menopausal woman in his 1970s best-seller *Everything You Always Wanted to Know About Sex But Were Afraid to Ask*. He describes postmenopausal women as being "castrated by Father Time" and menopause as a "defect in evolution." In other words, he implies women were never meant to live past reproductive age. Reubin tells us that this is a time when "a woman comes as close as she can to being a man . . . a tragic picture . . . Not really a man, but no longer a functional woman. . . . Having outlived their ovaries, they may have outlived their usefulness as human beings. The remaining years may be just marking time until they follow their glands into oblivion." Then he delivers his final blow: "Once the ovaries stop, the very essence of being a woman stops."[34]

This attitude in medicine persisted until very recently. In an article published in 1987 in the journal *Obstetrics and Gynecology Clinics of North America*, W. H. Utian writes "sufficient evidence now exists to confirm that the climacteric syndrome is a specific one that can be regarded as an endocrinopathy. . . . The human female climacteric represents a pathologic rather than a physiologic state."[35]

Fears of waning femininity fueled a demand for estrogen. Before Wilson's time, critics had referred to estrogen as a product in search of a market. Now, however, the advertising industry had discovered a most potent motivator for promoting this new miracle medicine. Advertisements by pharmaceutical companies during the 1970s showed "a sad and depressed woman, a burden to herself and her husband until she started to take estrogen."[36] Side effects and risks of estrogen were never mentioned.

Thus, the Western medicalization of what is essentially a normal transition in every woman's life was born. Women and doctors both, to varying degrees, had bought the notion that every woman's life would necessarily become meaningless and decline at menopause; that this was preventable and there was one remedy for all.

Menopause Now

The image of menopausal woman in the new millennium strikes a sharp contrast to that of her former counterpart. It's not that real women's experience of menopause has changed so dramatically. It is rather the *caricature* of the menopausal woman, created in the minds of advertisers, health providers, and their consumers that has evolved, thanks to persistent feminist writers, researchers, and outspoken baby boomers who have insisted on bringing menopause "out of the closet."

Menopause in Medicine

Modern texts on women's medicine now encourage physicians to regard the menopause as a normal transition. The current edition of *Gynecologic Endocrinology and Infertility*, considered widely to be one of the most authoritative medical text on women's reproductive health, directly contradicts the assertions made by authorities in the none-too-distant past. "It is time to stress the normalcy of this physiologic event," the authors state. "Menopausal women do not suffer from a disease (specifically a hormone deficiency disease)."[37]

By the mid-1990s, enough scientific evidence had been amassed to disprove the notion that menopause was generally a time of melancholy or depression for women. Today, several studies demonstrate that menopause is statistically the happiest time in women's lives. In a 1998 survey of 752 postmenopausal women, ages 50–65, performed by the North American Menopause Society, 51% reported that they were happiest and most fulfilled at this time in their life, as compared with only 10% who were happiest in their twenties, 17% in their thirties, and 16% in their forties. Also, most women reported that their sexual relationships had either remained unchanged or improved after menopause.[38] The Massachusetts

Women's Health Study found that women today report either neutral or positive feelings about menopause.[39] With the exception of women who had a surgical menopause, women in the study felt that the cessation of their menses had almost no impact on their physical or psychological health.

These studies echo the conclusion of Gabriella Berger after she had compiled her data on menopause in dozens of foreign cultures throughout the world. Berger consistently found that women's global menopausal experience "fails to support any negative image of this time." This finding prompted her to propose a new definition of menopause, as "a natural progression primarily unaffected by major physical and psychological trauma."[40]

Of course the menopause transition is not always a bed of roses. Just as we reject the idea that menopause must be a universally negative experience, it is equally important to criticize the perspective that every woman ought to be able to "sail through" menopause without any discomfort, for every woman's experience is unique. What these studies accomplish, however, is to reverse the overwhelming generalization that menopause signals a decline in quality of life for most women. In fact, menopausal women are, overall, the happiest women in our society.

Menopause in the Media

Advertising strategies for the pharmaceutical as well as natural supplement industries are quick to adapt to these new findings. Although scare tactics still exist (for example, the proverbial hunched-over osteoporotic woman image used to sell calcium supplements), the "new menopausal woman" is more commonly portrayed as the picture of health. One attendee of a recent convention of the Congress of the International Menopause Society noticed this change in the promotional photographs of women as she walked through the sponsors' display areas, where booths of pharmaceutical and medical product companies promoted their products. She wrote:

> Unlike the women shown in the pharmaceutical advertisements in the 1970s, this 1990s version of the menopausal woman does not look at all depressed, but is shown exercising, playing with grandchildren, lunching with friends, talking to a daughter, looking through a microscope. Usually smiling, glowing with fitness, with well-maintained teeth, hair, and skin, these pictures sometimes also suggest a discreet but well-enjoyed sexuality. Everyone looked far too fit to break a hip, have a heart attack or witness the slow destruction of their minds by Alzheimer's disease.[41]

Menopause in the Workplace

The face of menopause has changed, in part, because women's lifestyles have changed. First of all, women are having fewer children, and they're having them later. One of the most articulate commentators on the evolution of menopause in our culture, writer Gail Sheehy points out the dramatic change in the workplace because so many women today take jobs outside the home. In our mother's generation, women were much more likely to assume the role of "grandmother" as their predominant job. More often than not, today we're holding down a career or other large responsibilities. In fact, the number of women holding jobs outside the home in the United States jumped from 35.5% in 1960 to 54.3% twenty years later. Nearly 80% of women age 50–60 who graduated from college are still in the workforce today. Professional women may be just now hitting their stride, holding top positions. "The boardrooms of America are lighting up with hot flashes," Sheehy writes.[42] Grandma never dreamed that life at menopause could look like this!

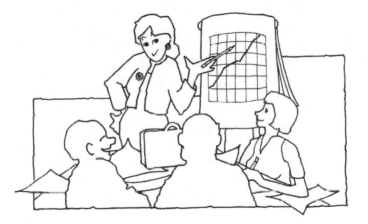

With women making up roughly half the workforce today, Sheehy asserts we now need the same type of workplace consciousness-raising around menopause as was accomplished in previous decades with pregnancy. In a survey of 100 professional women, she found that women are afraid they'll be perceived as losing their "edge" if their male counterparts learned they were in menopause. Nine percent of her respondents said their companies offered programs to educate staff about menopause and 80% felt their company could benefit from such education. Such initiatives, Sheehy asserts, will demystify this natural phase of life, and further dismantle lingering attitudes that cause women to be concerned about their male colleagues or co-workers' perceptions of menopause.

Lifestyle Changes in Menopause

It is no accident that many changes in lifestyle frequently occur for women around the time of their menopause. Family dynamics usually undergo some type of shift when a woman reaches 45 or 50. If she is a mother, she may be contending with children growing up and leaving home around this time. Her own parents or parents-in-law may be requiring care. A myriad of other potential variations on household transitions exist.

The French refer to this time as "le troisième age," or the third age, when a ripening maturity combined with changing family dynamics often leads one toward a deepening sense of self and mission. In some cultures, like that of Hindu people in India, this age is when yogis would give up material possessions and begin their pilgrimage up the proverbial mountain in search of enlightenment. In many cultures, spiritual life really begins in the climacteric.

In modern Western society, lifestyle transitions may look different, but be no less profound. A woman whose life has revolved around caring for a family might choose to redirect her energies into furthering her education or beginning a new vocation. Women who have been in the workplace often change jobs. Marriages or partnerships might shift. Both inwardly in their bodies and externally in life, "change" can be the order of the day for women in menopause or perimenopause.

Transition times are ideal opportunities for us to reflect upon where we've been, where we want to go, and how to get there. Most women know, by this time, what lifestyle changes they can make that will result in a better quality of life. The menopause presents a natural time for us to "pause" and consider how we'd like to live out our lives. In fact, according to the North American Menopause Society, three-quarters of menopausal women do reassess and make positive changes in their lives at menopause.[43] Over half of women make changes in diet or nutrition. Other frequently cited changes included stopping smoking, exercising more, increasing personal time, and incorporating alternative or holistic remedies.

Aided by the decline in estrogen, many women report an experience of feeling "life" more intensely—that their emotions as well as bodies seem to "speak" more loudly than before. Without the "buffering" effect of estrogen, some women say they experience more acutely the result that lifestyle choices, including diet and exercise, have on their bodies and minds. We can use this increased sensitivity to motivate positive lifestyle changes—and to see and feel more vividly their rewards.

Inspiring Women in Midlife and Beyond

Menopause is an important threshold to what could in reality be the climax of our lives as women; the decades in which we are finally able to apply our life's experience and fully bring our unique contribution to the world. Many great women have opened the eyes of the world to the wisdom and power which menopausal women possess. Great Britain's longest-serving prime minister of the twentieth century was a menopausal woman. Margaret Thatcher became prime minister of England at the age of 54, and held this post until age 65. The unparalleled contribution Catholic Albanian nun, Mother Theresa (1910–1997) made to humanity only escalated in her menopausal years until her death at the age of 87. Diane Feinstein became the first woman mayor of San Francisco at the age of 45, and later, became (and continues to be) a United States senator. Eleanor Roosevelt, visionary and composer Hildegard von Bingen, and Mrs. Gandhi, president of India, provide yet further examples of women whose greatest achievements were made in their full maturity. Susan B. Anthony fought for and achieved the women's vote, and essentially started the women's rights movement in the United States during her menopausal years. Georgia O'Keefe was not firmly established as an artist until age 59, after the death of her husband. She created her best known paintings in the years following and lived and painted to the ripe old age of 98. Late photographs of her strong, heavily lined face and soulful gaze illustrate just how beautiful a woman living her passion in her 90s can be.

Menopause in the New Millennium

Changing cultural views on menopause will continue to affect every aspect of women's experience of this time. As anthropologists Kaufert and Lock point out,

> How physicians and others think about menopause and treat the menopausal woman depends on whatever is the currently accepted model of the menopausal woman. This model also determines how menopausal women see themselves and how they are seen in the wider society, including how they are expected to look and to behave.[44]

Ninety percent of all women alive today will live through menopause. Most American women will live thirty years beyond this transition,[45] which means living over one-third of their lives as menopausal women. Yet, as we've seen, women are staying active, productive, and in the workforce well into these years. By necessity then, the image of life in and after "the

Change" is undergoing a complete revision. We are leaving the outdated and erroneous description of the depressed, passionless, and burdensome menopausal woman in the dust. In its place we are manifesting the image of a vital and wise woman who is relearning to use age as an asset.

Today's menopausal women are artists, board members, doctors, teachers, mothers, new grandmothers, scientists, musicians, hikers, and more, hardly "awaiting the judgment" as Hamlet supposed. To the contrary, women today are both reclaiming the respect that appropriately comes with age, and expressing their vitality in every aspect of their lives. Women can be found redefining this transition in women's groups, at retreat centers, and at lunch with friends. They are reaching out through their writings, through the arts, and even online, where dozens of Internet sites promote "conscious aging" and feature stories by and for women in midlife.

Some women, like Pamela, are celebrating menopause as a rite-of-passage. On her fiftieth birthday, Pamela invited female friends of all ages to her home, with instructions of bringing "a bead and a blessing." When they had gathered, each woman offered her blessing; a poem, song, story or memorable event that they had witnessed with or of Pamela. As they told their stories, each woman presented Pamela with the bead she had brought, as a representation of how Pamela had touched her life. By the end of the stories, everyone in the room felt like they had come to more fully know this unique woman—to honor her fifty years of life history and wisdom. The beads were then strung together, symbolizing the tales that, when strung together, form a continuous life story line. Pamela keeps her one-of-a-kind necklace as a reminder of that day and of the unique beauty of her own life.

Today, Pamela, 57, is a full-time, practicing physician. She thinks her fiftieth birthday party helped not just her, but those she invited, feel more

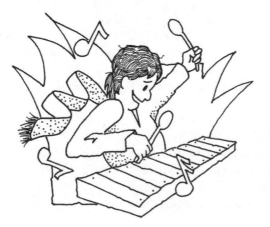

comfortable about growing older. Four years ago, she began pursuing a lifelong goal of learning to play a musical instrument, and surprised everyone in her family by joining a marimba band! "I have more energy now for my career, my practice, and for learning than ever before," she says. "When you're at this time in your life, you say 'you'd better just do it now. Quit procrastinating and putting it off 'til later.' There *is* no later!"

In subtle and profound ways, our society's views of life in menopause is evolving positively, and it's women themselves who have led this change. Suzanne Labarge, author of *The Metaphysics of Menopause*, describes menopause as a time in which women's creative energies are often freed from household activities such as child rearing, and are now available for her to use in other fulfilling ways. She calls this a transition "from *procreative to pure creative.*"

Women who take advantage of this shift of focus can find themselves embarking on all kinds of new adventures: learning a skill they've always wanted to have but didn't have the time for, taking a long-awaited trip, emersing themselves in the arts, or deepening a relationship with themselves or with others. As Sheehy proclaims, "The openings are numerous for women today as they enter the Flaming Fifties."[46]

The freedom to explore new dimensions of life comes as a welcome reward for those who have "put in their time," perhaps by raising families,

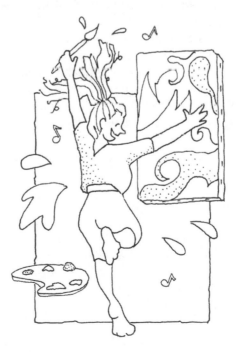

maintaining a home, punching a time clock, or otherwise spending much of their time responding to the necessities of daily life. Most menopausal-aged women have established more security in home, relationships, and financial status than they had in their twenties, thirties, and early forties. Their life experience is greater and they are wiser for it. They have established a stronger sense of self. This increased security creates an environment ripe for internal and external exploration.

The numbers of midlife women who are in fact drawn to some type of spiritual inquiry is propelling self-help books to the top of the *New York Times* best-seller list time and time again. Menopausal women today are interested in creating a life beyond merely subsisting (much less one of "decline")—but instead, one full of meaning and purpose. "Find your passion and live it," declares Oprah Winfrey, television's most influential personality, to her responsive and largely female audience. Challenges like these resonate with and are accessible to the new generation of empowered menopausal women.

Applying Our Knowledge

As Western women in the new millennium, we are at a unique and fortunate position in history and in society in terms of knowledge about menopause. From this vantage point, we can see clearly how menopause is affected by both cultural and historical beliefs—and we can use this to our advantage by altering our own beliefs.

Our cross-cultural study of menopause teaches us that women are not "locked in" to a certain physiological or psychological experience of this time. Rather, we have the power to dramatically influence our own menopausal experience. Diet, lifestyle, and beliefs can, and do, alter women's menopausal experience—and we have the power to change all three of these factors. Taking steps to free ourselves from negative expectations of what menopause and perimenopause will be like will give us much more freedom to create healthier lives, mentally and physically.

Likewise, a critical look into the history of how menopause was portrayed both in medicine and by the media can help us not "buy into" any image we don't want to make reality in our lives. The changing image of menopause promoted by these institutions—from "disease" to "natural transition," in little more than a decade, is just that—an image. It is not reality. And it will never be the exact replicate of your personal experience.

The Menopause Media Quiz

In a market-driven society such as ours, much of the image-of-the-day portraying The Menopausal Woman will be carefully crafted for one purpose: to sell you products. Try this little experiment the next time you see an advertisement targeting menopausal women in a magazine or on television. In doing so, you will start to see how commercialism influences (and in the case of menopause, confuses) the unsuspecting consumer. If you do it a few times, you will begin to learn how to take information from the advertisement, but remain more objective about whether or not that product would really benefit you personally.

It doesn't matter if this advertisement is for supplements, prescription drugs, or some other product targeted toward a menopausal consumer. Take a close look at the *model*, the woman supposed to be portraying *you*. Ask yourself the following six questions:

1. Does she look like you and your friends?
2. Does she have that ten or more extra pounds around the middle like most menopausal women do?
3. Does her hair show even a tiny bit of thinning?
4. Is her skin just like that of most women her age?

Ask yourself how realistic this image is. Now, *imagine how much money and time you could spend trying to achieve this image*. Would you ever get there? Finally, (these last questions seem particularly self-evident, but they're as effective as they are silly) ask yourself this:

5. Does this advertiser know *my* personal health needs?
6. In other words, is this company motivated by concern for my well-being?

The more "no's" you answered, the further away this advertisement is from portraying a realistic image of a menopausal woman—like you. You may still choose to take note of the information you heard or read and bring it up with your health practitioner if it interests you. Remain cognizant of the fact, however, that the message delivered may indeed have little to do with you.

In the past, media images of menopausal women were of sad, burdensome, withering women. Although this was not a realistic image, many women "bought into it," and bought products to avoid becoming what they most likely wouldn't become anyway. Currently, the commercial and,

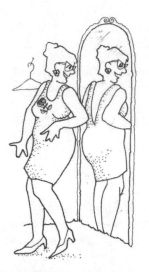

therefore, media image of the Western woman in midlife tends to be different, but no more realistic than her past counterpart. Today the "menopause" models are thinner and younger looking than what is realistically the case for most people. The very discrepancy between what is portrayed as ideal, and what is attainable for most women makes for a very effective marketing technique. The longer the baby-boom generation of menopausal women strive toward an unattainable goal, the more dollars we spend on the perfect wrinkle cream, diet program, pill or surgery to keep us young looking and skinny. (For a quick test to apply to advertisements, see "The Menopause Media Quiz" on page 35.)

Beyond the waste of time and money, a larger tragedy occurs when a woman's psyche becomes conditioned to battle against her own nature. Resenting the wrinkles that reflect back to us in the mirror is in fact a negation of the smiles, the concerns, and the days with sunshine it took to create them. Love your face! Upon it lies the story of your life. Decide to appreciate your body for all it's done for you. Investing in self-acceptance will create far greater wellness than will investing in antiaging products.

Your Menopause Is Unique

Whether it's drugs or supplements, exercise classes or beauty products, companies who market merchandise for menopause are in it for their bottom line—not yours. And they've got your number—meaning your age and your address. No doubt you've already received some kind of promotional product regarding how to address aging or health via the mail. Each supplier has a vested interest in convincing as many women as possible that their product is essential for your well-

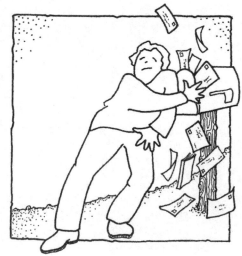

being. Unless you learn to discriminate, you'll end up with every conceivable supplement on your shelf, and feel more confused than ever. This is also where a careful assessment of your *unique* situation can help you edit out media messages that don't apply to you. That's what we'll spend the rest of this book doing.

Getting Support

You don't have to figure out how to handle menopause alone. Since an estimated 1,328,000 women in the United States actually hit menopause every year now, you have lots of company! Bouncing ideas off someone else and sharing your experience can be personally validating and offer insight. Randi held a tea party for all her friends who were entering perimenopause. She picked up a tasty blend of spearmint, chamomile, and motherwort herbs at a local herb store, and served this "soothing and cooling" tea to her guests, while they all shared stories about theirs and their mothers' experiences. "My husband tries to understand, but he just can't get it all," she said. "It was refreshing to just be able to relax and listen to other women's experiences. I also got some good information."

Nancy had a different approach to getting support. She found, quite by accident, that she had adopted a "menopause mentor" in a 60-year-old woman who has a garden next to hers in a community plot. "One day I got brave and told her that I was having some hormonal mood swings, and the next thing you know, we were chatting up a storm about menopause. I found out that I really liked the approach she had taken in her life, and it's been helpful to have a role model for that. So now she's my menopause mentor. We've gone out for tea a few times, too. It's helpful to have someone who I respect validating my approach."

Envisioning Total Wellness in Menopause

To some extent, we become what we believe. This journaling exercise will help you become an empowered architect of your menopausal years.

Get a blank piece of paper, a large note pad, or a journal if you have one. Ask yourself the following four questions aloud, and write out your responses.

1. What do I think I will experience in menopause, physically, mentally, and spiritually?
2. Where did I get these ideas?

Now, let's design a "new, improved" version. Even if you have a positive outlook on menopause, we can make it even better. Don't worry if you don't have a complete answer to question 4—that's what this book is for! Beginning to contemplate these questions and search for the answers is what's important for now. Respond to the following questions with abandon—as if the sky is the limit:

3. What would I like to experience in menopause, physically, mentally, and spiritually?
4. How can I facilitate this?

Activating Your Intuition

Most of this book will guide you in assessing your needs in and around menopause from a medical model, albeit one that integrates natural and conventional medicine. We will present the best available scientific data on each subject. However, it will always be important that you balance information gleaned from this book, as well as any source, with what feels right intuitively for you.

Somewhere, amidst our mix of memories, beliefs, and stored knowledge lies our intuition and a deep sense of what is right or wrong for our particular body. Intuition is often likened to a "gut" feeling, or a sense of knowing in our "bones" or "heart" (all places affected by female hormones, in fact!).

Many who provide health care advice to women do not mention this powerful authority in a woman's decision-making process. Nonetheless, we acknowledge that a woman's intuition has value and veto-power, whether the provider wants to acknowledge it or not. Intuition often has the final say in what therapies a woman chooses and sticks with.

After you've read all the books, met with the practitioners and conversed with friends over the question of "what to do?"—you need to then close the books, silence the conversations, and simply ask yourself "What feels right?" (For a journaling exercise to help with this, see "Envisioning Total Wellness in Menopause" on page 37.) However you contact your intuition—through gardening, walking, listening to music, writing, meditating or a host of other ways—following through with this final step will add the power of commitment to your choices. Also important, it will strengthen your own internal voice; the same voice that can rise over the media din and inform you about your unique experience of this time.

A woman who creates time and support for reflection during peri-menopause and menopause often finds this transition to be a powerful time of self-actualization. She can often be surprised by the depth and intensity of her knowledge. As Germain Greer declares in her groundbreaking book, *The Change:* "The climacteric marks the end of apologizing. The chrysalis of conditioning has once and for all to break and the female woman finally to emerge."[47]

3 Cycle Changes and Bleeding Problems

As we round the last bend in our reproductive years, our monthly cycles may present us with a few final challenges. In this chapter, we'll describe which changes are normal, which require more investigation, and best of all, what to do to make your ride through this time as smooth as possible, using either natural or conventional supports.

Changes in Bleeding Patterns

The only change that every woman encounters at menopause is a change in her periods. For some women, this means that her periods simply stop, without any fanfare whatsoever. For most women, however, a change in bleeding patterns will arrive anywhere from two to eight years before her periods end for good.

It's wise to keep track of your periods as they change. Use the "Menstrual Cycle Record" provided in Figure 3.1 for an easy, visual history that will help both you and your health practitioner in assessing your situation. Bring this record to any office visits in which you intend to discuss your periods.

As mentioned in Chapter 1, many women in their late thirties or forties say their periods are lighter than before. This change does not necessarily signal perimenopause. Likewise, it's common and normal to skip a period during perimenopause. While it's a good idea to keep your health practitioner informed about changes in your cycles, rest assured that the vast majority of these are normal.

Abnormal bleeding patterns for women in their 40s generally occur for one of two reasons: either cycles are changing as hormone levels change

YEAR

MENSTRUAL CYCLE RECORD

DAY	1	2	3	4	5	6	7	8	9	10	11	12	13	14	15	16	17	18	19	20	21	22	23	24	25	26	27	28	29	30	31
JAN																															
FEB																														■	■
MAR																															
APR																															■
MAY																															
JUN																															■
JUL																															
AUG																															
SEP																															■
OCT																															
NOV																															■
DEC																															

Enter appropriate letter in
proper calendar day square
as needed:

S - Spotting
B - Bleeding
H – Hot flashes
N – Night sweats

Figure 3.1. A simple chart to keep track of changes in bleeding patterns.

approaching menopause or, more rarely, something may be wrong with female structures (uterus or ovaries). Common structural problems at this age include polyps and fibroids. These are both benign conditions, but can cause bleeding problems and may require treatment, ranging from naturopathic therapies to surgery. The newest conventional fibroid treatment is *uterine artery embolization*, which shrinks a fibroid by cutting off its blood supply. Naturopathic therapies involving diet, lifestyle, and herbal treatments only rarely result in shrinkage of a fibroid, but are very good at decreasing problems like bleeding and cramping. For a good naturopathic resource for this problem, consult the *Women's Encyclopedia of Natural Medicine*, by Tori Hudson, N.D.[1]

In rare cases, abnormal bleeding can be a sign of abnormal tissue growth of the uterine lining. Below, we will discuss when it's important to check in with your health care provider for an evaluation.

Increased Bleeding

Many women report heavier bleeding or longer periods at the time of perimenopause. Although these bleeding episodes may be caused by the normal hormonal fluctuations at menopause, they can be uncomfortable, and in extreme cases, dangerous if blood loss is extreme.

"Flooding" refers to excessively heavy bleeding during a period. As a guideline, flooding means a menstrual flow greater than a super pad or super tampon each hour for more than eight hours in a row. This can occur during perimenopause, especially during an *anovulatory* cycle (one in which you didn't ovulate), where progesterone is absent.

If you experience flooding, or if you are fatigued by, or concerned about the bleeding, contact your health care provider immediately. If you

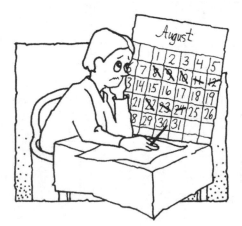

soak through a super tampon or maxi-pad every thirty minutes or less, for more than eight hours, you should seek medical attention.

Often, women in perimenopause have erratic cycles. This might mean having two periods in one month, skipping a month or more, and many other variations. Cycle lengths, which may have been consistent in the past, can fluctuate by several days. Many of these changes are normal and result from a tired ovary doing the best it can to hatch the last remaining eggs. If you are concerned by the lack of a familiar pattern, contact your practitioner. Also, if the bleeding pattern remains erratic for several months, especially if it involves more than one bleeding episode per month, seek medical guidance.

Decreased Bleeding

Many women experience less frequent and sporadic periods in perimenopause. It is common for periods to seemingly disappear, then reappear after several months. This is not a cause for concern. The notable exception is when a woman has vaginal bleeding after one year without a period. In these cases, it may be necessary for a health practitioner to obtain either a biopsy of the uterine lining or an ultrasound of the uterus and surrounding structures to rule out abnormal tissue growth or, rarely, uterine cancer. Keep in mind that you can become pregnant all the way up until menopause. If you are heterosexually active and not using a reliable birth control method, you may want to test for pregnancy if you skip a period.

When to Seek Help

Bleeding changes in perimenopause are usually normal. However, contact your health care provider if:
- your periods become very heavy or frequent.
- you develop spotting between periods.
- your periods begin again after six months without one.
- you have any vaginal bleeding after one year of no bleeding.

Remedies for Bleeding Problems

Several solutions exist to help your body maintain regular cycles as long as possible (until they eventually end) and to control heavy bleeding. Here, we'll present natural and conventional options in increasing order of strength and intervention for these issues.

Regulating Cycles

Although irregular cycles caused by hormonal fluctuations don't necessarily require treatment, you and your practitioner still may opt to regulate them. Some women decide to do this to avoid the inconvenience of periods coming at unexpected times. Several therapies can help you gain some control over perimenopausal bleeding irregularities. The following treatments are arranged in ascending order of intervention, and also from the more natural to more conventional options. Try these only after you and your health practitioner have assessed that your bleeding changes are hormonal in nature, and not due to fibroids, polyps or abnormal uterine tissue.

Vitex

Generations of herbal practitioners have relied on Vitex *agnus castus*, otherwise known as chaste tree berry. Vitex was employed as a treatment for uterine hemorrhaging as far back as the fourth century B.C., by Hippocrates, the father of medicine. German gynecologists have largely pioneered its modern research and use. Their studies demonstrated the effectiveness of Vitex in correcting abnormal or absent menses, and in treating PMS, infertility and hyperprolactinemia (an abnormal elevation of the pituitary hormone responsible for lactation).[2]

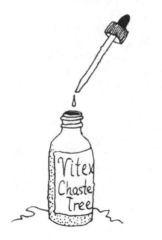

Vitex is most helpful for women at the beginning of their perimenopause, when periods may be irregular, but are still present. Its intended effect is to regulate both the timing and the quantity of bleeding for as long as possible, while viable eggs still remain in the ovaries. By itself, Vitex is not indicated for severe hemorrhaging.

Vitex seems to work by acting on the pituitary gland. Extracts of the berries are reported to increase LH production and mildly inhibit FSH, resulting in a relative increase of progesterone as compared to estrogen.[3,4] Recall that estrogen promotes growth of the uterine lining, while progesterone stabilizes it. Therefore, a shift toward progesterone production would produce a more stable endometrial lining.

Doses of Vitex commonly used in clinical studies are one 175 mg capsule, or 40 drops of a German standardized extract of the liquid, one time daily. Herbal practitioners in the United States and Canada typically prescribe anywhere from 15–60 drops of liquid tincture one to two times per day, depending on the strength of the tincture and its desired result. Always consult a practitioner experienced in herbal medicine when deciding on your dose. Side effects of Vitex are rare—noted in only 1 to 2 percent of patients. These most commonly include gastric complaints such as nausea and skin rash.

Progesterone and Progestins

Recall that progesterone is made by the body after ovulation to stabilize the uterine lining. If ovulation doesn't occur (which is common in perimenopause), progesterone won't be produced. As a result, the uterine lining will be unstable, and shed more, and perhaps at odd times.

To help with this, women and their health practitioners may choose to use synthetic forms of progesterone, known as progestins, to supplement their cycles and cause a predictable period each month. Women who have extended times between periods and then have flooding can gain some control over this pattern by using progestins for 7–14 days each month, depending on the timing recommended by their practitioner.

Today, we also have access to a more natural form of progesterone, derived from soy and wild yam. "Natural progesterone," available through specialized "compounding" pharmacies or through some natural practitioners as creams, pellets, or pills can replace progestins. The demand for natural progesterone has prompted even regular pharmacies to carry it. The only prescription brand currently available is Prometrium®.

Practitioners hotly debate how well our bodies absorb natural progesterone and how its side effects differ from that of progestins. Natural progesterone is generally more expensive and not always covered by health insurance. For a detailed discussion of the pros and cons of various forms of progesterone, see Chapter 10.

Birth Control Pills

Just as taking progestins or natural progesterone can help you to "cycle," oral contraceptives can also provide this cycle control. Instead of your body making some estrogen, and adding the progestins/progesterone from medication as above, "the pill" gives you both hormones at controlled times. Thus, it basically turns off your hormone cycles and replaces them. Some women choose to use oral contraceptives during the perimenopause to control not only bleeding problems, but also many other symptoms like hot flashes, night sweats, and mood changes.

Managing Heavy Bleeding Episodes

Menstrual hemorrhaging at worrisome levels is defined as soaking through a super tampon or maxi-pad every 30 minutes or less, for more than eight hours. If this happens contact your health care practitioner immediately. If she or he isn't available, proceed to the nearest urgent care center.

Fortunately, most heavy bleeding episodes can be managed at home. If you are prone to these, having a few remedies on hand can help shorten and lighten the bleeding. Following, you'll find treatments arranged in order of ascending strength and intervention. They can be combined for enhanced effect. It's wise to make decisions about which to use in conjunction with a qualified practitioner. And of course, if your bleeding is severe, be sure you've received an assessment and do not require clinical treatment before trying any of these "home remedies" to slow bleeding.

Cinnamon

Cinnamon is used by herbalists as a *styptic*, or a remedy that slows bleeding. Cinnamon hasn't captured the fancy of researchers yet, so we don't have placebo-controlled studies to prove its effectiveness. However, many women will attest to its ability to head off heavy bleeding, when taken orally in therapeutic doses. It certainly is one of the tastier options available! Sprinkle ½ teaspoon on toast or applesauce and ingest up to 3 times per day.

Yarrow

Yarrow derives its Latin genus name, *Achillea millefolium,* from the story that Achilles used this popular remedy to staunch the bleeding wounds of his soldiers.[5] Yarrow has been classically used by Chinese and Ayurvedic (the traditional healing system of India) medicine as a "drying" or astringent herb, both for external wounds, but also for excess uterine bleeding.[6]

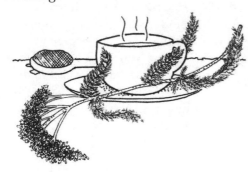

The white flowers of this herb—not the colored garden decorative varieties—can be infused in boiling water to make a tea. Alternatively you can purchase a liquid extract or tincture of the herb. To slow heavy bleeding, one cup of tea or 60 drops of tincture can be used every three hours, up to a maximum of 4 doses.

Yarrow *(Achillea millefolium)*

Progesterone or Progestins

Frequently, women bleed heavily when their bodies produce lots of estrogen, and less progesterone, relatively speaking. If you recall that estrogen grows the endometrium and progesterone stabilizes it, it's easy to see how this can result in heavier periods. Progesterone supplementation can, therefore, help correct excessive endometrial shedding.

As we will discuss in Chapter 10, progesterone and progestins come in a myriad of forms. The best form to take during an intense bleeding episode is the one that your practitioner knows best. The acute nature of the event makes experimenting with forms she or he may not be familiar with impractical. Once the bleeding event is under control, you may decide to discuss alternative forms to control potential future bleeding problems.

Side effects of progesterone and progestins can include PMS-like symptoms such as bloating, fatigue, and moodiness. Women with progesterone-sensitive breast cancer should not take progestins *or* natural progesterone.

Nonsteroidal Anti-inflammatory Drugs

Many women can control heavy bleeding with over-the-counter medications like ibuprofen (Advil®, Motrin®) or naproxen (Alleve®). If you are not allergic to these medications or to aspirin, it is okay to try 800 mg of ibuprofen every 8 hours or up to 600 mg naproxen every 8–12 hours to try to control heavy bleeding. Be aware that potential side effects of nonsteroidal anti-inflammatory drugs (NSAIDs) include gastrointestinal disturbance, and even ulcerations, if used in excess. In rare instances, kidney problems may develop from overuse.

Endometrial Ablation

"Can you just make it stop—so I don't have to worry about it any more?" Jean asked her gynecologist. For women who have ongoing problems with severe bleeding, or who have a concerning overgrowth of the lining of the uterus, *endometrial ablation* may be an option. There are several methods of either burning or freezing this layer of tissue and removing it, and *sometimes* this puts an end to periods altogether—depending on how close a woman is to her menopause. If other options have failed and you feel like you're going to wash away with unending periods, ask a gynecologist about this technique.

Remedies That Can Aggravate Heavy Bleeding

Some practitioners might suggest trying hormone replacement therapy (HRT) during the perimenopause, usually for help with symptoms such as hot flashes, insomnia or vaginal dryness. While this can dramatically reduce these symptoms, HRT may in fact aggravate or cause bleeding irregularities. The reason for this is because the doses of HRT are significantly lower than that of birth control pills, and may not be strong enough to "override" a woman's own hormones, which have their own agenda. As a result, HRT in the perimenopause is a less reliable way to provide cycle control and in fact, *can* make bleeding problems worse.

The drug warfarin (Coumadin®) and some natural supplements are blood thinners, and may intensify menstrual bleeding, especially if more than one are taken at a time. If you experience excessive bleeding, this is a good time to review your supplements to see if, inadvertently, they are contributing to your problem. If you take two or more of the products listed below, please consult with a practitioner versed in natural medicines to evaluate your doses and the potential effect they may have on bleeding:

- Vitamin E
- Omega-3 fatty acids (evening primrose oil, flaxseed oil, fish oil, black currant oil, borage oil, hemp oil)
- Ginkgo biloba
- Ginseng (Panax variety)
- Garlic
- Ginger

Anemia

Very long and/or prolonged bleeding can sometimes cause an iron-deficiency anemia. Women who are anemic from heavy periods may feel fatigued and listless. By no means are these symptoms universal, for it is possible to be anemic and not notice a change in energy. If excessive bleeding and/or fatigue with your periods occurs for you, ask your practitioner for a simple test for anemia.

Adding Iron

If in fact you are anemic, you can help your body recover by ingesting iron in your diet and in supplements. However, all iron is not created equal. Some forms are easily absorbed, and some aren't. This applies to both foods and supplements. If you are having a hard time keeping your blood measurements for anemia up, the following information is especially important.

Foods

Kelp (good in soups), brewer's yeast, and blackstrap molasses contain the most concentrated forms of dietary iron. Pumpkin seeds, wheat bran, red meat, sunflower seeds, almonds, and raisins are also good sources.[7]

Beef and liver have the most highly absorbable form of iron of all foods. The form of iron found in meat, poultry, and seafood is much more easily absorbed than that from vegetarian sources. Therefore, vegetarians who are anemic generally need to be more conscious of supplement doses and the factors affecting iron absorption.

Heme Iron Supplements

"Heme" iron supplements are the best absorbed form of iron next to actually eating meat because they are manufactured from animal products. They absorb at close to 35%, and do not cause the gastrointestinal side effects frequently experienced with synthetic iron compounds. According to naturopathic physician and nutritional expert Michael Murray, N.D., supplementing with 3 mg of heme iron provides the bloodstream with as much iron as taking 50 mg of the most common form of synthetic iron, ferrous sulfate.[8] Heme iron supplements are available from specialized vitamin stores. They are bulkier and less pleasant to take than ferrous sulfate.

Herbal Iron Supplements

Burdock, dandelion, yellow dock, and nettle are among the herbs most famous for their iron content. (For the iron content of these herbs, see Table 3.1.) Teas, capsules, or tinctures (liquid extracts) of the roots of these herbs can contain significant amounts of iron, and have been effectively used to treat anemia for generations. Like heme iron, herbal iron supplements are not associated with gastrointestinal side effects such as constipation. They can usually be found in stores specializing in natural health products and natural food stores. Ask the proprietor for an "herbal iron compound." One such product, Floridex, combines herbs and ferrous gluconate to provide 7.5 milligrams of iron per 10 milliliters. Locally made compounds, made from organic or wildcrafted herbs, will tend to produce the purest, freshest, and best remedies. In general, lower doses of herbal forms of iron work comparably to higher doses of synthetic forms. Tinctures are usually dosed between 1–2 teaspoons (5–10 mL) per day.

Synthetic Iron Supplements

Ferrous sulfate is the most popular form of iron supplement because it is inexpensive and non-bulky and, hence, easy to take. It is also the least absorbable. Ferrous sulfate has an absorption rate of less than 3%, and hence, high doses need to be ingested for enough iron to actually make its way into the bloodstream. This absorption problem contributes to ferrous

Table 3.1. Iron Content of Selected Herbs

Herb	Iron Content*
Nettle	41.8 mg
Yellow dock	76 mg
Dandelion	96 mg
Burdock	147 mg

*Milligrams of iron per 1,000 milligrams of dried herb, which equals approximately two single "0" gel caps.
Information adapted from *Nutritional Herbology*, Mark Pederson[9]

sulfate's side effects of nausea and, most commonly, constipation. Ferrous sulfate is now available with a stool softener additive to combat this problem.

About one-fifth of the total milligram content of ferrous sulfate is actually "elemental iron." To supply the 100–200 mg per day of elemental iron one needs to combat iron deficiency anemia, patients generally need to consume 500–1000 mg of ferrous sulfate divided up over the course of a day.[10]

Many conventional practitioners are turning to ferrous gluconate over ferrous sulfate when recommending a synthetic iron supplement to their patients. Enhanced absorption and fewer side effects make this remedy more attractive. It is bulkier than ferrous sulfate, however. One needs to take 800–1900 mg of straight ferrous gluconate to supply the needed 100–200mg/day of elemental iron in anemia.

Enhancing Iron Absorption

Iron is a picky mineral—meaning it dislikes sharing the digestive tract with several nutrients and foods in order to optimize its uptake into the system. For example, absorption of iron can be impaired by up to 50% by drinking coffee or black tea, because chemicals in these beverages, known as tannins, bind to iron and prevent its absorption from the gut. Likewise, carbonated soft drinks, aspirin, and alcohol, if ingested with iron, bind to it and form insoluble compounds which are not transported into the bloodstream. Even some foods, such as eggs, cheese and fiber, as well as minerals like calcium, magnesium and zinc can interfere with iron absorption.

Vitamin C, on the other hand, increases iron absorption. If your digestive tract can tolerate it, take iron supplements between meals. Adding a source of vitamin C will enhance its uptake into the system.[11] This is especially important for women choosing vegetarian sources of iron.

"Perimenopausal PMS"

Linda is 47 and prides herself on living a healthy lifestyle in her small town on Cape Cod. She takes care to exercise regularly, shops at a local natural foods store for her family, and strives to create balance between home, work, and community. For most of her life, Linda has been able to recognize and wait out minor PMS.

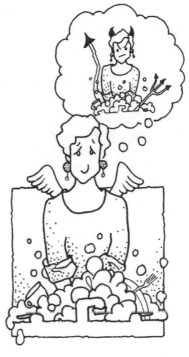

"I used to have about three days of breast tenderness and bloating before my period—and I was able to predict when it was coming," she says. "I'd get crabby one day before my period. Lately, however, the PMS seems to go on and on," she continues. "Now I can get those changes for two weeks or longer before my period shows up. It feels like my period should be coming, but it might not come for weeks. The hardest part is the mood swings. Last week my husband said, jokingly, 'Who are you and what have you done with my wife?' I don't know how much longer his patience is going to hold."

Stories like Linda's are common. As the menopausal years approach, changes in cycles can sometimes include changes in our experience with PMS. For many women, this means that premenstrual symptoms, which used to last for a short time, now can stretch out for days or even weeks, particularly during anovulatory cycles. Women with perimenopausal PMS feel premenstrual, but the period comes late, or doesn't show up at all. When this happens, PMS that was once relatively short (and therefore tolerable) can turn into an extended time of discomfort.

What Causes "Perimenopausal PMS"?

Much debate and study over the exact cause of PMS have turned up many theories—ranging from changes in brain chemicals and their function, to imbalances in female hormones, to social and cultural feelings about menstruation. The cause of PMS may turn out to be a combination of several interweaving factors.

Researchers generally see a significant placebo effect in the treatment of PMS,[12] which suggests that psychological factors do play a role. It also supports the theory that negative views on menstruation and menopause may indeed influence women's experiences during the days leading up to the menses.

Regarding a connection between PMS and perimenopause, women who have a history of severe PMS during their reproductive years tend to have more difficulties with the perimenopause.[13,14] In Chapter 9, we'll explore how fluctuating hormones in both PMS and in perimenopause can affect mental health in similar ways. It's likely that physical experiences such as bloating, food cravings, and headaches at perimenopause stem from hormonal changes much like that during PMS earlier in life.

Some researchers have demonstrated a decrease in progesterone and its breakdown products in women with PMS.[15,16] Other researchers refute these findings.[17,18,19] Similarly, studies have found both positive[20] and negative[21] results using either oral or vaginal progesterone in the treatment of PMS. Many practitioners espouse a theory that PMS at perimenopause is caused by an imbalance in the ratio of estrogen and progesterone, or a state of relative estrogen dominance. Preceding menopause, it is known that women's bodies experience an elevation in FSH and correspondingly, sometimes have slightly elevated levels of estradiol (estrogen).[22,23] If the theory of estrogen dominance contributing to PMS turns out to be true, the increase in PMS some women experience in perimenopause could relate to an increase in estrogen related to progesterone at this time. Certainly the observation made by many natural health practitioners and their patients is that progesterone-enhancing therapies can be a valuable tool in decreasing symptoms of PMS in perimenopause.

Help for "Perimenopausal PMS"

Besides the reassurance that PMS will one day vanish when cycles come to an end, there are things we can do right now that can help tremendously. In this department, natural methods, in particular, work well as frontline approaches.

Exercise

Anecdotal reports on the value of exercise for PMS symptoms are now being supported by research. Studies have found that mood disturbances are the premenstrual symptom that responds best to exercise. Ability to concentrate, pain and behavior changes were also improved.[24] In studies done in the United Kingdom and Australia, PMS symptoms improved the more women exercised—up to a point. Women who actually competed in athletics did not have a better time premenstrually than others,[25] which may lead us to believe that a more relaxed and less pressured form of exercise works best. Whether it's the release of natural "antidepressant" endorphins in the body, the speeding up of hormonal metabolism with increased circulation, or a host of other factors that are responsible for alleviating the discomforts of PMS, women who latch onto this nearly universally helpful remedy will all tell you one thing—it works.

Diet

Naturopathic physicians typically recommend a low animal-fat, high fiber diet with plenty of fresh fruit, vegetables, and fluids (minus the caffeine and alcohol) for their patients who suffer from PMS. Current research suggests that the effectiveness of this approach may be due to an increase in the type of protein which binds up estrogen, rendering it less active on tissues.[26] We'll discuss more about estrogen and this carrier-protein in Chapter 11.

Vitamin B₆

Vitamin B_6 is a favorite remedy for women suffering from PMS at any age. Scientific studies generally support its role in PMS,[27,28] although the existence of several negative studies also tells us that it's not necessarily the strongest remedy for this problem. Vitamin B_6 has been proposed to enhance the production of brain chemicals found to be decreased in women with PMS.[29] Recommended doses are 50 mg either once or twice per day. Vitamin B_6 taken long-term in excess (150–500 mg/day) can be associated with toxicity, manifesting as numbness, tingling or sensation loss in the hands or feet.[30]

Calcium

A review of all scientific data published on calcium in the treatment of PMS found that 1200–1600 mg per day can be considered an effective treatment for PMS.[31] These numbers are approximately the same as the recommended daily allowance for perimenopausal woman—and so most women should be getting this much calcium anyway. The problem is that most women don't. Chapter 7 includes a chart to help you figure out your daily average dietary consumption of calcium. To treat perimenopausal PMS then, you can supplement enough to bring your daily intake into the 1500 mg/day range.

Researchers are just beginning to understand the relationship between calcium intake and PMS. It is known that estrogen affects the body's absorption, usage, and breakdown of calcium; therefore, normal cycle fluctuations in female hormones affect calcium blood levels. It has also been pointed out by researchers at Columbia University that PMS symptoms look remarkably similar to those of people who suffer from calcium deficiency. They hypothesize, therefore, that PMS actually results from an underlying calcium deficiency that is "unmasked" when ovarian hormone levels go up.[32]

Vitex

A recent German study of 1,634 patients with PMS found vitex to decrease symptoms in 93% of these women.[33] The herb's effectiveness for PMS has also stood up to randomized, placebo-controlled study (the "gold standard"), as reported in the British Medical Journal in 2001.[34] If you recall from our discussion about regulating cycles on page 43, vitex seems to work by favoring the body's production of progesterone by mildly increasing LH and inhibiting FSH. This mechanism lends support to the theory that a predominance of estrogen, relative to progesterone, may contribute to PMS.

Because vitex is such an excellent herb for both regulating cycles and for PMS, it is one of the most valuable remedies for women in early perimenopause. Frequently, this one herb can take the place of several remedies—which is a relief for women who feel they're taking too many pills. Doses are the same as for regulating cycles (see page 43), and in some cases, the herb can be taken during the last half of the cycle only. A knowledgeable practitioner, trained in herbal therapies, can help you decide when and how much to take.

There will come a time in the perimenopause, when follicles are getting fewer and farther between, when vitex will no longer be effective. At that time, you and your practitioner can choose a subsequent therapy. This is an illustration of the fact that perimenopause is an evolving process, which means that your treatments should be reevaluated as you progress through this transition.

Herbal Combinations

Many herbs, in addition to vitex, have historically been employed for women for relief from symptoms of PMS. Some examples include dandelion leaf for water retention, valerian or skullcap for anxiety[35] and don quai, black cohosh, and wild yam for the more elusive reported action of "hormone balancing." While research is beginning to provide us with some understanding of these herbs, we are far from understanding their exact action on the body and on PMS symptoms in particular.

Herbal companies frequently combine a number of these herbs into one product—some with knowledge of how the herbs work synergistically, and some out of a more or less "shotgun" approach. In addition, herbs are widely variable in potency and, therefore, effectiveness. Thus is it important to obtain the recommendation of someone knowledgeable about herbal medicine before bringing one of these combination PMS remedies home. Better yet, working with a practitioner who can pull together a combination of the herbs most indicated for you specifically will greatly increase your chances for success in treating "perimenopausal PMS" with herbs.

Natural Progesterone

The widespread popularity of over-the-counter natural progesterone creams mandates a discussion of this topic, which we will begin here, and continue in Chapter 10. Women are arriving at their practitioners' doorsteps, armed with a copy of a popular book about natural progesterone in one hand and a tube of the cream in the other—seeking a professional's advice. They have read or heard that natural progesterone will cure everything from PMS to hot flashes to osteoporosis—will increase bust size, enhance libido, treat fibroids, and more . . . all without side effects or risks!

Aggressive marketing of the product has turned an important tool for women's medicine into a controversial topic, and put it in the hands of thousands of women who are taking this hormone without the supervision of a health practitioner. Natural progesterone is a hormone, and carries with it potential side effects and risks, including promoting depression and some more rare, progesterone-sensitive breast cancers. (Yes—just because it's "natural" doesn't mean it has no effect on cancer risk.)

Used with appropriate supervision, natural progesterone can be quite helpful. Many natural and integrative health practitioners, including gynecologist and popular author Christiane Northrup, M.D., have reported quite a bit of success treating PMS, before and during perimenopause, with various forms of natural progesterone, based on the theory of "estrogen dominance" as a cause.[36]

A review looking at all the studies done to date on progesterone for PMS, however, found no benefit over placebo (BMJ).[37] Yet many women and practitioners swear by this remedy. If we look closer, it seems that the effectiveness of progesterone cream for PMS probably depends upon which PMS symptoms a woman has. Anxiety, insomnia, rage, and irritability (which some practitioners feel are signs of estrogen dominance) may respond well to progesterone. Depression and bloating, on the other hand, can get worse on natural progesterone. If you are interested in looking into this method for treatment of perimenopausal PMS, your best bet is to locate a well-trained practitioner who has considerable clinical experience in this area, and can supervise your use of this steroid hormone.

Birth Control Pills

Many women will find relief of PMS symptoms by using birth control pills, but others will not. If you intend to use oral contraceptives for control of bleeding, then PMS may be improved as well. The theory behind this action is that birth control pills provide a rather consistent level of hormones throughout the cycle. This can be a relief to women whose hormones fluctuate widely.

How to Choose Your Best Approach

So now you've learned a lot about the cycle changes possible during the perimenopause, and have been handed a list of treatments for their potential challenges. But how do you know which one to use?

Ah . . . this is where the art and science of medicine come together. Obtaining an accurate assessment of your situation with your clinician can narrow down your choices. For example, if your periods have begun to get less predictable, but bleeding isn't much heavier or longer, you may appropriately use natural medicine, such as vitex, if you desire to regulate your cycles. On the other hand, if you experience regular severe flooding or even hemorrhaging, you should promptly see a primary care provider for an assessment.

Many problems can be approached from both a conventional and a natural perspective. For example, anemia must be diagnosed and followed using conventional laboratory testing by a qualified practitioner. If not severe, you can opt to use a natural treatment for it, such as an herbal iron compound and diet. When you are using both natural and conventional practitioners, it is best to get them talking to one another, sharing information regarding your treatment.

When providers from different disciplines work collaboratively, it is called "co-management," and it promotes receiving safe and effective therapies that fit your situation and desires. As a patient, you have a right to request that your practitioners respect and work professionally with one another, on your behalf. You can facilitate this by asking that they each

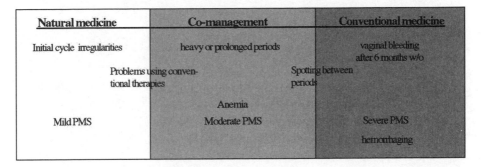

Natural medicine	Co-management	Conventional medicine
Initial cycle irregularities	heavy or prolonged periods	vaginal bleeding after 6 months w/o
	Problems using conventional therapies	Spotting between periods
	Anemia	
Mild PMS	Moderate PMS	Severe PMS
		hemorrhaging

Figure 3.2.   Continuum of therapies for menopausal changes

copy their notes from your visit to send to one another, or by granting them permission to exchange information about you via telephone, if appropriate. Besides getting the best of both worlds, you will be furthering the integration of worlds of medicine which have long been separate.

Figure 3.2 provides a rough guideline showing when to seek conventional intervention and when natural approaches are appropriate. It includes an overlapping section where both might be used collaboratively. (Arguably, the overlapping section could well be extended in either direction.) As with most things, there are always exceptions to these guidelines; so if you aren't sure, speak with your practitioner about which approach she or he feels would be appropriate for you. These guidelines are intended to help point those unfamiliar to this arena in the right direction.

4   Vasomotor Changes

Mention the word *menopause* and most Westerners immediately associate it with the hot flash. Hot flashes, or flushes as they are sometimes called, fall under a category of physical symptoms known as *vasomotor changes*. Vasomotor changes are alterations in circulation that cause temperature fluctuations. Hot flashes and night sweats, as well as insomnia and, possibly, heart palpitations are all a result of vasomotor changes. In this chapter, we'll address the causes, contributors, and solutions for all of them.

Hot Flashes and Night Sweats

There is substantial variability in how women experience hot flashes and night sweats. The following example of Jane and Rosemary illustrates this point. Jane, a 51-year-old social worker, was not actually sure if she was having hot flashes. "I'm not aware of feeling flushed or sweating or anything like that," she recounts. "It's just that I feel, overall, warmer than before. This is the first winter where I don't have to wear a sweater all the time. Actually, it's a welcome change."

By contrast, Rosemary, 49, wonders if she'll ever stop sweating. "One hot flash just seems to roll right into another," she says. "I can't even count them. The sleep is the hardest part. I'm up no less than four times per night."

Jane and Rosemary are experiencing two ends of the spectrum of vasomotor changes. While some women, like Jane, have mild or even unnoticeable symptoms, others, like Rosemary, may experience significant discomfort. Rarely, in severe cases, hot flashes can occur every few min-

utes, or last for up to an hour.[1]
Typically, the severity of vasomotor
symptoms for women who do have
them fall somewhere between the
two extremes. Hot flashes end naturally, for most women, after one
or two years. For some women,
however, hot flashes and night
sweats can last up to five years or
more.

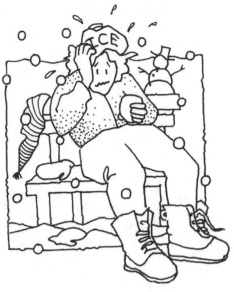

Even though the hot flash has
come to be known as the hallmark
of menopause in this country, a significant percentage of women do
not have hot flashes. Remember—
there are cultures that don't even
have a word for this experience. In
other words, hot flashes are not
obligatory!

What Causes Hot Flashes and Night Sweats?

Despite much study, the exact cause of hot flashes and night sweats
continues to elude doctors and scientists. Like PMS, many causes are proposed, and the real answer may turn out to encompass several contributing factors. Pulses in leuteinizing hormone (LH) from the pituitary have
been implicated. So has the interaction between several different chemicals—neurotransmitters and endorphins—in the brain and bloodstream.
The quest is on to understand just how the delicate orchestration between
these and other potential players results in a hot flash. No doubt, the
search will keep menopause researchers busy for a long time.

We *do* know that the decrease in estrogen somehow causes the temperature regulating centers of the brain, located in an area known as the hypothalamus, to behave differently. Sudden signals from the hypothalamus
alter the body's blood flow, causing arteries near the skin's surface to di-
late. This produces a sometimes visible "flush" and brings heat to the
skin's surface.

Environmental temperature changes, stress, diet, exercise, smoking,
body weight, and other factors can affect hot flashes. We can learn a lot
about these and other factors by observing the diet and lifestyle habits of
women in cultures where vasomotor symptoms are more rare. When we
discuss treatment options later, some of these lifestyle changes will get top
billing.

More and more frequently nowadays, my hot flashes have begun to feel like urgent communiques from the interior of a vast, dark continent—fast breaking news, items from my heart of darkness. Sometimes hot flashes trigger sudden insights into previously obscure experiences. Other times, in reverse fashion, a rush of revelations will release the heat like thunder after a flash of lightning. Either way, I have come to trust the wired insight that hot flashes produce. Because I believe in epiphanies, I record most of these illuminations in a notebook I carry in my purse. Since hot flashes are often cryptic, I try to decipher their meanings as soon as possible.

Barbara Raskin[2]

What Happens During a Hot Flash?

The body's physical changes during a hot flash includes a rise in body temperature on the skin surface—by as much as four degrees. While the

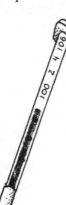

skin's temperature goes up, meanwhile, the temperature in the core of the body (i.e., in the organs) goes down. This decrease in core temperature causes *chills* for some women, which therefore count as vasomotor symptoms. Our pulse can increase by nine beats per minute or more during a hot flash. Blood pressure, typically, does not change.[3]

Night sweats are caused by a stronger version of the same mechanism which causes hot flashes. They range in intensity, sometimes causing profuse perspiration. The same therapies offered for hot flashes also will apply to night sweats.

Perimenopausal Insomnia

While Jane barely noticed hot flashes or night sweats, she did have one annoying perimenopausal symptom: "I wake up at 3 A.M., like clockwork. Then I'm up for at least an hour." Although she never sweats, she says her husband notices the rise in her body temperature. "He say's I'm like a furnace. He has to move to the opposite side of the bed."

Research shows that perimenopausal insomnia is the result of the same vasomotor fluctuations in blood flow and temperature that cause hot flashes and night sweats. In many cases, a woman may be aware that she woke up during a night sweat or a temperature elevation. In other cases, her temperature probably fluctuated enough to wake her, but not enough for her to notice, or to cause her to perspire.

Most perimenopausal patients with insomnia report little to no trouble getting to sleep. Instead, they awaken in the middle of sleep, often between 2–4 A.M. (and with surprising frequency near 3 A.M.) Therefore, one

helpful way to differentiate insomnia caused by stress or anxiety from one attributed to
perimenopause is to note
whether you have trouble
falling asleep or if you wake in
the middle of the night.

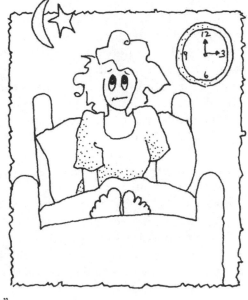

Another common pattern is
to wake up very early, such as
4:30 or 5 A.M. and not be able to
get back to sleep. Nancy, an educational consultant, describes
her experience of this pattern
succinctly. "I'm up!" she exclaims. Eyes wide open, Nancy
comically illustrates her early
morning alertness. "I'm up!
There's no use trying to get
back to sleep. I'm up for the day."

Some women find that they seem to actually need less sleep beginning
at menopause than they did before. A few will report using these quiet
early morning hours productively, engaging in activities such as writing,
exercise, or meditation. This quality is not shared by women who suffer
from depression (which can also cause an early wake-up pattern), and is
therefore one distinguishing factor between these two causes of insomnia.
Commonly, women find that an extended time of little or interrupted
sleep becomes exhausting. Whether a woman awakens rested and re-
freshed, or groggy, may have to do with how deeply she slept during her
shortened sleep time, as well as the general demands of her life.

Many women find they need to get up to urinate during the night and
wonder if it's their bladder that wakes them up. In Chapter 8, which covers
urinary health, we will discuss the effect of dropping estrogen levels on
the urinary tract, which may become more sensitive to urinary urgency.
Waking easily to use the bathroom is probably caused by the combination
of increased bladder sensitivity and the fluctuating temperatures that lead
to a more superficial sleep.

Heart Palpitations

Normally, we are not aware of our heart beating. During a heart palpi-
tation, we "feel" our heart. Palpitations are a sense of rapid or irregular
heartbeat and may feel like a fluttering, a pounding, or just an increased
sensation of the heartbeat.

Many women entering the menopausal years report these sensations.

Sometimes, they happen in tandem with a hot flash or night sweat. Episodes may occur rarely or several times per day. Clinicians do not unanimously agree as to whether heart palpitations which occur at this time are truly related to menopause. Furthermore, research to settle the dispute is scant. We do know a little about what happens to the heart during a hot flash, however, and this knowledge is the basis for some practitioners' belief that palpitations are, in fact, vasomotor symptoms.

First of all, we know that the heart beats faster during a hot flash—as we learned, up to nine beats per minute or more. In addition, one study has found that the sympathetic (also known as the "fight-or-flight") portion of the nervous system is more active at menopause.[4] It is possible that this increase in sympathetic nerve output, which increases heart rate, may trigger an actual irregular beat. At the very least, experiencing a faster heartbeat is a known vasomotor change.

The vast majority of heart palpitations around the time of menopause are benign and don't require treatment. It is important, however, to be aware that causes unrelated to menopause, such as thyroid problems, anxiety, caffeine, or indeed actual heart abnormalities, can trigger palpitations. For this reason, it is not safe to assume that palpitations are benign without an evaluation. As a precaution, if you have palpitations and are unsure of their cause, please see your practitioner. If you experience shortness of breath, chest pains or anxiety with them, see someone immediately.

Remedies for Vasomotor Changes

Many women have tolerable vasomotor changes and choose to let nature take its course in this regard. For those who find these symptoms disruptive or sometimes debilitating, the following approaches can be very helpful. As before, we've arranged them in increasing order of strength and intervention.

Diet

Although science has yet to sufficiently study the dietary triggers of hot flashes, many a perimenopausal woman doesn't need a study to confirm that a particular food can set off a hot flash for her. "One sip of alcohol is all it takes for me!" says Peg. "I light up like a Christmas tree." In one study of 334 menopausal women, alcohol intake was suggestive, but not proven, as contributing to hot flashes.[5]

Other anecdotal reports from individual patients include triggers such as caffeine, hot liquids, spicy foods, and sugar. Dietary triggers may be unique to each woman. You can easily and safely test your own response to these foods by avoiding them for two weeks, and then introducing one at a time, paying attention to whether or not they provoke a hot flash for you. Nutritionists and naturopathic physicians can help you create a specific schedule for doing so if you'd like guidance.

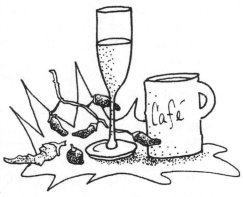

Also for hot flashes and night sweats, try adding "cooling" foods and beverages to your diet. Iced peppermint, spearmint or hibiscus tea, cucumbers and watermelons all have the reputation, particularly in warmer climates, of having a cooling effect on the body. With "cooling" foods, expect modest, not dramatic, results.

Most menopausal women are familiar with the recommendation to add soy to the diet. Soy has enjoyed the spotlight for its health benefits for several years. This attention has fortunately resulted in a multitude of studies of this famous legume. Today we have much data on soy's impact on menopausal symptoms, heart disease, osteoporosis, cancer risk, and more, yet we have much more to learn. We will revisit soy in several chapters in this book, as we address each area individually. For now, let's find out what is true about soy's effect on vasomotor symptoms.

Studies routinely find that soy protein reduces hot flashes. The part of soy responsible for this action is its isoflavone content. Soy contains several isoflavones (genestein and diadzein are the best studied), in addition to other compounds, which have the remarkable ability to act like weak estrogens in the body. Any plant constituent that mimics the effect of estrogen is known as a *phytoestrogen*. Thus, when we consume soy products when our estrogen levels are low, the isoflavones in soy give our bodies a phyto-

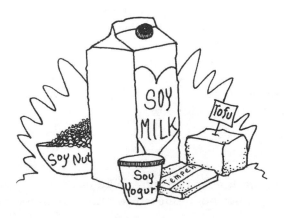

(or plant) estrogen boost. Soy isoflavones do not seem to induce growth of the endometrial (uterine) lining, like estrogen can, however. This finding leads many experts to suggest soy is a potentially safe alternative to estrogen replacement.[6]

A recent study found 76 mg of soy isoflavones per day superior to placebo in decreasing menopausal hot flashes.[7] To replicate this amount of isoflavones in your diet, you could include, for example, one cup of soy milk and one-half cup of tofu. Alternately, you could put one-eighth cup of soy flour in your pancake batter and munch on one-fourth cup of soy nuts during the day. Table 4.1 gives you a quick reference to help you calculate isoflavone content in your diet. These are average amounts—certain brands may vary.

Table 4.1. Isoflavone Content of Selected Soy Foods

Food	Serving size	Isoflavones
Cooked soybeans	½ cup	150
Roasted soy nuts	¼ cup	60
Textured soy protein	¼ cup	60
Soy milk	1 cup	40
Tofu	½ cup	35
Tempeh	½ cup	35
Soy flour	¼ cup	25
Soy yogurt	6 oz	25
Roasted soy butter	2 tbsp	15
Miso	1 tsp	5

Many Americans have difficulty digesting soy products. This may be due to differences in preparation methods of soy foods between the Orient and the West. Japanese and Chinese soy foods are traditionally fermented and, therefore, easier to digest. If you have a problem digesting soy products, try starting out with the two fermented items on this list: miso and tempeh. Helpful cookbooks in learning how to prepare tasty (yes—tasty!) soy dishes include *The New Soy Cookbook* by Lorna Sass and *The Whole Soy Cookbook* by Patricia Greenberg.

Lifestyle

The way we live our lives can actually make us more or less susceptible to vasomotor changes like hot flashes. If you have room for improvement in any of the following elements of lifestyle, instituting a change here could make a significant difference for you.

Stop Smoking

Smoking in thin women (but not in overweight women) is associated with an increased frequency of hot flashes.[8] Hot flash relief, of course, is just the tip of the iceberg when it comes to the health benefits of not smoking. We will revisit the detrimental effects of smoking in our chapters on osteoporosis, heart disease, and cancer.

If you smoke and are ready to quit, most providers of natural and conventional medicine can help you. Inquire about prescription or over-the-counter nicotine substitutes from your conventional provider. These come as gum, patches, or inhalers, and decrease the physical discomforts associated with smoking cessation. Ask about referrals to smoking cessation programs in your area. These programs can include behavioral medicine referrals, acupuncture, hypnosis, and herbal therapies. Because "company is stronger than willpower,"[9] a support "team," consisting of your practitioner, friends or family, and a smoking cessation program (if available) can help you stay on track and win the battle against this most addictive of substances.

Reduce Stress

Studies routinely find a correlation between stress levels and increased hot flashes.[10] Relaxation techniques such as meditation, guided visualization, and listening to relaxation tapes have been promoted to reduce stress and therefore potentially help relieve hot flashes.

Researchers have found that a stress reduction technique of deep abdominal breathing, borrowed from yoga, resulted in a 50% reduction of hot flashes.[11] "Women who've been trained to use this technique as soon as they feel a flush coming on are often able to abort the flash or at least reduce its severity," the study concluded. Try a relaxation method, such as *the Abdominal Breathing Technique* presented on page 73 to head off or decrease the intensity of a hot flash. Moreover, regular practice of abdominal breathing, even when we're not having a hot flash, may prevent future ones.

Different people will be attracted to different types of relaxation methods. Try out a few and see what works for you. Reading, napping, yoga, t'ai chi, massage, and meditation are just a few of the many options. For more ideas about stress reduction techniques that may reduce hot flashes, consult the book *Healing Mind, Healthy Woman* by Alice Domar, director of the Center for Women's Health at Harvard Medical School's Mind/Body Medical Institute.

Marilyn's Halloween Costume

Marilyn took the humorous approach to dealing with her hot flashes. One Halloween, in the middle of her perimenopause, Marilyn dressed as a *hot flash* for a costume party! She donned a red skirt, blaze orange blouse, and a red plastic apron she had found in a discount store. In the apron's see-through pocket, she placed a flashing bicycle night-light. She fashioned a hat of red netting, and arranged it so that it looked like a flame leaping out of her head.

When the other partygoers learned what her costume represented, they inevitably burst out with laughter. "It had everybody talking about menopause," Marilyn remembers. "It was great fun. And most of all, it broke the stigma attached to menopause and hot flashes. I think everyone at the party was changed by it."

Exercise

A 1998 Swedish study of over 1,300 women ages 55 and 56 found that sedentary women were three times more likely to experience hot flashes than physically active women.[12] Likewise, a second Scandinavian study found that sedentary women were more than twice as likely to have hot flashes when compared to active women. What's more, researchers found that the more women exercised, the fewer and less intense their hot flashes were. Women in this study who exercised 3.5 hours per week had an average of zero hot flashes.[13] No one knows exactly how exercise decreases hot flashes. Scientists theorize that it may have to do with the production of *endorphins,* the same molecules which contribute to mood enhancement. So if you're feeling blue and have hot flashes to boot, an exercise plan could help in both ways.

Turn Down the Heat

There are some pretty simple measures that many women use in coping with hot flashes. Layered and cool clothing, so you can pare down as needed during the day is often essential. Keeping the thermostat lower, especially at night, is important. Lighter bedclothes, lighter blankets, and sleeping with the window cracked open are yet other coping tactics.

Nutritional Supplements

If diet and lifestyle measures don't take care of your vasomotor symptoms, try the next category of treatments: supplements. You can also double up on lifestyle, dietary, and supplement approaches, such as eating cooling foods, cutting out coffee and sugar, and using one of the remedies below.

Vitamins E and C

Vitamin E has a reputation for treating hot flashes that dates back to studies performed during the 1940s[14] and has received very little attention from researchers since. Therefore, we don't have current data on the use of vitamin E for hot flashes in the general menopausal population. (There was a study recently done with breast cancer survivors, which we'll mention in Chapter 9.) The recommended dose is 400–800 IU. Note that vitamin E is a blood thinner and should not be used in conjunction with Coumadin®, aspirin, or other blood thinners without supervision by a provider who can monitor this potential problem. Also, stop vitamin E supplements two weeks before any surgery, even minor dental surgery, to prevent bleeding complications.

Vitamin C, along with compounds known as bioflavonoids, has been shown to decrease hot flashes.[15] The recommended dosage is 1,200 mg vitamin C, combined with 900 mg hesperidin, a bioflavonoid which can augment its effect. Vitamin C derived from rose hips contains this bioflavonoid, and can be found at most health food stores.

Realistically, vitamins E and C each have only a modest impact on vasomotor symptoms at best, and the research is scant. Because their action is relatively weak, it makes sense to use these remedies only in cases where hot flashes are mild or there is another, stronger indication to use one. Vitamin E, for example, may be a good choice for a woman who has mild hot flashes along with some cardiac risk factors. (Vitamin E is well indicated to decrease some forms of cardiac risk, as we'll discuss in detail in Chapter 6.)

Soy Supplements

Many nutritional product companies have jumped on the soy bandwagon and now offer us pill-popping Westerners an easy way to consume the "miracle food." Soy supplements do work for vasomotor symptoms, and they are more effective for this than vitamins E and C. They are dosed according to their isoflavone content, and range from around 40 to 150 mg of isoflavone content per day.

Most researchers agree that women who consume these amounts of soy isoflavones *in the diet, and over a lifetime*—such as the Japanese—are generally healthier for it. However, at present, no data exists regarding the long-term use of concentrated soy supplements in menopausal women.

Therefore, as a general precaution, experts generally recommend that women not consume more than 150 mg isoflavones per day, which is the upper limits of that found in a traditional Japanese diet.[16] At 150 mg of isoflavones, Western women are already consuming 50 times that found in a traditional American diet!

Herbs

Black Cohosh

Unlike drugs or supplements, herbs have enjoyed a history of use in women's health for hundreds of years. Modern research that explains the actions of herbs continually refines our understanding of nature's pharmacy and allows for more sophisticated and appropriate prescribing. For many women, these gentle remedies are important allies along their menopausal journey.

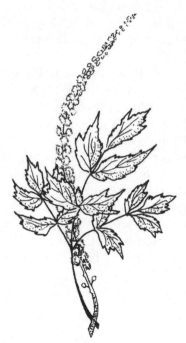

The most well known and well studied herbal medicine for relief of vasomotor symptoms is black cohosh. A native to North America itself, black cohosh (*Cimicifuga racemosa*) was used by native peoples of Canada, Wisconsin, and Missouri to treat pain during menses and childbirth. Westerners recorded its use for relief of menopausal discomforts beginning in the mid-1700s.[17] We find this herb listed in the pharmacy "bible" of the United States, the *United States Pharmacopoeia*, since its first edition in 1920.[18]

Black cohosh
(*Cimicifuga racemosa*)

Germans are responsible for black cohosh's modern popularity, and most of its Western scientific backing. Herbal historian Steven Foster chronicles its use in Germany during the 1930s, 1940s and 1950s in gynecology,[19] where great debate among physicians regarding its effectiveness led to several studies of the herb's use for menopausal complaints. Most of these studies yielded good results for effect and safety.[20]

Foster points out that as scientific rigor improved between the 1960s and 1990s, a series of double-blind, placebo-controlled trials in Germany on a standardized version of black cohosh known as Remifemin® were conducted. These studies led to black cohosh becoming established as a menopausal "therapy of choice" among a large percentage of German physicians, particularly in cases where estrogen was contraindicated.

Black cohosh has compared favorably in head-to-head studies with estrogens. In one study, 60 women with vasomotor symptoms following hysterectomy (without ovary removal) were randomly divided into four groups and blindly given either black cohosh, estriol (an estrogen that we'll say much more about in Chapter 10), conjugated estrogens (like Premarin®), or estrogen plus a synthetic progesterone. Black cohosh therapy lowered the intensity and number of symptoms at the same rate as the estrogens.[21]

Currently under investigation, the exact mechanism of action of black cohosh is far from understood. Previous reports of black cohosh acting like a plant form of estrogen, or "phytoestrogen" have not been reproduced. In fact, researchers are now reversing their original thoughts that black cohosh acted as phytoestrogen.[22] Black cohosh does consistently test as being able to suppress LH (leuteinizing hormone). However, it does not affect levels of other hormones (estrogen, FSH, and others), which researchers believe would be affected if the herb contained significant quantities of phytoestrogens. Animal studies have shown a lack of estrogenic activity that led to the conclusion that black cohosh's effects do not exert themselves via estrogenic stimulation.[23]

Black cohosh has been applied to breast cancer cells in laboratory experiments and found to actually suppress cancer growth.[24, 25] This preliminary data has led many practitioners to feel more comfortable recommending this herb for menopausal women who have a high risk or personal history of breast cancer. At the moment, the evidence looks good, however, we look forward to more studies being done to absolutely confirm its safety in breast cancer survivors.

Pure black cohosh is available in capsule, tincture, or tea form. The propriety product brand Remifemin (which is simply black cohosh) was recently purchased by a large pharmaceutical company, and is available at chain stores. A practitioner trained in herbal medicine can guide you toward an appropriate dose for you.

Red Clover

In the 1940s, Australian sheep farmers who had planted red clover (*Trifolium pratense*) in their fields to feed their sheep became the unlikely folks to discover phytoestrogens. Many of their sheep, it turned out, became infertile in the years following the clover plantings. It took two years of research to learn that a chemical named *formononetin*, found in the clover, was largely to blame. Formononetin, researchers learned, had the ability to bind to estrogen receptors in the sheep's bodies in the same way that their own estrogen did. Consumed in enormous quantities over a whole day, these chemicals were actually able to interfere with the sheep's own hormonal system. In other words, the red clover acted like a contraceptive!

Later, scientists learned that red clover actually contains four phytoestrogens: *formononetin, diadzein, genestein,* and *biochanin.* (You may recall that soy contains diadzein and genestein.) All these compounds can bind

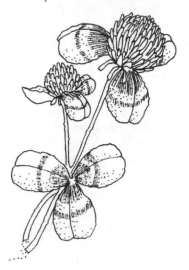

Red clover
(*Trifolium pratense*)

to estrogen receptors and therefore act like weak estrogen molecules. This fact has led to much marketing and development of red clover supplements aimed at the menopause market.

The problem is, very little data support red clover's use in vasomotor symptoms. One Australian (appropriately enough) study involving 50 women over a six month period of time failed to report a decrease in hot flashes with red clover extracts. On the plus side, the study showed that red clover raised HDL (good) cholesterol by 28%. In fact, the cardiovascular benefits of red clover have shown up consistently in studies, while its use for hot flashes, night sweats, heart palpitations, and insomnia have not.[26]

One word of caution is in order regarding red clover. A 1998 laboratory study demonstrated that breast cancer cells multiplied and grew when red clover was applied to them. In fact, the red clover extract had an equally strong effect as did estrogen itself, in this study.[27] Red clover's chief phytoestrogen, formononetin, may be responsible for this. In 1995, another study showed that formononetin promoted growth of breast cancer in mice when given in extremely high quantities (40 mg/kg formononetin = 1 mcg/kg/day of estradiol).[28] Therefore, if you are a breast cancer survivor, it is best to avoid red clover.

Other Herbs and Combinations

Many other plants contain phytoestrogens and are often included as ingredients in combination menopause formulas. Fennel, anise, alfalfa, flax, ginseng, and licorice all contain chemicals which bind to estrogen receptors. [29, 30, 31, 32] Other popular herbs used historically for vasomotor symptoms include don quai, wild yam, motherwort, and vitex.

In the area of vasomotor symptom relief, these herbs have enjoyed considerable historical use and have not yet been widely studied from a Western medical perspective. (However, one recent double blind study on wild yam cream found no benefit over placebo for daytime or nighttime flushing.[33]) The reason for such little scientific data on herbs has been lack of interest in the past from the general medical research community and from the pharmaceutical industry that funds most research on medicines in the United States. However, with the surge in popularity of herbal medicine in this country, we will probably see more research aimed at understanding, proving or disproving the effectiveness of such popular historic menopausal herbal remedies.

Estrogen and Progesterone/Progestins

Both estrogen and progesterone/progestins are effective for treating vasomotor symptoms. Of the two, estrogen generally works better. While the less invasive suggestions outlined previously in this chapter work in the majority of cases, in our clinical experience, hormones frequently provide more symptom relief than diet, supplements, or herbs in "tougher cases" of vasomotor symptoms. Therefore, we generally recommend HRT for women who either have extreme symptoms, and/or for women who have not found adequate relief taking more natural supplements—provided there is no contraindication to HRT. Women who have had a surgical menopause will likely need HRT to ease symptoms.

HRT has come a long way from its start at the beginning of the twentieth century. Today the choices of strength, forms, natural versus synthetic and delivery method are myriad—so many, that we've dedicated a whole chapter to discussing all the options. So if you find yourself looking seriously at using hormones to treat hot flashes, night sweats or insomnia, turn to Chapter 10. There you'll find a complete guide of the different forms of hormones to treat vasomotor symptoms.

For perimenopausal women, many practitioners will suggest oral contraceptive pills for treatment of vasomotor symptoms. This option may provide the additional benefit of cycle control, which is welcome for women who have erratic periods.

Selective Serotonin Reuptake Inhibitors

Rarely, chills and sweating can be caused by depression, rather than by low estrogen levels. If you suspect that you may be depressed, see a practitioner trained to diagnose this condition. If indeed it is determined that your "vasomotor" symptoms are due to depression, selective serotonin reuptake inhibitors (SSRIs), like Prozac®, Paxil®, and Zoloft® may benefit you and can even help with hot flashes. You'll need to consult a qualified practitioner to make this determination.

In Chapter 10, we'll discuss the potential use of SSRI medication for breast cancer survivors who have hot flashes.

Additional Remedies for Insomnia and Heart Palpitations

If you experience insomnia or heart palpitations, and if you and your clinician are reasonably certain that your problem is related to menopause, it is usually most effective to start with one of the remedies already mentioned. The therapies above all address the vasomotor changes that probably underlie insomnia or palpitations.

On occasion, however, one remedy just isn't enough. It is often appropriate to combine approaches, for added benefits. For example, eating soy products and exercising augment one another for relief of hot flashes. Likewise, HRT can be augmented by employing relaxation techniques to help with sleep. These are examples of appropriate integration of different therapies.

In other cases, "doubling-up" on remedies can be redundant, or even decrease each other's effectiveness. For instance, it doesn't make sense to take phytoestrogenic herbs along with HRT because they work by the same mechanism. At best, you'll be wasting your money on the herbs. At worst, it's conceivable that the herbs will in fact dilute the effect of the hormones.

If you are unsure of whether it makes sense to take two or more remedies for the same problem, talk it over with your practitioner. Whether or not she or he is familiar with the exact combination in question, she or he can most likely help you understand how each work. Together you have a good shot at determining the wisdom of using multiple remedies.

Outside of the realm of treating vasomotor changes, a few additional remedies can prove helpful for insomnia and palpitations. The treatments below do not address hot flashes or night sweats, and neither do they correct the hormonally related causes of insomnia or heart palpitations. However, they can be added to your plan if you need that extra bit of help.

For Insomnia

Many natural and conventional sleep aids are available. Sometimes, it's purely a matter of trial and error to see which one will work best for you. The following are some that we've found to be particularly useful for our patients.

Valerian

The herb valerian has been shown in several studies to have mild sedative effects and enhance sleep in people suffering from insomnia. The dose which has been shown to produce this result is 400–450 mg liquid extract before bedtime.[34, 35, 36, 37] Herbal practitioners will caution that valerian may cause drowsiness in the morning, which occurs in a minority of people. Milder herbal sleep aids include chamomile, hops, skullcap, and passion flower, which are available as teas or tinctures at health food stores.

Conventional Sleep Remedies

If sleep deprivation becomes a major problem, some practitioners may suggest over-the-counter sleeps aids, like Benadryl® (diphenhydramine). Taking 25–50 mg thirty minutes before bedtime allows for minimal drowsiness upon rising. On rare occasions, prescription sleep medications may be indicated but should not be used long-term as some may cause addiction. These include the benzodiazepines Ativan® (0.5–1.0 mg) or Klonopin® (0.25–0.5 mg), both taken at bedtime. Side effects of these medications can include daytime sedation and impaired coordination. Benzodiazepines should never be mixed with alcohol.

Trazodone (Desyrel®) is a sedating antidepressant sometimes used to help with sleep. It is dosed at 25–100 mg at bedtime, but may be taken earlier in the evening if sedation extends into the daytime. Zolpidem tartrate (Ambien®) taken in doses of 5–10 mg at bedtime has been shown to have side effects of mental status changes in addition to daytime fatigue and for this reason is less desirable.

For Heart Palpitations

If your clinician has ruled out serious causes of palpitations, you may decide to treat them if they bother you. This is purely a matter of comfort, for benign heart palpitations do not lead to problems down the road if left untreated. Try the following gentle remedies, which can be used safely along with any other therapies.

Deep Abdominal Breathing

One way to decrease output by the sympathetic nervous system and therefore decrease heart rate is through deep abdominal breathing. Use the diaphragm to move the belly *out* as you inhale, and *in* as you exhale. This activates the *parasympathetic* portion of the nervous system, which governs our digestive and reproductive organs and is in charge while we rest. By activating our parasympathetic nerves, we in fact redirect our nerve impulses from "fight-or-flight" into relaxation mode.

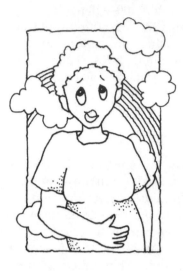

Most of us fill just the top part of our lungs when we take a deep breath. Sometimes we actually hold the belly in when we inhale, preventing full use of our lung capacity. These habits are ingrained, and require patience and persistence in order to unlearn. The following exercise will teach you how to breathe from deep in your belly, using the diaphragm.

Find a comfortable position, either sitting up straight or lying down. Uncross your legs. Take a few deep breaths and let them out. As you do this, notice what part of your torso moves when you breath. Does the chest rise and fall? Are the shoulders rising and falling? Is the belly moving in and out?

Now place your hands on your belly. Take a deep breath in, and as you exhale completely, use the abdominal muscles to pull the belly in toward the spine. Even press the belly in with the hands to accentuate the outbreath. Now, relax the belly, relax the hands, and fill the belly up like a balloon with the breath. Keep the shoulders relaxed, and the upper chest as still as possible. Breathe with the belly. When you've filled the belly, then relax it again, and then exhale all the air, pulling the navel in toward the spine, using the hands to press the belly in. Then inhale, filling the belly like a balloon.

Repeat this breathing twenty times. Allow yourself to be a beginner, and to practice diaphragmatic breathing in a relaxed environment once per day. As you become comfortable with it, you can use it then when you need to calm heart palpitations, relieve anxiety, or even head off a hot flash.

Motherwort

Motherwort is an historic herbal remedy used specifically for treating heart palpitations during menopause. Even the plant's Latin name, *Leonorus cardiaca*, refers to its use for heart complaints. Folklore describes motherwort as a remedy which "gladdens the heart."

Like many herbs, motherwort enjoys a long-standing tradition of use, and also there have been no Western scientific double-blind studies to prove its effectiveness in treating palpitations. Fortunately, motherwort has very low toxicity, no known drug interactions, and is deemed universally safe by knowledgeable herbal practitioners. For palpitations, 30 drops of tincture, or one cup of tea (using 1 teaspoon of dried herb) is recommended three times per day.

Reducing Caffeine Intake

Many a woman—whether she be perimenopausal, menopausal, or of childbearing age—see a practitioner for heart palpitations or insomnia and leave the office with an initial recommendation: "See what happens if you quit coffee." It seems like too simple an answer for some. Simple, yes—easy, no.

"I only drink one cup a day, and it's at breakfast. Well, sometimes I have black tea at work. But that can't be doing it, can it?" asked Katherine. You'd be surprised at what one little cup of coffee can do! (Especially for a woman who's low on sleep, high on stress, or for other reasons has a nervous system that is more strung-out than usual.)

If you drink coffee, or have any amount of caffeine (in tea, chocolate, sodas, too), and you are having problems with vasomotor symptoms, try going three weeks without it, just as an experiment. We recommend tapering slowly so as not to initiate a withdrawal headache. Caffeine is a powerful, and psychologically addicting drug. If you doubt that you're hooked, notice your reaction to the thought of giving it up!

Choosing the Right Remedy for You

As you can see, you have many choices regarding how to manage vasomotor symptoms like hot flashes. This is a good thing, because no one remedy can fit all situations. With so many choices, however, you may feel a little intimidated. You may wonder "How do I know which remedy to choose for myself?"

There are a few principles to keep in mind when deciding on an approach for your situation. First of all, vasomotor changes come in all sizes. As Jane and Rosemary illustrated for us at the beginning of this chapter, some women have mild hot flashes and some have severe ones. You can pick a mild, moderate, or strong remedy to correspond with the intensity of your symptoms. Jane's barely noticeable hot flashes would probably respond to mild remedies such as vitamin E or soy products. If this were the only thing she wanted to treat, anything stronger would be unnecessary. Rosemary, on the other hand, is more likely to require hormones in some form for her severe hot flashes.

Although each woman's response to a remedy will depend on many variables—including diet, general health status, and genetics—in general, you can let the intensity of your symptoms guide which treatment to try first. Are your hot flashes mild, moderate or severe? Mild and moderate hot flashes are more likely to respond well to lifestyle, herbal, and nutritional therapies. Very severe hot flashes are more likely to require HRT (of course exercise and diet improvement is still encouraged!). In Figure 4.1, the treatment options presented in this chapter are arranged in a pyramid that places the gentlest remedies at the base, and arranges others in order of strength as they head toward the top. Natural remedies, in general, are well-suited for mild and moderate symptoms. Severe symptoms often require pharmaceutical therapy or more than one remedy.

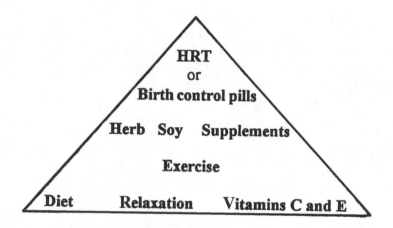

Figure 4.1.   The continuum of therapies for vasomotor changes.

A second principle to guide you in choosing the right remedy for you, is to "simplify." If you have more than one symptom, try to find one remedy that will address them all. For instance, exercise can address both hot flashes and the "perimenopausal PMS" we learned about in Chapter 3. Likewise, perimenopausal insomnia is often corrected with the same remedy that works for a woman's night sweats and an additional sleep aid may turn out to be redundant. We'll revisit this point as we discuss other issues in subsequent chapters.

It is possible to overdo supplementation of vitamins and herbs, just as it is possible to take more drugs, or stronger drugs than you actually need. Because the potential for side effects goes up as intervention increases, we recommend using the least amount of either natural or conventional medical intervention that will do the job. In other words, taking HRT for mild hot flashes only, when something gentler would work, is excessive and adds unnecessary risk of side effects from the drug. In a similar vein, taking three separate supplements for hot flashes wastes money at the least, and could potentially lead to adverse interactions.

Keeping Up With Your Changing Body

If there's one thing you can count on during the menopause, it's change. You will eventually note that the intensity and frequency of hot flashes will change (sometimes within a few weeks) even without treatment. Perhaps, for example, eating more soy controlled your vasomotor symptoms for a while, but that doesn't seem to work anymore. Conversely, you might go through a period of intense hot flashes that then lessen for no apparent reason. Both of 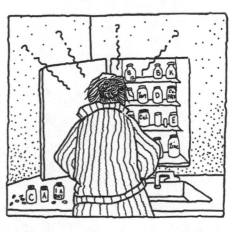 these scenarios are reminders that your ovaries have their own agenda. In addition, environmental forces beyond our control, like summer weather or emotional stresses, can turn up the heat on vasomotor changes. Just when you think you've got perimenopause tackled, your body may come up with another surprise.

Because of these natural fluctuations in symptom intensity, any treatment plan addressing symptoms should be reassessed periodically, as you and your provider ascertain. Expect that as your body moves through this transition process, your treatment plan will evolve with it. If you maintain follow-up visits with your health care provider, together you can track your body's unique journey toward menopause and respond to your needs as they inevitably change.

 **5** Our Changing Bodies

A popular national magazine published a recent cover article entitled "Staying Sexy." In this feature, "fabulous" 40, 50, and 60-year-olds pose in skin-tight evening gowns, showing off figures that don't look a day over 20. The women chosen to "represent" sexy older women were supermodels and famous actresses. One exhibited her hourglass figure in a bikini with the word "Grandma" written over the bust line. Another paraded the body that has resulted from literally making a career out of creating exercise videos. A 60-year-old supermodel, after who knows how many face-lifts, didn't look a day over forty.

While articles like this may inspire a minority of women to make healthy lifestyle changes, they are probably more effective at alienating women from their changing bodies. Despite its absurdity, we still can buy into the suggestion that women should somehow wind up with the same shape they had 30 years ago. Whole industries have cashed in on women's elusive pursuit of the physique they once had (or wish they had). From the corsets of the early 1900s to today's "new" weight-loss programs, these industries live off of the dollars women shed (whether or not we shed pounds) in our pursuit of an unrealistic standard of beauty.

A "tyranny of slenderness" as writer Kim Churnin calls it, effects most women in Western culture, and at very deep levels. Author Hillel Schwartz chronicles the evolution of body image as controlled by society during the twentieth century in her book *Never Satisfied: A Cultural History of Diets, Fantasies and Fat*. "The hostility toward fat extends far beyond physiology," she asserts. "Americans have taken the protocols of slimming as the protocols for social and spiritual renewal."[1]

Thanks to our culture's insistence that a woman should strive to maintain the body of a supermodel or exercise guru, Western women can end up with serious self-esteem challenges as we age. Modern mental health practitioners now recognize that body image issues are not reserved for young, anorexic girls, but rather can be just as important for midlife women. Feminist psychologists Joan Chrisler and Laurie Ghiz point out that our "beauty culture," which tends to define beauty as having a youthful appearance, sets women up for developing a body image disturbance as we age. Media sources, they explain, "drive home the message that women should grow old gracefully by hiding the signs of aging." They point out that the television industry is guilty of erasing age from the face of America by depicting only *3% of television characters as older people*, despite the fact that we live in an aging population, where *50% of all Americans will be of menopause age or older by 2015.*

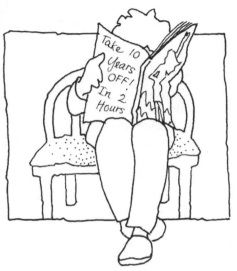

Neither do we see a realistic face of a mid-age woman on the covers of magazines targeted to this group. Not only do the faces of teenage girls grace the covers— but *retouched* photographs of these models, airbrushed to erase any sign of age (or *real* beauty, one might argue) show us what we're supposed to look like. Is it any wonder that women in midlife have a distorted view of their changing bodies?

The only healthy alternative is to reject these crazy notions that the media portrays as desirable or even attainable. The body of a twenty-year old is an unrealistic benchmark for anyone over, well, twenty. We need to seriously re-define health and beauty in midlife.

It's time for a new beauty standard; one which reflects and incorporates our maturity. Can we shift our admiration away from the unlined faces and adolescent figures to bodies that tell the stories of children borne, holidays enjoyed, and crises handled? Fifty-two year-old Kay did just that when she decided to stop coloring her hair. "I realized that I like the age I am—and there's no reason to hide it." Chrisler and Ghiz encourage women to consider their wrinkles and gray hair as "outward signs of inner wisdom, having been born out of surviving life's challenges."[2]

If anyone does, it's the baby-boom generation that has the *chutzpah* to redefine beauty in menopause. If we succeed, we will reclaim more of the self-esteem that women of our age and life experience deserve. We can also leave a better model of healthy, beautiful, empowered women as a legacy for future generations.

Reshaping the Beauty Standard

On what, then, will we base more enlightened parameters regarding the best body we can have in midlife and beyond? What definition of beauty will best serve our quality of life, on all levels? The following guidelines are a good place to start.

- *Be realistic.* First of all, we need a solid understanding of the real changes that occur in women's bodies at menopause. In this chapter, we'll describe the changes in metabolism, fat distribution, hair, and skin that *normal* women encounter at this time. The image of our "best body" then, must certainly be one of a "real body."
- *Focus on well-being.* Our body is the vehicle that carries us into this game of life. A healthy body allows us the freedom to fully participate in the activities that bring us fulfillment. We lose track of its real purpose if we think of the body as an end unto itself. Our "best body," therefore, will be one healthy enough to allow us to do that which makes us happy.
- *Every woman is unique.* Just as one approach to menopause does not fit all, one woman's optimal body will be different from another's. For one woman, a great body might be one that allows her to keep hiking into her 80s. Another woman might prioritize keeping her weight down to prevent a genetic tendency toward diabetes. Yet another might define "well-being" as possessing a mind that remains sharp into old age. It really doesn't make sense for all women to strive for one ideal.

To help you define what physical characteristics will make up your ideal body beyond menopause, do the following simple journal exercise. Take a piece of paper and fold it in half vertically. On the left side of the paper, list five things in which you would like to be able to fully participate in as you get older. On the right side, next to each item, write the most important physical capability or quality that you will need to possess to be able to do the activity. For example, if you would like to be able to hike when you are older, you might write "in shape" in the right-hand column. If you would like to paint, you might write "good eyesight." Essentially, what you are doing with this exercise is defining what wellness in the menopausal years means to you. The qualities you list on the right side of the paper can serve as your goals in achieving *your* best body. (Out of curiosity, will any of the capabilities or activities you listed require you to look like a teenage supermodel?)

Once we each know what we want from our bodies during our menopausal years, we are on the way to creating that. The next step will be to evaluate whether or not the expected, normal changes in weight and metabolism would likely put us at higher risk for real health problems later on. If so, there may be valid, health-related reasons to gain some control over how our bodies reshape themselves as we age.

Striking a Balance

And now for a twist: How our bodies can change in midlife may effect mental, as well as physical well-being. We've all had an experience of feeling good when we know we look good—or conversely, being told we look good when we are feeling good. Our mental and physical health are tied together in inextricable ways.

Depending on our own personal histories, the normal changes in hair, skin, and weight as we age will be easier or harder to appreciate. Sometimes, even the most outwardly self-assured woman can look in the mirror and wish her wrinkles away. While it is important to challenge and try to change the impact our culture has on our body image, we also must acknowledge that it is virtually impossible to escape its influence altogether. Some of us have culturally influenced beliefs that we won't ever be able to completely overcome. Thus, there may come a point for some women where the best thing to do is to *accept one's inability to accept* some changes in appearance. Modern medicine has made it often possible, for those who can afford it, to change what they can't accept about their appearance.

Say some aspect of your appearance is making you miserable. You've tried to embrace it, with no success. You've done affirmations, read self-help books, done therapy—and you still berate yourself every time you look in a mirror. Suppose you can change this aspect of your looks, and that would allow you to move on, feeling more confident, powerful and beautiful. Could Weight-Watchers, Rogaine®, or even cosmetic surgery be a healthy choice?

You bet.

The unifying theme in this seeming paradox—whether to accept our bodies as they are, or change them using the technology available—is the same that underlies all recommendations in this book: there is a unique choice, available to each woman that is right for her. One woman may come to feel completely comfortable with her changing body, while another may ultimately need medical intervention to feel healthy—physically or emotionally. Only you can decide what feels right for you. *You—*

not the television commercial, nor your husband, nor your mother—get to decide what's right for you.

Real Women, Real Bodies

The nature of life is change. Our metabolism and weight are not immune to this fact—especially at menopause. When we understand the forces of Mother Nature, it becomes easier to accept our changing bodies. Let's see what's in store for us.

Metabolic Changes at Midlife

There's no question that metabolism slows with age. In fact, after age 18, our metabolic rate declines by about 2% per decade.[3] That is why few of us can get away with the food portion sizes that we could eat/put away

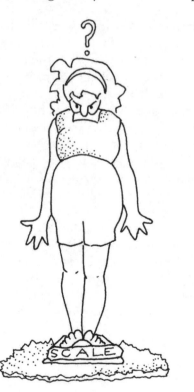

in past years. Many women notice body weight accumulating in their forties. This occurs because our resting metabolic rate—that is, the amount of fuel (as calories) our body needs for essentials like breathing, digesting and blood flow—declines as we get older. The thyroid gland, which controls metabolism, is slightly less active as we advance in years. Though normal, we can easily put on weight if we don't make the dietary adjustments to compensate for this change.

If thyroid function drops below a certain level, however, this can become a medical problem. If you have gained a lot of weight or experience a significant loss of energy without explanation, talk to your practitioner about whether your thyroid is indeed underactive. Hypothyroidism, or an abnormally low-functioning thyroid gland, sometimes first appears in midlife, but is not driven by menopause.

Recent evidence points to a separate, menopausally related drop in metabolism in addition to the normal age-related decline. Researchers and colleagues of ours at the University of Vermont studied the metabolism of 35 sedentary, healthy premenopausal women as they went through menopause. As the women entered menopause, their resting metabolic rates declined more quickly.[4] They also experienced an increase in central or abdominal fat. This is a reality that most menopausal women share. The link between abdominal fat and metabolism is so strong that some researchers have actually found they can predict a woman's metabolic rate at rest by measuring the amount of abdominal fat tissue she has.[5]

Our Bodies Rearranging Themselves

"Yep—it's right around the middle," says Ann, pointing to her belly. "There's nothing extra on my thighs, or breasts—which is where I would have gained weight in the past. I used to *think* I had a belly, but now I *definitely* have one."

Experiences like Ann's are the rule, rather than the exception. Women's bodies change in perimenopause—both in composition and in distribution. Although not all studies agree,[6] there is significant evidence that lean muscle mass decreases and total body fat increases in menopause. [7, 8]

One change that is undisputed is the increase in intra-abdominal fat that occurs for almost every woman at menopause. In a separate study, the research group at the University of Vermont indeed found that postmenopausal women had 49% more intra-abdominal fat when compared to premenopausal women.[9] This refers specifically to the internal fat that cushions our intestines. Similarly, Japanese researchers found the trunk-to-leg ratio in 545 pre- and postmenopausal women increased after menopause.[10] Dozens of researchers have confirmed this finding. It appears that throughout the world, *an hourglass figure is an unnatural and unrealistic image for women in menopause.*

Why does this shift toward more intra-abdominal fat occur for women at menopause? The answer has yet to become crystal clear, but it may have to do with the location of estrogen receptors in our bodies. There are actually estrogen receptors on our fat tissue, which means fat will be affected at menopause when estrogen declines. Our abdominal fat tissues decide whether to accumulate or release fat based on instructions from local chemicals called enzymes (lipases). According to Dr. Eric Poehlman, one of the leading researchers from the Vermont group, it appears that low estrogen levels affect how these enzymes behave. In menopause, enzymes essentially direct abdominal cells to hold onto their fat!

Or if you prefer, there's also a less technical and more philosophical way to understand this transition: Menopause is basically the reverse of puberty. If you remember what probably happened to your body during puberty, when your estrogen level just started to take off (for example, you may have suddenly developed hips and breasts), you can see why those areas don't "stand out" so much when the estrogen spigot slows down. Our bodies are no longer bent on reproduction, and our physiology will reflect this fact.

A Cultural Reality Check

It may be helpful, at this point, to put all this discussion about "fat" into perspective. During our mothers' generation, the average fashion model weighed approximately 8% less than the average woman—which is unrealistic enough. Today, however, that figure is 23% less. This destructive message misleads most women into believing that they are overweight—to the extent that 45% of even underweight women believe that they are too fat.[11]

Despite the fact—or, perhaps, due to the fact that a tiny waist for women in midlife (or at any time) is mostly a myth, the pursuit of this fallacy has fueled the garment, cosmetic, and even medical industries for generations. It's a great marketing strategy: simply capitalize on a cultural obsession (thin-waisted women) that just so happens to be a physical impossibility. Don't fall into the commercial trap of battling physiology without good reason.

Insulin Resistance

Fat redistribution at menopause affects metabolism in other ways. Levels of insulin, a necessary hormone that transports glucose from our bloodstream into our cells, rises for women at menopause, even if they don't consume more calories. This occurs because our ratio of fat to lean tissue determines insulin levels. When this ratio changes in favor of more fat, as it does in menopause, insulin levels rise.

When insulin levels go up, one of two things may happen. In the first scenario, more glucose gets transported into our cells. That would be no problem if we used it up—but as we saw, both resting and exercise metabolic rates go down in menopause. Guess what results? The glucose that isn't used up gets stored in the cells as fat. Because of these local enzymes in the abdominal area that we just learned about, this fat lands, mostly, right around our waist.

The second scenario occurs more frequently in women with higher amounts of central abdominal fat. For some of these women, insulin rises, but the body's cells begin to act like they're immune to it, not using it as readily to carry glucose from the bloodstream into the cells. Blood sugar levels then rise, causing a phenomena known as "insulin resistance." This is a major factor in the development of non-insulin-dependent diabetes, which itself is on the rise in postmenopausal women.[12] Because diabetes can bring a whole host of problems with it, women at risk for developing diabetes after menopause[13] should seriously try to limit the amount of abdominal fat they accumulate.

So you see, there's a vicious circle that can occur here, especially if a woman keeps eating the same amount of calories after menopause that she did in past decades. Increased fat will increase insulin levels—which can lead to increased fat—and on and on. Low estrogen levels will concentrate this fat in the abdominal region.

Effects of Body Composition Changes on Bone and Heart

We do have some good news in all of this. *Women who have more abdominal fat have stronger bones.*

A Swedish study comparing 71 hip fracture patients with 51 controls, found that having less body fat specifically made women more susceptible to fractures. A higher percentage of body fat was actually more protective than a higher actual weight, for these participants.[14] In addition, Japanese researchers have found that more body fat improved the bone density of not only women's weight-bearing bones (hips, legs, and spine), but also non-weight-bearing bones such as in the arm.[15] Both of these studies tell us that fat does more for our bones than simply putting more weight into our "weight-bearing exercises." As we saw in Chapter 1, fat also produces estrogen. This estrogen can have a real impact on bone density—but only if a woman has enough fat tissue!

There even seems to be a greater benefit to bone density to women whose fat tissue centers around the abdomen, rather than the hips. American and Japanese studies have both found the same connection between bone density and body fat distribution. Women with more central or abdominal fat had higher bone densities than women with more lower-body fat.[16] Therefore, if osteoporosis is a concern for you, there appears to be good, scientific reason to appreciate your belly!

On the downside again, a woman's risk for heart disease rises after menopause, approaching that of men, and the shift toward more abdominal fat is partly to blame. In Chapter 10, we'll describe in detail how to evaluate and minimize these risks, and define how much fat is too much.

Exercise and Weight

Remember that age-related decline in resting metabolic rate? It doesn't happen for everybody. Women who maintain a high fitness level keep their metabolism up at menopause. In one study, pre- versus postmenopausal endurance-trained swimmers and distance runners had no difference in metabolic rate.[17] Now, in case you're wondering if you have to be training for the Boston Marathon in order to keep your metabolism up in menopause, the answer, fortunately, is "no." Women who are not endurance athletes yet exercise aerobically are found to have higher resting metabolic rates than sedentary women.[18]

Also, moderate exercise does work to decrease fat tissue after menopause. In a study at the University of Texas, menopausal women who performed moderate activity for 60 minutes, three times per week (for example, walking or jogging plus light weight training) lost just as much fat as premenopausal women when compared to sedentary counterparts. What's less certain is whether or not exercise can prevent the *redistribution* of fat that Mother Nature has in store for us.[19] So realistically, we can expect to limit total body fat (abdominal fat included) with exercise, but not necessarily regain the hourglass figure.

Weight Loss Approaches Using Supplements

Several natural supplements have been employed by persons seeking to lose weight or alter body composition. Some of the most notable of these include fiber supplements, chromium, and ephedra (Ma Huang)-containing compounds. The following is our take on these approaches.

Fiber Supplements

Fiber is the indigestible starch found in foods such as vegetables, fruits, grains and legumes. Fiber produces weight loss in a couple of ways. First, according to nutrition expert Michael Murray, N.D., water-soluble fiber forms a kind of "gelatinous mass" that causes a sense of fullness.[20] Hence, a person taking a water-soluble fiber supplement before meals will probably eat less. Second, fiber can actually bind to foods and prevent their absorption, resulting in less calories consumed per day.

The problem with this approach to weight loss is that supplemental fiber (especially wheat bran) can prevent more than just calories from being absorbed. Fiber can indeed interfere with the absorption of certain minerals and drugs. Also, in a British study of overweight postmenopausal women, high fiber weight loss diet resulted in a loss of 4.8% of lumbar spine density, as compared with a 2.5% loss in controls.[20a] Therefore, we don't recommend fiber supplements as a keystone in a weight reduction program. Note that only excess *supplemental*, and not dietary fiber, can cause these problems.

Chromium

Chromium is an essential nutrient that has important effects on blood sugar, insulin, and regulation of fat and carbohydrate metabolism. Many studies show that chromium, in the form of chromium picolinate, helps with not only weight loss, but also in muscle gain.[21, 22] Not all studies, agree, however.[23]

Whether or not chromium helps with weight loss may have to do with a person's chromium status in the first place. Many people consume sub-optimal amounts of chromium in their diet. Safe supplemental amounts of chromium are between 200 and 400 micrograms. Toxicity, including anemia, low platelet count, and liver dysfunction has been noted if chromium is consumed in excess (1200–2400 micrograms) over a several month period of time.[24]

Ephedra

Ephedra is the perfect example of a good herb that has been given a bad name through commercial abuse. Ephedra—or Ma Huang, as the Chinese call it—is a potent herb which has been used successfully for generations for respiratory health. Its ability to both act as an antihistamine and also to open air passageways makes it an effective adjunctive treatment for asthma, allergies, bronchitis, and pneumonia.

The alkaloid, ephedrine, gives Ma Huang its broncho-dilating effect. Ephedrine acts on the *sympathetic*—or "fight or flight"—portion of the nervous system. This can increase heart rate and blood pressure, even in normal adults.[25] For this reason, it should only be used under supervision with someone knowledgeable about this herb.

Unfortunately, some supplement companies have exploited the potential ability of ephedra to increase metabolism, and have marketed it to people trying to lose weight. These are often the same people who can suffer the worst effects from an increased heart rate or blood pressure. Overdoses of ephedra have resulted in multiple problems, including death.

Currently, studies are under way concerning the safe use of ephedra for weight loss. Until they are in, and unless your practitioner has a very good handle on its use for this purpose and can monitor you closely, we do not recommend using ephedra for weight loss.

Weight Loss Using Hormone Replacement Therapy

Contrary to popular belief, hormone replacement has not been proven to induce weight gain in most women. In fact, just the opposite is usually true. Many studies have shown that HRT actually counteracts the

weight gain many women experience at menopause.[26] In a study performed at Boston Medical Center, 169 healthy postmenopausal women actually lost 4.8 % of their overall body fat by taking HRT.

In another study, obese women who were on HRT were able to lose an
average of 2.1 killigrams (4.6 pounds) by being on HRT for three months
as compared to women not on HRT. Additionally, the waist-to-hip ratio
can be decreased for both obese and healthy women on HRT.[27,28] In
Chapter 6, we'll discuss how this leads to HRT's effect on insulin.

Skin Changes

Both internal and external factors affect our skin's aging process.
Undoubtedly, genetics will play a major role in how our skin will change
with time. Since we can't do anything about our genes, let's take a look at
some of the influences on skin health that we *can* alter.

Hormones and the Skin

Skin cells have estrogen receptors on them. These receptors appear to
have a role in the amount of collagen our skin has, as well as determining
skin thickness.[29] This is why many women notice more wrinkles appearing
when they go into menopause.

Many studies have looked at whether or not taking hormones at
menopause can slow down the skin's aging process. One study found that
estrogen replacement not only prevented loss of collagen, but actually re-
stored skin collagen that had been previously lost.[30] Other studies have
not been so positive. A review of several previous studies by Scandinavian
researchers in April 2000 found that while topical estrogens may have
some benefit, oral estrogens taken for one year had no conclusive benefit
in skin thickness, or collagen.[31] Yet, many women report anecdotally that
hormone replacement and also herbal phytoestrogens improve skin moisture and appearance.

Environmental and Lifestyle Factors Affecting the Skin

Estrogen isn't the only thing that affects our skin. The next two factors,
both imminently controllable, have an enormous impact in its health and
appearance.

Ultraviolet Radiation

Ultraviolet (UV) radiation, found in sunlight and tanning beds, is the
single most important, controllable factor associated with the aging of the

skin.[32] UV radiation produces "free radicals," which damage the proteins in the skin that keep it elastic. (They are aptly named *elastins*.)

Avoiding UV damage by not sunbathing and by steering clear of tanning salons is perhaps the single most important way to avoid creating more fragile, sagging, or wrinkling skin. Wearing sunscreen with a *sun protective factor*, or SPF (a number representing the ratio of how much time it would take to get a sunburn with and without the sunscreen), of at least 15 is another good way to protect the skin. According to the National Institute on Aging, it's never too late to start.

Smoking

Now, an appeal to vanity: here's yet another reason to stop smoking. People who smoke have significantly more wrinkled and damaged skin than nonsmokers.

The exact mechanism of skin damage from smoking is currently under investigation. It appears that smoke damages collagen-producing cells, and that the formation of—once again—"free radicals" may have something to do with this.

Antioxidants and the Skin

Free radicals are highly reactive and destructive molecules formed when stable molecules are split apart. As we learned, they can be created by cigarette smoke and UV radiation. Many chemicals can cause free radicals too. Unchecked, they can bump into and severely damage the DNA, or genetic material, inside of a cell. On the skin, free radicals can damage collagen and elastin-forming cells, and profoundly contribute to the effects of aging. "Antioxidants," then, are the antidote to free radicals. Antioxidants bind up free radicals, rendering them harmless. Mother Nature actually equipped the skin with an antioxidant system which functions as our first line defense against free-radical attacks.[33]

A form of one famous antioxidant, vitamin E, has been shown to both inhibit the formation of free radicals from UV radiation and also to enhance antioxidant clean-up of UV damage.[34,35] Similarly, another popular antioxidant, coenzyme Q_{10}, has shown some promise in preventing damage from UV light when it was applied topically to skin in humans. In another experiment, skin cells treated with forms of vitamins C and E were spared the ravages of cigarette smoking.

The obvious advice here, in terms of slowing down the skin's aging process, is to not smoke, and to stay out of the sun or wear sunscreen. At the same time, it's probably not a bad idea to have some antioxidants on board for the times we can't control exposure to radiation or chemicals.

Fresh fruits and vegetables are replete with antioxidants, and skin health may turn out to be another in the long list of benefits from supplementing with 400–800 IU of vitamin E.

Dermatological Options

In some cases, women decide to seek the advice of a dermatologist to reverse the visible effects of skin aging. A continuum of options here range from the slow-acting topical creams to more dramatic chemical "peels" and even laser surgery.

Topical tretinoin, a relative of vitamin A, is a prescription cream which has been shown to reduce fine wrinkles, skin roughness, and age spots. It requires daily, long-term application to produce and maintain results. Mild to moderate dermatitis is a common adverse side effect. Very little, if any, gets absorbed into the body. Tretinoin is thought to be safe even in pregnancy.[36]

Chemical peels are relatively common procedures in cosmetic dermatology. The most common chemicals used for chemical peels—phenol and croton oil—have been combined for this purpose since the 1920s.[37] During a "peel," chemicals penetrate all the way down to the deeper layer of skin, or *dermis*, creating a controlled chemical burn as they go. The burned skin then peels away, leaving younger-looking skin on the surface. Very little of the chemicals actually enter the body, and toxicity and/or allergic reactions are rare, although they do exist. Most of these may be caused by the highly toxic phenol or derivatives of it.[38]

Carbon dioxide laser "resurfacing" is a technique where a dermatologist applies carbon dioxide via a laser, again to obliterate the top layer of skin and bring younger skin to the surface. The ultimate effect is to reduce the appearance of wrinkles. About half of patients undergoing laser resurfacing can expect areas of redness to be visible for up to two months after the treatment.[39]

For both laser resurfacing and chemical peels, corticosteroids are prescribed after the procedure to control swelling. Patients often experience effects such as prolonged redness, burning sensation, dermatitis, and the appearance of visible blood vessels on the skin surface after these procedures. These problems are thought to being partly due to dependency on the corticosteroids.[40]

Hair Changes

Let's be realistic. It is normal that both men and women lose some degree of hair as we get older. In most cases, there are no medical abnormalities that cause this, and to be honest, little in the way of permanent antidotes to hair loss. Be assured that you will not go bald!

Genetics and hormones play the biggest roles in determining hair loss. Rarely, hair loss can be due to serious hormone disorders involving the thyroid gland, adrenal glands, or ovaries. If your hair loss seems extreme to you, or you are worried about it, your practitioner can test you for these problems.

The most common cause of hair thinning for women, however, *androgenic alopecia* [41] is not due to an abnormality. Androgens are male hormones, like testosterone, and "alopecia" just means hair loss. This type of thinning is caused by the influence of male hormones in our bodies, which are more prominent when our estrogen levels drop at menopause. The dwindling ratio of estrogen compared to these androgens also accounts for the hairs that crop up on our chin, nipples, abdomen and other places that can challenge one's notion of femininity.

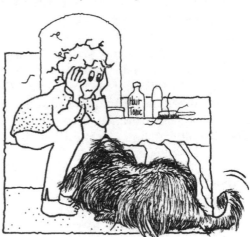

A gradual, diffuse, thinning from the top of the head is the hallmark of androgenic alopecia. How fast hair actually falls out may have to do with the genetically inherited way our hair follicles respond to normal hormonal changes.[42] In almost all cases, the hormonal changes are too subtle to be detected by a laboratory as abnormal.[43] About 40% of women experience androgenic alopecia by age 50.[44]

Most health practitioners recognize that stress is a major contributor to hair loss. A pilot study found that women who experience high stress are *11* times more likely to experience hair loss.[45] Stressful events can include marriage, divorce, death of a loved one, career crisis, problems with kids, and even overwork. When menopause coincides with a major stressful event, hair loss can be dramatic.

For some, hair loss is harder to accept than others. After all, this is the generation that invented the phrase "bad hair day"! Cultural focus on our tresses has led to the invention of all kinds of versions of the old fashioned "hair tonics." If hair loss presents a significant psychological burden for you, the following options may be of interest. Below you'll find information on the most commonly used therapies, along with a realistic critique of their success and side effects.

Hair Growth Medication

Minoxidil (Rogaine®) was discovered as a hair-growth remedy by accident. Originally, it was tested as an oral blood pressure-lowering drug, and found to have the side effect of unwanted hair growth in various places. Drug companies then got the bright idea to test its topical use to induce desired hair, and voilà, the modern hair tonic was born.

The drug works. Although Rogaine® is most beneficial to men between ages 20 and 30 who just began losing their hair, it has been proven to help at least some women. Results of a 32-week trial of minoxidil showed 44% of women using it had new hair growth compared with 29% in the placebo group.[46]

Here's the bad news: you must apply minoxidil twice daily forever, or you'll lose all the hair you gained. Side effects may include itching, dizzy spells, and in 40% of users, headaches. Overdosing can lead to heart complaints. Also, a month's supply of Rogaine® costs about $30, and is not usually covered by insurance. If you're frantic about hair loss and committed to your coiffure, however, minoxidil is a viable option.

Anti-Androgen Therapy

Cyproterone acetate or spironolactone are drugs that decrease the effect male hormones can have on hair. These drugs are generally reserved for women who actually have abnormal elevations in male hormone, or androgens. Up to 50% of patients see improvement after 6–12 months of treatment, and dermatologists usually recommend at least 12 months of treatment. These anti-androgens will only decrease *rate* of hair loss, and will not cause new hair growth, unless begun very early in the hair loss process. Spironolactone may have the unwanted side effect of inducing unwanted uterine bleeding.

Hormone Replacement Therapy

Deeper study shows us that androgenic alopecia seems to involve not only androgens, but actually a subtle interplay between these and other hormones, such as estrogen, progesterone, cortisol (from the adrenal gland), and thyroid.[47] Needless to say, there is still a lot we don't know about this most common cause of hair loss.

There is little other than anecdotal evidence that HRT slows hair loss. Among its proponents for this, there is debate between whether the estrogen or the progesterone component is working to hold on to your hair. If you have other indications for being on HRT, it may be worth a try, but by no means is it guaranteed.

Serious Relaxation

As mentioned above, women can experience hair loss during times of stress. If hair loss doesn't coincide with the onset of menopausal symptoms, it's more likely that stress, rather than waning hormones, is to blame. If you find yourself in this boat, it might be time to get serious about getting relaxed.

There's an adage that states "It's best to dig the well when the house isn't on fire." It refers to the comic image of someone trying to find water during the crisis. If we have well-established methods of handling stress already in place, we will be better equipped to handle situations as they arise. This is why it is not only a good idea, but actually *important* to have some kind of stress reduction plan, in addition to a nutrition and exercise plan, as part of our overall approach to wellness—starting as soon as possible. Yoga, meditation, t'ai chi, biofeedback—all of these and many others cultivate an ability to weather life's storms with equanimity.

What to Do About This Changing Body?

Contrary to Sartre's claim that after forty we get the face we deserve, women after forty get the face they have the courage to present.

Jo Anna Isaak, *Feminism and Contemporary Art*[48]

So there it is. Our bodies will naturally change as we hit menopause and beyond. We get a little thicker around the waist, put on some more wrinkles, and see hairs disappear from the top of our head, only to crop up elsewhere. Is this a problem?

Before you answer this question, turn back to page 80, where you listed the physical attributes you needed to achieve your "best body." Are any of these changes realistically going to prevent you from doing what will make you happy and fulfilled as you age?

For some women, normal changes may in fact, be useful. For example, if you have big risk factors for osteoporosis (we'll show you how to calculate this in Chapter 7), putting on a few pounds, and especially in the abdominal area, might actually be healthy for you. On the other hand, women at risk for heart disease or diabetes, will want to take measures to minimize this weight gain.

Hair and skin issues, on the other hand, don't effect physical health—but can affect mental health. Are you able to welcome age courageously, as one writer exclaims, "repossessing our purloined faces and wearing them unrepentantly."[49] Or, would you be happier defying the effects of age, and using whatever means available, like 47-year-old Natalie? "I say, if you can change it—do it, and stop complaining about it," she states emphatically. For Natalie, an eyelid tuck made a huge improvement in her self-esteem. "My other option was to feel self-conscious," she explained. "I have no regrets."

However you approach dealing with a body in transition, if you make decisions that support your own definition of well-being, you'll be able to live comfortably with the results. And regardless of what we can change with supplements, exercise, hormones or more intense intervention, we'll never be able to escape aging altogether. Women in midlife can always benefit from a hefty dose of self-acceptance.

"Look at yourself as you are now," says noted beauty expert, Bobbi Brown,[50] "not in comparison to how you used to be. You may be surprised at your beauty." Writer Veronique Vienne points out that the "intelligence of a mature face" possesses beauty, with more definition, more expression in the eyes and an easier smile.

Vienne points out that we often cringe when looking at old photographs of ourselves, and feel grateful to have outgrown the old hair and makeup styles of the past. "If you could see the changes in your appearance objectively," she asserts, "not through the harsh light of agism, but through the natural glow of real life—you would be surprised to discover that you do indeed look better than you ever have."[51]

Weathering

My face catches the wind
from the snow line
and flushes with a flush
that will never wholly settle.
Well, that was a metropolitan vanity,
wanting to look young forever, to pass.
I was never a pre-Raphaelite beauty
and only pretty enough to be seen
with a man who wanted to be seen
with a passable woman.

But now that I am in love
with a place that doesn't care
how I look and if I am happy,
happy is how I look and that's all.
My hair will grow gray in any case,
my nails chip and flake,
my waist thicken, and the years
work all their usual changes.

If my face is to be weather-beaten as well,
it's little enough lost
for a year among the lakes and vales
where simply to look out my window
at the high pass
makes me indifferent to mirrors
and to what my soul may wear
over its new complexion.

Fleur Adcock[52]

6   Heart Health

Cardiovascular disease claims more American women's lives than the next 14 causes of death combined.[1] It is by far a greater threat to the health of women in menopause than breast, or any other kind of cancer. In 1997, for example, twelve times as many women died of cardiovascular disease as did from breast cancer (the numbers were 502,938 and 41,943, respectively). Currently, more than one in five women in the U.S. have some type of heart or blood vessel disease.[2]

These statistics are not meant to scare you. Rather, we've included them to put into perspective the importance of heart health as a menopausal issue. Many a woman's fear of breast cancer overshadows her attention to heart health—which may in fact be a more significant concern.

Now, while the numbers above are sobering, they say nothing about you as an individual. Each woman has a unique set of circumstances which determine her likelihood of having future cardiovascular problems. The importance of an individual assessment, again, cannot be underestimated. You will only know whether or not you should be concerned about heart disease when you have undergone a careful assessment.

In this chapter, we will help you do just that. First, we define the risk factors for heart disease. Next, we will help you assess your own risks. The final portion of the chapter presents options in prevention and treatment. Your degree of cardiac risk will obviously determine how important the final portion of this chapter is for you. As usual, we'll list the gentlest, most natural approaches first, and lead into more conventional options for more serious cases. We will include information alongside the treatments that help you ascertain if they may be appropriate for you.

Defining Cardiovascular Disease

Cardiovascular disease (CVD) refers to disorders of the heart and/or the blood vessels. It is a broad category of problems, many of which can contribute to others, and all can result in major impairment to blood flow and oxygen to important tissues. The most common forms of CVD are high blood pressure, coronary artery disease, stroke, congestive heart failure, high cholesterol, and atherosclerosis.

We are finally realizing that CVD is not only a man's disease. In fact, after age 65, CVD is actually more prevalent in women than in men.[3] Its impact can be dramatic. CVD is a major cause of disability in women.[4] A total of 42 percent of women who have a heart attack will die within the next year.[5]

Understanding the Process

Atherosclerosis is a major cause of chest pain (angina) and, ultimately, heart attack. In atherosclerosis, the arteries harden and narrow. Understanding how this process happens, and how cholesterol, blood pressure and other factors influence it, better equips us to prevent atherosclerosis.

The damage starts when influences such as high blood pressure or free radicals (from things like smoking, air pollution, and certain chemicals and drugs) injure the blood vessel walls. Using a sort of band-aid approach, our bodies attempt to patch up damaged arteries by putting down a "plaque" made of cholesterol and other components such as calcium. (Don't worry—taking your RDA of calcium will not cause this!) One such band-aid is no problem. But if the assault on blood vessels continues, our body has to keep patching them up. A buildup of these plaques over time

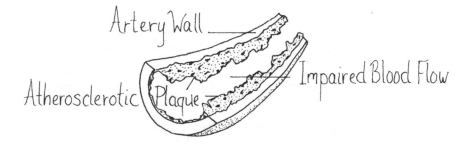

Figure 6.1. Cross-section of artery narrowed due to buildup of plaque.

causes our arteries to progressively narrow. (See Figure 6.1.) Some people have arteries which have narrowed by 90% or more.

As the accumulating plaques forces blood to flow through a tightening tube, the chances that a blood clot can get stuck and shut off blood flow goes up. Deprived of blood (and therefore oxygen), the tissues that depend on that particular blood supply have nothing to "breathe." When this happens, we call it an *infarct*. If it happens in the brain, a stroke ensues. If it happens in the blood vessels that supply oxygen to the heart, a heart attack occurs. These tragic events are the end point of atherosclerosis.

Cardiovascular Disease Risk Factors We Can't Change

Some risk factors for CVD are not within our power to control. One of these is our ethnic heritage, or *race*. For example, Chinese people have lower cardiac risk factors than whites.[6] Afro-Caribbean women have more hypertension and diabetes, but a better lipid profile.[7] Genetics have the largest say in determining these kinds of differences. Black women have a 14.6% higher incidence of coronary heart disease (blocked arteries to the heart) and 31.4% higher incidence of stroke as compared to white women.[8] This is partially due to the fact that blacks, on average, have higher blood pressure than whites.

People of South Asian heritage tend to have a higher blood pressure, more diabetes, and less favorable blood lipid profiles than Caucasian people. One proposed explanation for this is that, on the whole, this population has a higher proportion of abdominal fat than whites. As we learned in the last chapter, more abdominal fat can cause problems with insulin. Increased abdominal fat can also adversely affect cholesterol levels.

Family history is another heart disease risk factor we can't change. Women who have a parent who died of CVD before the age of 65 have the greatest risk of developing it themselves. If a woman's mother died of CVD, she also has a high risk herself. If her father died of CVD, she again has increased risk, but less so.[9]

Cardiovascular Disease Risk Factors We Can Change

Fortunately, we do have control over many areas that affect heart health. By maximizing positive changes in these areas, we can go a long way toward keeping our heart healthy.

Smoking

Simply put, smoking is the "single most preventable cause of death in the United States."[10] Although smoking also contributes to deaths from many cancers (lung, mouth, larynx, esophagus, urinary tract, kidney, pancreatic, and cervical cancers) its deadliest impact is in the area of heart disease. Women who smoke increase their risk of stroke and heart attack—and this risk goes up with the number of cigarettes consumed per day.[11] Long-term exposure to secondhand smoke also increases cardiac risk.

Blood Pressure

Our blood pressure naturally rises with age. After age 55, in fact, over half of all women have high blood pressure, or *hypertension*. High blood pressure is the greatest risk factor for stroke, and causes three out of every five cases of heart failure in women.[12]

Blood pressure refers to the amount of force created by the blood as it is pumped through the arteries by the heart. The ability of the artery walls to relax helps determine blood pressure. As we learned above, constant or frequent high blood pressure, or force on the artery walls, can lead to damage there and initiate atherosclerosis.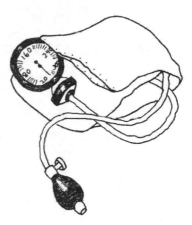

Normal blood pressure is expressed as 120 over 80 millimeters of mercury (120/80 mmHg). The top number (systolic pressure) is the force exerted on the arteries at the time the heart contracts. The bottom number (diastolic pressure) is this measurement between beats, while the heart rests. In the past, doctors believed that mainly diastolic blood pressure determed cardiac risk. We now know that systolic pressure is also very important. Uncontrolled systolic blood pressure increases risk of heart attack and stroke. To determine if your blood pressure is normal or elevated, see Table 6.1.

New information obtained from a large, ongoing trial involving 6,859 people and known as the Framingham Heart Study indicates that even women with "high normal" blood pressure, as defined in Table 6.1, had an increased risk for cardiovascular disease. Women between the ages of thirty-five and sixty-four had a 4 percent increase and those sixty-five to ninety years old had an 18 percent increased incidence of disease.[13]

Weighing 20% over a healthy weight for your size and build is a predictor of high blood pressure. (You can refer to Figure 6.2 on page 102 to see where your weight falls.) In some women, birth control pills can cause high blood pressure. Near the end of this chapter, we will discuss lifestyle,

Table 6.1. Blood Pressure Categories for Women[14]

Status	Systolic Pressure/Diastolic Pressure
Optimal	<120/<80
Normal	<130/<85
High Normal	130–139/85–89
Elevated—Stage 1	140–159/90–99
Elevated—Stage 2	160–179/100–109
Elevated—Stage 3	≧180/≧110

Note: If your systolic and diastolic pressures fall in different categories, the higher category determines your status.

dietary, supplemental, and medical remedies for keeping your blood pressure at healthy levels.

Cholesterol

Almost *half* of American women between the ages of 20 and 74 have a cholesterol level above the normal benchmark of 200 milligrams per deciliter (mg/dL).[15] Cholesterol is one of the most important markers of heart disease. Elevated cholesterol, especially LDL cholesterol, increases the chance of forming blockages in the arteries. Here's how it works:

LDLs are the bad cholesterols. They transport cholesterol that we eat or make to the arteries. The good cholesterol (HDLs), on the other hand, pick up cholesterol in the blood vessels and bring it to the liver, which can ship it out via the digestive tract. A race between the cholesterol dumpers (LDLs) and the cleanup patrol (HDLs) is occurring every minute of the day in your body—including now!

Healthy cholesterol levels are under 200 mg/dL. More importantly, however, it's best to keep the HDLs over 60, and the LDLs under 130. If you can do this, you will have a favorable ratio of HDL to total cholesterol. Practitioners like to keep an eye on this ratio, because it gives us an idea about your cardiac risk. The average total cholesterol/HDL ratio for Americans is 4. Given that half "average" Americans develop heart disease, we like to see our patients maintain a ratio that's well under 4.

Weight

While our acceptance of the normal, physiologic changes in our body can contribute to our overall sense of well-being, we must know when to draw the line on body fat—and know the problems with crossing this line. An astonishing one-third of American adults are obese. Among women only, 25% are considered overweight, and an additional 25% are obese. The implications of this epidemic in our relatively affluent society cannot be overestimated. The Nurses' Health Study, which for twelve years observed the health behaviors and status of more than 75,000 women between the ages of 38 and 63, estimated that 23% of all deaths in nonsmoking women in midlife are due to the problem of our weight.[16]

To find out if you are overweight, see where you land on the chart in Figure 6.2. Or, assess your weight by calculating your body mass index (BMI). Plug your height in inches and weight in pounds into the following equation to see if your weight (adjusted for height) puts you at risk for cardiovascular problems:

$$\underset{\text{weight}}{\underline{\qquad}} \times 700 \div \underset{\text{height}}{\underline{\qquad}} \div \underset{\substack{\text{height} \\ \text{(again)}}}{\underline{\qquad}} = \underset{\text{BMI}}{\underline{\qquad}}$$

A BMI of 25 or less means you have a lower risk for CVD.

The BMI of Americans now averages 26.3.[17] While this level may be healthy for athletes and some large-boned or heavily muscularized women, it is too high for most of us. Obesity is defined as having a BMI of 30 and higher. Obesity strongly predisposes women to high blood pressure, elevated cholesterol and triglycerides and diabetes—all of which can lead to atherosclerosis. Being moderately overweight (BMI over 25 and under 30 unless you are athletic) increases risks for these problems as well.

As we learned in Chapter 5, menopausal women normally put on fat right around the waist. This accumulation is one of the main reasons why our cardiovascular risk increases at this time. Too much of this abdominal fat can lead to high blood pressure and high cholesterol. It can also raise our risk for diabetes, which, in turn, drastically increases cardiovascular risk. So while a little is okay, more isn't necessarily so. Another way to determine whether you have an increased risk of CVD is to measure your waist circumference with a tape measure, then compare this measurement with your hip measurement. You have increased risk if you waist measures 35 inches or more, or if your waist is larger than your hips.

Adolescent Weight

Practitioners and researchers have noted that a woman who was overweight as an adolescent has a greater risk of having more central fat as an adult—along with the increased risk for diabetes and heart disease that it

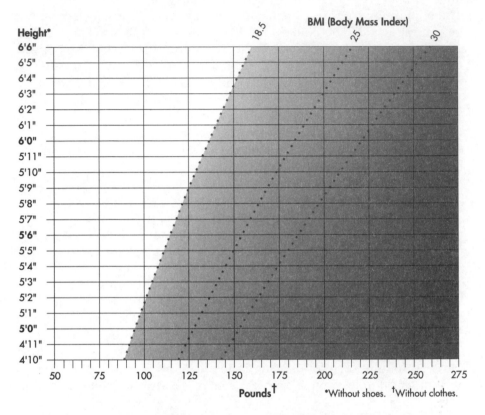

BMI measures weight in relation to height. The BMI ranges shown above are for adults. They are not exact ranges of healthy and unhealthy weights. However, they show that health risk increases at higher levels of overweight and obesity. Even within the healthy BMI range, weight gains can carry health risks for adults.

Directions: Find your weight on the bottom of the graph. Go straight up from that point until you come to the line that matches your height. Then look to find your weight group.

    Healthy Weight BMI from 18.5 up to 25 refers to healthy weight.

    Overweight BMI from 25 up to 30 refers to overweight.

    Obese BMI 30 or higher refers to obesity. Obese persons are also overweight.

Source: Report of the Dietary Guidelines Advisory Committee on the Dietary Guidelines for Americans, 2000, page 3.

Figure 6.2.   Are you at a healthy weight?

brings. The reason for this is that the fat we put on in adolescence goes mainly to the abdomen.[18] When our metabolism slows down in old age, we deposit the energy we're not burning up into the same areas in the form of fat. We can help our children and grandchildren to maximize their long-term health by encouraging exercise and maintenance of normal weight in adolescence.

Activity Level

According to the Surgeon General's Report on Physical Activity and Health, 60% of all American women do not get the recommended amount of physical activity. Over 25% are not active at all. Besides contributing negatively to other cardiac risk factors like weight, cholesterol, and blood pressure, inactivity directly increases heart disease risk. Inactivity can also increase stress levels and depressed mood—two factors that can negatively impact heart health. In the latter part of this chapter, you'll learn just how healthy exercise is for your heart and blood vessels, and why.

Stress

Many Americans have no trouble believing that emotions can affect heart health. After all, we use the metaphor of the heart in describing many intense feelings: as in receiving "heartbreaking news," delivering a "heartfelt thanks," or in describing someone as "heartless," or alternatively, as a "sweetheart."

The National Institutes of Health (NIH) have taken an interest in the relationship between emotional stress and heart disease. Citing that "studies have found that the most commonly reported incident preceding a heart attack is an emotionally upsetting event, particularly one that involves anger," the NIH is now calling for more research in this important area. In addition, the NIH recognizes a role for relationships in heart health. "Studies also suggest that having emotionally supportive relationships lessens the chances of developing heart disease and prolongs life following a heart attack."[19, 20, 21, 22]

We're beginning to have a scientific understanding of just how emotions affect the heart. Some studies suggest that a negative interaction with another person makes blood levels of our stress hormones rise. This in turn increases the load on the heart and blood vessels. Just the opposite happens when we have positive interactions with others.[23]

Based on preliminary data that emotions of anger and hostility actually cause blood vessels to constrict, researchers at the University of Maryland wanted to find out if there was any link, conversely, between humor and heart disease. To do this, they looked at 150 patients who had cardiovascular disease, and compared them with 150 controls. Each person answered a questionnaire, asking them how much humor they found in 20 hypothetical situations. According to lead researcher, Dr. Michael Miller, "Patients with heart disease had a 40–45% decreased likelihood of responding with laughter" to the situations in the questionnaire. With a second questionnaire, Miller and his associates found that "those who responded with laughter had the lowest likelihood of anger and hostility." Miller explained that laughter releases opioid compounds from the brain that produce euphoria, and that it also lowers pulse and blood pressure.[24]

Stress and Blood Pressure

"Yes, but I only have high blood pressure at the doctor's office," exclaims Jan. "Whenever I take it with one of these machines at the drugstore, it's fine." What about Jan, and people like her who spike a high blood pressure under stressful situations? If you have high blood pressure when a doctor or nurse are coming after you with a blood pressure cuff, what do you think is happening in heavy traffic? While having a difficult conversation or argument? While paying bills, or during any other potentially stressful situation? If you think about all the moments in your day that might cause an elevated blood pressure, you might see how even these "situational" elevations might

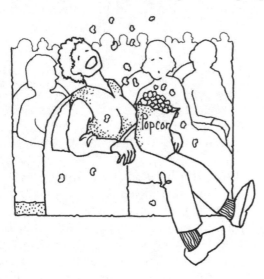

have an impact. Unless you do enough activity to work off the adrenaline the situation produced, your blood pressure may stay high long after the stressful situation has passed.

Researchers at Duke University wanted to see if mildly overweight people with elevated blood pressures could actually prevent the further elevations that come with stressful situations. They put 99 men and women with stage 1 and 2 hypertension through a bunch of stressful situations (cold temperatures, public speaking, and recall of an event that made them angry) and then measured their blood pressures—which, of course, went up. Then, they divided the participants into three groups. The first adopted an exercise plan. The second not only exercised, but also participated in a behavioral weight loss plan. The third group made no changes. After the six months, everyone went through the same "stress" tests. Those who exercised, and particularly people on the weight loss plan, maintained significantly lower systolic and diastolic blood pressures during stress than did those who didn't.[25]

Diabetes

Usually of adult onset, non-insulin-dependent diabetes is hereditary and weight related. Most commonly, this type of diabetes is highly preventable. Proper diet, exercise, and weight maintenance can usually prevent, and can even reverse or cure adult onset diabetes. By contrast, insulin-dependent diabetes, which usually comes on earlier in life, is often impossible to prevent, and is not as strongly related to family history.

Both types of diabetes wreak havoc on the cardiovascular system. Women with diabetes are three to seven times more likely to develop heart disease or have a heart attack than nondiabetics. This occurs because high blood sugars are one of the things that can damage blood vessel walls, which as we know, leads to atherosclerosis. If you have a family history of adult-onset diabetes, the best thing you can do for your heart and blood vessels, is to eat healthfully, exercise, and prevent this disease.

Assess Your Heart Health

To assess your risks for cardiovascular disease, check the box next to any that are true for you:

___ I smoke
___ I have diabetes
___ My basal metabolic index is over 30 (see page 102)
___ I have high blood pressure
___ My HDL cholesterol is under 60
___ My LDL cholesterol is over 130
___ A parent, sibling or offspring had a first heart attack before age 60
___ I am of African descent
___ I exercise fewer than two times per week
___ I have significant stress and no routine relaxation program
___ I am over 60

If you have *any* of the above risk factors, you have an increased risk for cardiovascular disease. The more factors you checked, the higher your risk, and the more intervention you will need to maintain a healthy cardiovascular system. Take this list with you the next time you see your practitioner. It will help you both focus on which areas need attention.

A Heart-Healthy Lifestyle

If you have high normal blood pressure (130 to 139 over 85 to 89) or stage one hypertension (140 to 159 over 90 to 99), you may have a good chance of lowering your blood pressure through lifestyle interventions and natural remedies. Particularly if you are overweight or if your diet or exercise program could stand some improvement, changes in these areas could go a long way toward controlling your blood pressure. Herbs, which we'll discuss later, can also be effective in this blood pressure range.

If you have stage 2 or higher hypertension (160 or higher systolic over 100 or higher diastolic), you should first get these pressures under control with conventional medicines (see page 120), while working on diet and exercise. Later, with healthy lifestyle changes solidly in place, you may be able to decrease your medication, make a transition to a natural treatment, or go off "meds" altogether, as long as you work closely with your health practitioner and monitor your blood pressures several times per week.

Diet

The American Heart Association's (AHA) October 2000 revision of its dietary guidelines showed a look very different from past versions. The goals—to help Americans achieve healthy eating patterns and maintain appropriate body weight and desirable cholesterol and blood pressure levels—didn't change. However, the approach to foods took on a much more user-friendly slant. Gone is the focus on calculating percentages or milligram amounts of various dietary components one ought to consume. In its place is this simple concept: *Eat nutrient-dense foods without adding empty calories.*

"In the past, we have focused rather heavily on the percent of calories as fat and amounts of cholesterol," says Ronald M. Krauss, M.D., principal author of the new guidelines. "These are still important considerations, but the emphasis has shifted to allow consumers to understand the importance of an overall eating plan." The new streamlined guidelines, Krauss explains, urge people to eat "a diet rich in fruits, vegetables, low-fat dairy products, and leaner cuts of meat in smaller portions." In this way, Krauss believes that Americans will end up limiting saturated fats and cholesterol naturally, without needing to count calories or focus on the numbers.[26]

The standard heart-healthy foods remain the same: fruits, vegetables, legumes, whole grains, lean meats, and poultry. New on the menu is the addition of two weekly servings of fatty fish, such as tuna or salmon. These fish dishes are included because of the beneficial effect that their *omega-3 oils* have on cholesterol. Also, for the first time, the AHA recommends the substantial reduction of *trans fatty acids* found in hydrogenated oils and many margarines. These unnatural forms of fatty acids stick to blood vessel walls more easily and can even hold on to cholesterol, which might otherwise just flow by. As you might imagine, trans fatty acids, therefore, can contribute to the further formation of an atherosclerotic plaque.

Studies focusing on cardiovascular health in women parallel the AHA's general dietary recommendations. Low-overall-fat, as well as low-saturated-fat, diets definitely bring down LDL (bad) cholesterol levels for women—often enough to keep some of them off medications.[27]

A study published in the December 2001 issue of the *British Medical Journal* found lower cholesterol levels in people who ate five or six small meals per day, rather than three large meals. The researchers proposed that lower spikes in insulin levels accounted for the difference, because physical activity, weight, and smoking habits had been factored out of the equation.[28]

Whole Grains

Findings from the Nurses' Health Study show that higher intake of whole grains independently reduced the risk of stroke.[29] Likewise, in a study of nearly 40,000 women, eating more fruits and vegetables protected the women against heart attacks.[30] The more servings, the better.

Whole grains include both the interior and exterior of a grain. (See Figure 6.2.) Examples of grains include wheat, oats, corn, barley, millet, rice, spelt, and quinoa. Processing takes the outer germ layer from the grain and strips grains of fiber and important nutrients.

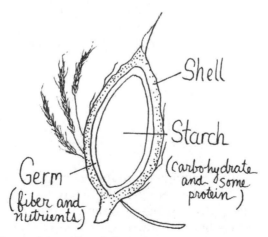

Figure 6.2.   Cross-section of a whole grain.

It is easy to think that you're eating whole grains, when in fact, you may be consuming processed ones. Labels that read "Honey Oat," "Multi-grain," or "Country Wheat" do not guarantee you're getting a whole grain. The same is true for ordering "wheat" bread at a restaurant. In fact, the Western palate is so used to processed flour, that most of what "looks" like brown bread to us contains but a fraction of whole grain flour. When buying bread, it's important to turn the loaf over and read the list of ingredients. Only if the bread lists "*whole*" grain only, are you getting a complete food.

Oat Bran

Eat more cookies and lower your cholesterol? That's exactly what a group of Mexican researchers found—provided the cookies included oat bran.[31] King of the cholesterol-lowering grains, oat is distinguished as the first food sanctioned by the FDA to claim a health benefit. Oat bran incorporated into a diet can lower cholesterol, and in particular, those nasty LDL cholesterols.[32]

For women in particular, it appears that oat bran has its best effect on cholesterol after the age of fifty.[33] Amounts that are effective are 28 grams (1 ounce), twice daily.[34] Best of all, you can mix it into cookies, muffins, and bread, also on cereal, and obtain all its benefits.

Soy

In addition to calming hot flashes, menopause's most famous food has another claim to fame. In all categories of lipids, soy does the right thing. In a large review of thirty-eight controlled clinical trials published in the prestigious *New England Journal of Medicine,* soy protein proved to lower total cholesterol, LDLs, and triglycerides, without negatively affecting HDLs. Specifically, 47 grams of soy protein per day had the following effects on blood lipid values:[35]

- Total cholesterol decreased by 23.2 points or 9.3 percent
- (Bad) LDL cholesterols decreased by 21.7 points or 12.9 percent
- Triglycerides decreased by 13.3 points or 10.5 percent
- (Good) HDL cholesterols increased by 2.4 percent

In an offshoot of the Framingham Study on cardiovascular health that looked at the diets of 939 postmenopausal women, those eating the highest amounts of dietary phytoestrogens (mainly from soy) had not only lower triglyceride levels but also lower waist-to-hip ratios, which we saw correlated with lower cardiovascular risk.[36] These results and others have convinced the U.S. Food and Drug Administration to also approve heart-healthy labeling claims on soy foods. It is generally accepted that the constituents of soy that benefit heart health as well as menopausal symptoms are its isoflavones.

In addition to improving lipids, soy exerts its beneficial effect on the blood vessels at least four more ways. First, soy increases the ability of the arteries to relax, a quality known to practitioners as *arterial compliance.*[37] Second, soy's isoflavones inhibit the formation of potentially dangerous blood clots.[38] Third, one of these isoflavones that we have seen before, *genestein,* kicks off antioxidant reactions, which may prevent damage to LDLs. This action, along with soy's fourth one—that of being an actual antioxidant itself—may likely decrease the formation of atherosclerosis, which relies on oxidation of LDLs to form plaques.

The majority of soy studies used about 47 grams of soy protein powder per day to achieve the results listed above. That's equivalent to about one block of tofu. If tofu isn't a big hit in your household, or if the quantity of tofu seems daunting, take heart. Soy protein can be eaten in many, varied ways (see page 64), and amounts as little as 20 grams per day or less may still reduce risk of heart disease.[39, 40]

Alcohol

Although, as health care practitioners, we hate to admit it, moderate alcohol intake does show cardiac benefits. The data is pretty clear that a low intake of alcohol, and red wine in particular[41,42] is cardioprotective. Alcohol lowers blood pressure and increases the good HDL cholesterol.[43] Alcohol, and in particular the *polyphenols* in red wine, also appears to decrease the ability of platelets to stick together and form clots,[44,45] which can result in blockages. A mild to moderate alcohol intake reduces deaths from coronary heart disease.[46]

It's tricky business to go about thinking that drinking is good for you, however. Expert in women's natural healthcare Tori Hudson, N.D., points out that alcohol increases risk of "depression, pancreatitis, liver cirrhosis, gastritis, degenerative nervous system conditions, fetus damage, substance abuse, and cancers of the mouth, pharynx, larynx, esophagus, and liver," in addition to adding to the risk of breast cancer.[47] Add in alcohol's impact on automobile accidents, abusive behaviors, and serious drug–alcohol interactions, and it looks like even less of a wellness remedy. When it comes to recommending alcohol intake for health, therefore, let's keep the big picture in mind.

At least one study has suggested that the cardiac benefits of alcohol can be obtained with as little as one glass of red wine per week.[48] Also, more than two daily drinks actually increases the risk of stroke and infarct (blockage), the two main causes of death from heart disease.[49]

Please note that *all* of the benefits of alcohol on the heart can be achieved in ways that do not add to other health risks. Diet, exercise, relaxation, and many natural remedies can optimize cholesterol ratios while improving our overall health. Many foods, such as grape juice, squash, sweet potatoes, and many berries contain high amounts of the same flavonoids thought to increase red wine's protective properties.

Salt

Dietary salt has been the subject of seemingly conflicting studies regarding blood pressure. Large population studies point to a significant benefit over a lifetime in people with low sodium intakes. Smaller, controlled studies have not been so consistent. A review of many of the studies done has made some sense out of apparent conflicts. It seems that certain individuals have more salt-sensitivity than others, and that genetics or acquired factors may play a role in determining if you are salt sensitive or not.[50] The best way to tell if you are one of these people is to actually try it out. Cut out the salt—and see what happens to your blood pressure. Keep in mind that salt is a very common additive: to canned foods, baking soda, carbonated beverages, and even antacids.

Weight Loss

Weight loss remains the most important thing an overweight woman can do (besides smoking cessation) to support her heart health. The most successful way to do this is to participate in, or create, some type of structured program, which includes support on many levels. Weight is an issue tied not only to genetics, biochemistry, and nutrition, but also to powerful mental, emotional, cultural, and social factors.

"I've never met a plate of food that turned me down," says Ann, a 45-year-old mother of three who suffers from bouts of binge eating between diets. Although she knows the health implications of being overweight, issues of low self-esteem have consistently sabotaged even her most determined efforts to lose weight. For Ann, and women like her, addressing the emotional attachments to food in a supportive way will be an essential part of any successful weight loss plan.

Key components of a weight loss plan are: (1) a goal, (2) close supervision, (3) a diet plan, (4) exercise, and (5) support. Losing weight takes a truly concerted effort. If you're serious about taking and keeping off some pounds, make sure that you address all five of the above areas—and that they support one another. Also, how you fulfill the five key components of a weight loss plan will be very individual. One woman, for example, may find Weight-Watchers or Overeaters Anonymous to be most helpful. Another woman, however, may prefer to see a nutritionist, and have two or three exercise buddies lined up.

In addition to support, there are a couple of key concepts to know about weight loss. The first is a simple equation: "*calories in* must be less than *calories out*." This means that whatever you consume must be less than what you burn up. This is why exercise is essential to any healthy weight loss.

Second, take things "slow and steady." Weight loss of one—or at most—two pounds per week is optimal. Crash diets almost always result in women putting weight back on—and usually more than what they lost. The reason for this is that the body actually interprets fast weight loss as starvation. As soon as food is plentiful, we put on more weight in order to survive the next "famine." By contrast, slow, gradual weight loss gives the body time to adjust, and to actually change its metabolism over the long term. It also gives one's *mind* time to adjust to the new foods. *Sustainable* weight loss almost always comes from a gradual and permanent shift toward healthy eating.

Take some time, and be creative in setting up a structured plan for yourself. (For help, see page 112.) Anticipate what issues may be most challenging for you, and structure a solution before you even begin. For example, if finding time for exercise is an issue—make a decision about what you can cut out of your schedule and replace the time with exercise. Similarly, if you can foresee getting stumped about how in the world to cook healthy food that actually tastes good, sign up for and begin a cooking class before you actually begin your "program."

Remember, you don't have to do this on your own. If you truly want to succeed, recruit some help. Round up a friend who also wants to lose weight. If you think emotional issues are likely to surface when you change your diet, schedule some visits with a therapist in advance. If you live in a cold climate and dislike winter sports, think about joining a gym. Whenever possible, get your health practitioner on board, and schedule a few "check-in" visits to monitor your progress and receive moral support.

Most naturopathic physicians, nutritionists, and many conventional primary care providers can help you in setting up a safe weight loss plan. See page 289 for referral sources of practitioners near you who can help you. Ultimately, however, the most important person in your plan will be you. The more foresight you have in planning to overcome inevitable challenges, the more success you can count on.

Optimal Weight Plan

If you determine that weight loss will make you healthier, a structured approach will help you achieve and maintain a healthy weight.

Step One: After each of the following five key elements, write down how you can fulfill it.

(1) A Goal (this can be anything: a feeling, a fit, a specific weight) _____
_____

(2) Close Supervision (Who will you ask to help monitor you? A practitioner? A group?)
_____

(3) A Diet Plan (How will you choose one and put it together?) _____
_____
_____

(4) Exercise (actually scheduling this works best) _____
_____

(5) Support (Are there friends or family members who would also like to join you in this endeavor? Can you think of books, tapes, groups, a therapist, or other support?)
_____
_____

Step Two: Putting the plan into action.

Choose the best time to enact your plan. (November and December holiday months are not advised!) Share it with at least one person you've designated as a supervisor (see number 2 above).

Put the pieces above into place—taking as long as you need to set up your plan. The key to success is in the preparation. Gear up for success, and vow to be kind to yourself when you slip—as we all do. Remember the principle of "slow and steady," and when you're ready—Go for it!

Stress Reduction

Many of us think of diet and exercise as important components to heart health—but how many of us are just as mindful to include stress reduction into our wellness plans? Ours is a society focused on doing, rather than being. The question seems to be—will we make the time for relaxation?

The Center for Natural Medicine and Prevention, located at the College of Magarishi Vedic Medicine in Fairfield, Iowa, has done some intensive study on the results of one stress reduction technique, Transcendental Meditation (T.M.), on heart health. They found that African American patients could actually reduce the amount of atherosclerosis in the arteries in their neck through meditation.[51] They also found that T.M. lowered cholesterol and blood pressure, as well as reduced smoking as a behavior.[52]

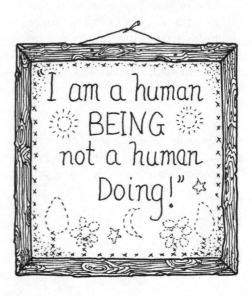

Stress reduction doesn't have to mean taking a T.M. class, signing up for biofeedback, or anything fancy. Any activities that we enjoy can activate the relaxation responses in our bodies. Playing with pets, doing our hobbies, and talking with friends are great stress reduction activities. More organized approaches, like taking a yoga class or getting a massage work too. Prioritizing ourselves by making time to engage in regular, relaxing activities can do our heart good, on many levels. Susun Weed, author of *Menopausal Years, the Wise Woman Way* says, "Give yourself plenty of nice strokes so you won't have a bad stroke."[53] It's quite possible that by enjoying your life more now—you'll actually be around longer to live it.

Exercise

Scientists have become excited recently because they believe they have discovered precisely how weight loss lowers blood pressure. Sensitive blood tests have shown that obese people have more *noradrenaline* in their bloodstream than do non-obese people. Noradrenaline is a chemical that induces the "fight or flight" response in the nervous system, raising blood pressure and heart rate (presumably so that we can either fight or run away from a dangerous situation). Of course, if there is no actual danger and we don't use up the noradrenaline, our blood pressure remains elevated. Weight loss, and the drop in blood pressure that comes with it, is correlated with a decrease in noradrenaline levels.[54]

Endurance exercise training has been shown to reduce both systolic and diastolic blood pressures approximately 10 points each in 75 percent of people who have high blood pressure.[55] Less intense regular exercise also lowers blood pressure and may lower diastolic levels as much as endurance training does.[56] The surgeon general of the United States has concluded that as little as thirty minutes of moderate activity per day, such as walking, biking, raking leaves, or gardening, is good preventive medicine for the heart. If you—like many women—are "too busy" to fit in thirty minutes, you can divide it up into ten-minute intervals, three times per day.

In choosing an exercise plan, there's one crucial guideline to keep in mind: it *must* be enjoyable! If it's not, you won't stick with it for long. Be creative and open-minded as you contemplate adopting or resurrecting a fun activity. Many choices can "do our heart good" in ways well beyond the cardiovascular benefits.

Dancing of all kinds (ballroom, country, contradance, classical, African dance, and more) can be fun, social, aerobic, and weight-bearing at the same time. Inviting someone to play tennis, golf, canoe, or hike can help you find time for friendships and exercise both, allowing you to socialize while you're getting fit. Winter sports, like skiing, snowshoeing, and ice-skating all provide benefits for heart, bones, and often lift our spirits when daylight is short. Practices like yoga, t'ai chi, and martial arts cultivate equanimity and self-confidence in addition to being heart-healthy.

When envisioning an exercise plan, it's sometimes helpful to schedule in one or two activities during the week, then fill in the other days with easy-to-incorporate ones, like walking or biking. Varied, scheduled and supported (with another person, a group, or even an exercise video) plans are a great way to ensure you can really follow through with exercise. Neighbors Jan and Sally, find this expecially true for them. "We were talking one day about needing to get more active, and decided to make a pact," explains Sally. "Sometimes I feel lazy, and probably wouldn't do it, but since Jan's counting on me—I get up and go. She probably says the same thing!"

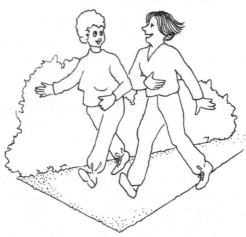

The Ornish Program

University of California cardiologist Dean Ornish has been investigating the effects of serious changes in diet, exercise, and other factors as an actual alternative to coronary bypass surgery for people in advanced-stage cardiovascular disease (CVD) for over ten years now. Ornish's patients embrace a 10% fat, whole foods vegetarian diet, regular aerobic exercise, and stress management training. They also quit smoking and participate in psychosocial support groups. He has consistently found that sticking to this regimen can actually result in reversing artery blockage.[57]

In a three-year study of 333 patients, Ornish showed that patients on his program who had significant coronary blockage could avoid bypass surgery without jeopardizing their health. Chest pain in these patients fell to levels akin to what bypass achieves. Not surprisingly, a lot of money was saved in the process.[58]

Several hospitals offer Ornish's, or similar programs to cardiac patients. These structured programs are usually intended for highly motivated, seriously ill people who want an alternative to bypass surgery. And while the program is not for everyone, the lessons learned from its success can be. Ornish simply pulled together several recognized treatments for heart disease, packaged them in one comprehensive plan, and added the key element of group support. As such, the Ornish program gives us an image of a heart-healthy lifestyle to work toward. Whatever level of changes one can integrate from this model can keep our hearts healthier.

Natural and Conventional Remedies for Heart Health

When diet and lifestyle measures aren't enough, it's time to consider supplements or medications. Ultimately, keeping our risk factors for heart disease at a minimum, through whatever means necessary, is one of the smartest things we can do for our health in the long run.

Nutritional Supplements

Most studies find significant links between adequate nutrient intake and heart health. The majority of large studies point out that *dietary* nutrient intake (from food, rather than supplements) is most important for the general population. Some supplements are worth mentioning, however, because of the volume of research and attention that they garner, and because they may be important for certain individuals.

B Vitamins

The B vitamins may play an important role in the prevention of cardiovascular disease. Deficiencies in vitamins B_6, B_{12}, and folic acid may lead to elevated levels of a compound known as *homocysteine*. Homocysteine, just like free radicals from smoke and other chemicals, can damage blood vessels, which can lead to atherosclerosis.

Although vegetarians usually have lower cholesterol levels than meat eaters, they usually have higher homocysteine levels. Vegans (those who also avoid eggs and dairy products) are most susceptible, because animal products are our biggest sources of B vitamins. In one study, 26 percent of vegetarians and 78 percent of vegans were shown to be deficient in B_{12}, as compared with 0 percent in meat-eaters.[59] While this information isn't meant to suggest vegans or vegetarians should go out and eat animal products, it does indicate they need to be especially mindful of getting enough vitamins B_{12}, B_6, and folic acid from other sources.

Citrus fruits, tomatoes, vegetables, whole-grain products, beans, and lentils are good sources of folic acid. Meat, poultry, fish, fruits, vegetables, and grains are good sources of vitamin B_6. Food sources of vitamin B_{12} are meat, poultry, fish, and milk products. Vegetarians may opt for brewers yeast, blue-green algae, and/or oral supplements as alternative sources of vitamin B_{12}.

As a tangential benefit to cardiac health, one of these B vitamins, vitamin B_6, has been shown to inhibit platelet aggregation, thereby reducing the incidence of blood clots. In this way, B_6 works similarly to aspirin as a blood thinner, although it has not by any means been as extensively studied for this purpose. Vitamin B_6 has also demonstrated the ability to lower blood pressure, possibly by toning down the "flight or fight" mechanism that kicks into gear when we encounter stress.[60]

Vitamin E

Vitamin E, one of the most famous antioxidants, is perhaps the first vitamin to be accepted into the repertoire of mainstream medical providers, and many recommend vitamin E for their patients with cardiac risk. Current, vigorous research has illuminated some helpful trends, although we expect more conclusive results on the cardiac benefits of vitamin E within five years.

The Cambridge Heart Antioxidant Study (nicknamed CHAOS, for short), tested the results of giving patients with known heart vessel blockage either 400 or 800 IU of vitamin E daily. Results demonstrated a 47% reduction in heart attack among vitamin E users, although no real change in lifespan was noted. Other studies of this kind, known as "observational" ones, have found similar reductions in cardiovascular disease risk. Some suggest that patients must use vitamin E for at least two years for this benefit.[61] An analysis of four large "randomized" studies (where vitamin E is compared to placebo), however, failed to show a benefit in terms of heart attacks.[62]

Some clinicians worry that vitamin E, which acts like a blood thinner, could actually increase risk of certain kinds of stroke. However, a study of over 34,000 postmenopausal women found that women taking the larger amounts of vitamin E in their *diets* had the lowest number of deaths from all types of stroke.[63] We're less certain about *supplemental* vitamin E and stroke risk. Certainly, if you have bleeding problems, are on blood thinning medication, or have a surgical procedure planned, you need to remain cautious and inform your clinician about your vitamin E intake. Talk to your health practitioner about your personal risks for cardiovascular disease and stroke. For most women, a dose of 400 IU/day may be considered as potentially preventive for the majority of cardiovascular problems.

Niacin

Niacin, or vitamin B_3, is one supplement that straddles the fence between natural and pharmaceutical agents, in both its strength and risks. It is quite effective at lowering total cholesterol, LDL, and triglycerides while raising HDLs. An early, large-scale clinical trial looking at the effects of various interventions on heart disease, the Coronary Drug Project of the 1970s and its fifteen-year follow-up showed an 11 percent long-term improvement in death rates for the participants who had previously taken niacin.[64,65] Compared to lovastatin, a popular prescription drug, niacin has slightly weaker effects in decreasing LDL, but stronger effects in elevating HDL.[66] Additionally, niacin decreased the levels of another risk factor for coronary heart disease, Apoprotein A. Niacin has also been shown to work well together with some statin drugs.[67,68]

The problem with niacin is that useful levels often cause patients to flush intolerably. This is not a welcome side effect for many menopausal women! Also, niacin therapy must always be monitored by a clinician, as long-term use can potentially lead to liver problems in some individuals. Gastric irritation and nausea are also occasional side effects of niacin.

Supplement manufacturers have found what they feel is a solution to the side effects of niacin. *Inositol hexaniacinate* (sometimes referred to as "non-flushing niacin") is a safer and more tolerable form of this vitamin. Taken in this form, more patients can tolerate the doses of up to 1–1.5 g/day that are required for niacin to work.

Omega-3 Oils

A significant body of evidence has amassed that points to the benefits of omega-3 oils in heart health. Omega-3 oils are the reason why the American Heart Association now recommends 2 servings weekly of fatty fish. Fish oil is a prime source of these beneficial fats. Flax, borage, evening primrose, black currant, and hemp oil also contain omega-3 fatty acids.

Omega-3 fatty acids lower total cholesterol and triglyceride levels.[69,70,71] A study of postmenopausal women showed that those taking fish oil had improved blood lipids than those on placebo—whether or not the women were on hormone replacement therapy.[72] Omega-3 oils have an additional benefit too: arterial compliance, or flexibility, which protects the vessels from damage, increased on both fish and flax oil.[73]

Omega-3 fatty acids are generally thought to increase (good) HDL levels. But some studies have found that the detrimental LDLs can also increase. There is some question, too, about the possibility of these LDLs actually being oxidized,[74] which would tend to make them stick to arteries more readily.

Once again, when it comes to taking supplemental omega-3 oils for cardiovascular health, we'll need to await more data before making definitive statements. Little doubt remains about the benefits of these oils taken in food form, however. Furthermore, when they were, in fact, compared head-to-head, omega-3 oils from actual food sources connoted more benefit than the same amount of the oils from supplementation.[75] Vegetarians, who can develop deficiencies in essential fatty acids more easily than women who consume flesh foods, should consider supplementation.

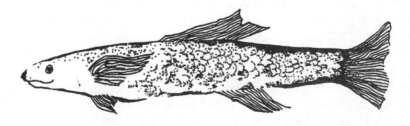

Phytonutrient Supplements to Lower Cholesterol

The following medicines from the plant world have varying effects on cholesterol and other parameters of cardovascular health. We've arranged them in increasing order of effectiveness.

Garlic

Garlic gained popularity as a cholesterol-lowering remedy after a first round of studies showed a beneficial effect. Unfortunately, subsequent attempts to repeat these results have failed. While garlic does have a blood-thinning effect that may be useful, it is not reliable as a cholesterol-lowering supplement.

Red Clover

Although red clover has yet to be proved definitively as a reliable remedy for hot flashes and other menopausal symptoms, its cardiovascular benefit has stronger support. Red clover has shown the ability to improve arterial compliance.[76] This is something that estrogen, soy products, and as we saw above, omega-3 oils also do, and it contributes to their actions in maintaining heart health.

Red clover has other beneficial effects on the heart too. A 1999 study printed in the journal *Atherosclerosis* found a red clover extract to increase (good) HDL cholesterol by 21 percent in 60 premenopausal women over six months. Additionally, the cholesterol that was still floating around in circulation were not as easily oxidized and, therefore, presumably less apt to be incorporated into plaques.[77]

Another good piece of news from this study is that red clover extract does not induce growth of the uterine lining. It, therefore, should not contribute to any risk for uterine cancer. (In Chapter 10, we will talk about the risk of uterine cancer with estrogen.) We may not be able to be as confident about its safety in women with a known history of breast cancer, however. For more information on that topic, see Chapter 9.

Gugul

A resin from the Indian tree, gugul (*Commiphora mukul*), shows promise in lowering cholesterol. One of India's most famous herbs, gugul, lowered total cholesterol by 11.7% in one Indian study. Additionally, LDLs went down by 12.5% and triglycerides by 12%.[78]

Practitioners familiar with gugul generally find it to be helpful for women who have mildly elevated total cholesterol levels or LDLs. Don't expect miracles—but in conjunction with good diet and exercise, gugul may help you drop the few points that could mean the difference between normal and mildly elevated cholesterol.

Note that gugul may render blood pressure medications propranolol and diltiazem less effective. One small study found that patients taking gugul with either of these medicines had lower-than-expected blood levels of the drug.[79]

Red Yeast Rice

A natural product derived from fermented red yeast rice and marketed as Cholestin is very effective at lowering cholesterol levels. In a placebo-controlled study, researchers at UCLA School of Medicine found 2.4 grams per day of Cholestin to lower cholesterol levels in volunteers from 254 to 208, on average, after eight weeks. The decrease appropriately came out of the LDL (bad) cholesterols.[80]

Although naturally occurring, the active ingredient in traditional Cholestin looks chemically similar to that in Mevacor (a prescription drug that we will learn about below) and works in the same fashion. The natural supplement is also several times cheaper than Mevacor. In 1998, the FDA ruled that Cholestin was actually a drug and should be regulated as such, and ongoing court battles threaten its over-the-counter availability. While it remains available, we suggest using this remedy, or any containing extracts of red yeast rice, only under the supervision of a health professional who has considerable knowledge about this remedy and experience with its use.

Conventional Medications to Lower Cholesterol

Sometimes, even the best of diet, exercise, and natural medicine isn't enough to keep cholesterol under control. This is particularly true for people who have a very strong familial predisposition to high cholesterol. In these cases, stronger conventional medications can often afford women the protection they need.

The most commonly used cholesterol-lowering medications are called *"statins."* They have names like atorvastatin, simvastatin, and lovastatin. You may have heard of these via their commercial brand names: Lipitor®, Zocor®, and Mevacor®. Statins typically reduce (bad) LDLs between 20–60%, lower triglyerides by 10–40%, and produce a smaller, but still significant 5–10% increase in (good) HDLs. These medications work primarily by blocking an enzyme in the body that helps make cholesterol. Preliminary data suggests they may also stop constriction of the heart's own blood vessels, prevent the oxidation of LDLs and also act as a blood thinner, preventing blood clots.[81]

Most people tolerate the statin family of drugs with few side effects. Muscle aches or, more rarely, liver problems can occur, however. Your practitioner should monitor your liver function with periodic blood testing if you are on one of these drugs.

The statins have really taken center stage for cholesterol lowering of late, because of their effectiveness and relative lack of side effects. Other types of medications are also available, however, and may be appropriate in certain situations. Resins, which work by acting on bile acids, effectively lower LDLs. Examples include cholestyramine (Prevalite® or Questran®) or colestipol (Colestid®). Since bile helps us digest our food, resins can cause side effects like abdominal distress, constipation, and bloating.

For people with high triglycerides, a third type of fat-lowering medicine may be important. Clofibrate (Atromid-S®), gemifibrozil (Lopid®), and fenofibrate (TriCor®) are derivatives of fibric acid, a chemical which effectively lowers these free floating blood fats. These medications can cause trouble with gallstones or bowel complaints.

Herbs to Regulate Blood Pressure

A comparison of traditional Chinese herbal medicine and Western medications, done at the University of California, Irvine, found that mild hypertension could be controlled with the traditional Chinese herbs, but that Western therapy was more effective for those with higher blood pressures.[82] This pattern is the general rule regarding herbal medicines for blood pressure. With one exception, herbs are considerably weaker than pharmaceuticals for hypertension. The notable exception, rauwolfia, is a strong and potentially toxic herb that should only be prescribed in tiny drop doses by very well trained practitioners. The two herbs listed below can subtract a few points from your blood pressure and possibly make the difference if you are on the edge of needing conventional medication, particularly when combined with diet, exercise and weight loss.

Dandelion

To understand how herbs and medicines work on blood pressure, it's often helpful to use the analogy of water pressure inside a garden hose. One of the ways to lower pressure inside the hose is to actually have less water running through it. Diuretics are remedies that work in just this way.

Dandelion (*Taraxacum officinale*) leaf is a diuretic. As such, it is a popu-

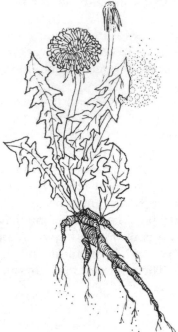

Dandelion (*Taraxacum officinale*)

lar herbal remedy for water retention in the body. Dandelion leaf works on hypertension in the same way that conventional diuretics do. In fact, in one animal study from the 1970s, dandelion leaf was found comparable to the diuretic furosemide (Lasix®) in action.[83] Hopefully, as interest in herbal medicine continues to grow, research dollars will become available to update research like this and validate its effect on humans.

Conventional diuretics are often associated with depletion of potassium from the body. In a perfect example of nature's wisdom, dandelion leaf is found to be rich in potassium. This may be why dandelion leaf is not associated with the side effects of conventional diuretics.

Hawthorne

Hawthorne (*Crataegus oxycantha*) is a Western shrub whose heart-shaped berries and small pink and white flowers have provided key historic cardiac remedies for centuries. Hawthorne's effects on the heart are many and gentle.[84] It has been described as an overall "heart tonic" by herbalists, and used for complaints as varied as angina, arrythmias, improving cholesterol, and preventing atherosclerosis.[85] Hawthorne is perhaps best known for its ability to enhance blood flow to coronary arteries,[86] a quality that probably explains its ability to have improved cardiac performance and symptoms in an eight-week German trial of 136 patients with congestive heart failure.[87]

In addition to its other cardiac effects, hawthorne has very modest blood pressure lowering abilities. It works in this way similarly to some of the newer blood pressure drugs on the market, known as angiotensin converting enzyme (ACE) inhibitors, by decreasing the ability of blood vessels to constrict.[88] Doses can range from 300 to 500 mg daily in capsule form, given in three divided doses.

Because hawthorne is such a weak blood pressure lowering herb, it is usually most effective if it is combined with other herbs by a well-trained herbal practitioner. The only drug interaction to watch out for is the possibility that hawthorne can potentially lower the dose needed of conventional cardiac medications—so work with your prescribing practitioner if you are thinking of adding hawthorne. Hawthorne has been creatively made into jams, jellies, flavored brandy, and other foods, which attests to its safety as a gentle heart "tonic." Side effects are almost never reported.

Conventional Medications to Regulate Blood Pressure

As with high cholesterol, sometimes diet, exercise, and natural medicine aren't enough. If you've given these a try for high normal or Stage 1 blood pressure (see page 106) and still aren't able to get your blood pressures in the normal range, it's time to think about conventional medicines.

Women with Stage 2 or higher blood pressure (systolic over 159 and/or diastolic 100 or more) need to be on conventional medication. If you're just being diagnosed with high blood pressure at this level, and you haven't tried natural means of controlling it, you may be able to switch to these in time, with supervision. However, while you're getting the diet, weight loss, exercise, and natural therapies well established, you should rely on conventional means to keep high blood pressures from damaging your arteries or increasing your stroke risk.

The aim of conventional therapy is to use a single medication at the lowest possible effective dose, while keeping side effects to a minimum. Over 50% of women will get good control with only one medication. Some women, however, will require a combination of two or more drugs to control blood pressure.

Diuretics

Conventional providers often start with diuretics, for a person with newly diagnosed high blood pressure. Diuretics are commonly known as "water pills" because they remove fluid, as well as sodium, from the body. Removal of excess fluid lowers the amount the heart needs to push around. Also, when sodium is flushed out of the blood vessels, they open wider. The combination of wider vessels and less fluid simply equals lower blood pressure. Conventional diuretics include Dyazide® and hydrochlorothiazide.

Losing a lot of fluid relatively quickly can result in dizziness—a reversible side effect. Also, in contrast to dandelion, conventional diuretics may need to be supplemented with potassium, because of potassium loss with all that fluid. Elevation in blood sugar is another potential side effect to diuretics.

Beta-Blockers

Beta-blockers decrease nerve signals to the heart and blood vessels. As a result, the heart beats less often and with less force. Using our garden hose analogy, it's as if we turned the spigot down, allowing less water to flow into the hose. Atenolol and propranol are popular beta-blockers. Side effects include depression, fatigue, and sleep disturbance. These medications are generally not good for diabetics.

Calcium Channel Blockers

Calcium channel blockers work by blocking the normal fluctuations of calcium in and out of cells in the body that cause blood vessels to contract. As a result, the vessels open up, allowing us to pump the same amount of fluid, but the added width will decrease the pressure. Examples include diltiazem, verapamil, and nefedipine. Watch out for side effects of dizziness, headache, constipation, and flushing.

Angiotensin Converting Enzyme Inhibitors and Angiotensin Antagonists

Another family of drugs for blood pressure are the angiotensin converting enzyme (ACE) inhibitors and angiotensin antagonists. ACE inhibitors work a bit like calcium channel blockers in that they prevent our blood vessels from constricting, an action which increases blood pressure. They do this by preventing a buildup of angiotensin II, a chemical that causes blood vessels to narrow. The more relaxed the blood vessel, the lower the blood pressure.

Enalapril, lisinopril, and quinapril are types of ACE inhibitors. These drugs, like diuretics, can cause a potassium imbalance. Another fairly common side effect is a cough, which can limit the tolerability of ACE inhibitors for some people.

Other Blood Pressure Medications

Several additional categories of drugs are sometimes, although less frequently, used as compared to those above. Alpha blockers (such as Minipres®, Cardura®, and Hytrin®) reduce nerve signals to blood vessels, which causes the vessels to constrict less. Alpha-beta-blockers such as labetalol (Normodyne®) and carvedilol (Coreg®) combine the actions of alpha-blockers and beta-blockers, thereby slowing heartbeat and reducing blood vessel constriction. Vasodilators, like hydralazine, relax the muscles that line the blood vessels to allow for dilation. Finally, nervous system inhibitors, such as clonidine, control nerve impulses coming from the brain that direct constriction of blood vessels.

Hormone Replacement Therapy and Heart Health

Now, for the controversial issue of using hormone replacement for heart protection. Since the early 1940s, estrogen replacement therapy has been considered a possible protective measure against coronary heart disease in postmenopausal women. Several recent studies have questioned HRT's benefit for overall women's heart health. Two of the most famous have been the PEPI trial and the HERS study.

The Postmenopausal Estrogen/Progestin Intervention (PEPI) trial reported that estrogen alone helped increase HDL (good cholesterol), decreased total and LDL cholesterol, and *increased* triglycerides. When progestins (synthetic progesterone) or natural progesterone were added, the positive effects of estrogen on the blood fats was blunted but not reversed (progestin faring than natural progesterone). The PEPI trial, along with several other prior studies, led health care providers to suggest that hormone replacement therapy would provide a "cardioprotective" or beneficial heart effect by positively effecting blood lipid levels. More studies at the time suggested other positive effects of estrogen on the heart and blood vessels. The assumption was made in 1995 that since estrogen had a beneficial effect on cholesterol and blood vessels, that HRT reduced actual incidence of heart disease for women.

In 1998, another study called the Heart and Estrogen Progestin Replacement Study (aptly named the "HERS" study) virtually stunned the medical community with findings that refuted the dominant belief about HRT and heart health. The HERS study was the first large study of its kind to investigate what actually happens when women with established heart disease took HRT. After all, these events (heart attacks and strokes) are the real problems we're trying to avoid by improving our risk factors like cholesterol.

The HERS study evaluated 2,763 women, randomized to receive either Prempro® (synthetic estrogen and progestin) or placebo. While cholesterol did improve in the women actually on medication, that didn't translate into decreased heart attacks or deaths. In fact, during the first year, 50% more cardiac events (especially blood clots and stroke) occurred for women on HRT. Later, after two years of HRT, cardiac events decreased for these women. By the time the study was over, after 4.1 years on Prempro®, no detectible difference between postmenopausal women on HRT for their cardiovascular disease could be found.[89,90,91] Subsequent investigation has confirmed these findings.[92]

Understandably, medicine has hit the breaks with regard to the question of HRT for heart health. Especially in women with known, established heart disease or high risks, starting HRT is not proven to provide any heart benefits—and may even cause more problems. Women who have recently had a heart attack or stroke should not initiate HRT—because early use actually *increases* the chance of having another one of these events.[93]

Researchers are still busy at work on this issue, so you can expect to hear more in the future. It is true that HRT improves blood lipids and flexibility of blood vessels, and so you may still hear it recommended for cardiac protection in women who don't have heart disease—which seems pretty unnecessary to us. Also, HRT slightly increases risk of blood clots in virtually every study. On the other hand, proven lifestyle changes such as diet and exercise can be considered more effective and less risky than HRT for preventing heart disease. If you do have high blood pressure, high cholesterol or other risk factors, natural and conventional medicines directed at your specific situation are better options than HRT. Until more convincing evidence comes available, we recommend sticking to other approaches for heart health, whether you currently have heart disease, risk factors, or not.

7 Bone Health

Our bones are alive. They are living, breathing, changing tissue, just like our skin, our blood, our organs. Every day, new bone cells begin again the process of building our foundation, and simultaneously, others remove the old parts, making room for the new. (See Figure 7.1.) Our bones constantly remodel themselves, vigorously and continually doing their part to revitalize our body.

We call the cells that actively create bone *osteoblasts*. An osteoblast is a young, active cell which lays down a mix of calcium and other minerals that harden into bone. It is like a cement worker who pours cement for a foundation. These busy cells get so involved with their work, that they end up cementing themselves in! To access the bloodstream for food, oxygen, and waste product exchange, osteoblasts have to then extend long, tentacle-like arms to the nearest capillary. Using these arms, osteoblasts also form communication bridges with their nearest neighbor cells. By the time they've reached this state, these bone cells have taken on a new name and function: the mature, bone-maintaining *osteocyte*.

After several years of work, the osteocyte is ready for retirement. Thankfully, relief is in sight. A third bone cell, called an *osteoclast*, comes along and dissolves the osteocyte along with the surrounding bone it was maintaining, making room for another osteoblast to build new bone and set up residence. This process of dissolving bone tissue is known as *resorption*.

The cycles of birth, growth, maintenance, death, and dissolution occur for bone more slowly than for practically any other tissue. We like this fact about bone. We count on its stability as the framework for our entire body. By contrast, it takes just three months to create a fresh batch of red blood

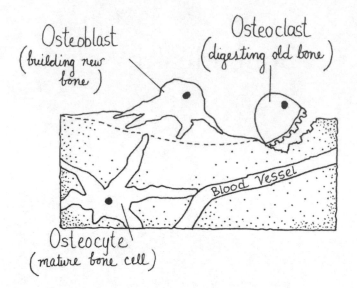

Figure 7.1.   Osteoblasts build new bone, while osteoclasts digest old bone to make room for the new bone.

cells, and only three days for the lining of the stomach to completely re-place itself. Just imagine how unstable we would be if our bones were that changeable!

Nonetheless, bone does transform. Your skeleton today is made up of entirely different cells from the cells of seven years ago. Are there ways we can then influence the characteristics of the bones we'll have seven years from now? You bet.

Your bones today reflect the forces of diet, lifestyle, medications, exercise, hormones, and genetics that were in place during the last seven years, while os-teoblasts and osteoclasts literally remodeled them. While we cannot (yet) control the expression of our genes, we can control many of the other variables that can influence bone. What an opportunity! With proper foresight and support, we can go a long way to creating the set of bones that will literally carry us into the coming decades.

What's Up With American Bones?

We learned in Chapter 2 that women in some cultures, like that of Mayan Indians, maintain strong bones into old age. This is unfortunately not true for most women of Western, developed nations. Between 15 and 20 million women in the United States alone have osteoporosis, leading to 1.3 million fractures per year. A total of 40% of women age 50 will experi-ence an osteoporotic fracture during their lifetime.

Perhaps more alarmingly, *over one-fifth of the women who break a hip will die within one year* as a direct or indirect result of the fracture. People who break a hip become dependent on others for care. Relative immobility carries with it a whole host of health problems associated with lack of exercise: heart problems, infections, arthritis, and very importantly, depression. Chances are, you already know of someone who suffered a hip fracture, and declined significantly or perhaps died by the time one year had passed.

Why are Western women encountering osteoporosis in epidemic proportions? Should we blame our genes? Our diet? Our lifestyle? Is there something we're doing—or *not* doing—that is causing our bones to literally vanish? Are there lessons from traditional cultures that we ought to incorporate in order to keep our bones strong and healthy? Does an optimal medical solution exist?

The answer to whether or not we can influence our risk of osteoporosis is a resounding "Yes!" We can influence many of the factors that determine bone health. Later in this chapter, you'll learn how. Today's prevalence of osteoporosis is due simply to the fact that we're aging as a population. We are now witnessing the effects of genetics and lifestyle on our bones.

Before discussing the factors that affect bone, it's helpful to understand something about the anatomy and physiology of this amazing tissue. The next section will make it easy to understand not only how bone works, but also how it responds to various treatments. You will get all the knowledge you need to make intelligent decisions about the health of your bones.

Bone Architecture

When we look at bone through a microscope, we notice that it doesn't appear solid, like a rock. If it were solid, we would be very heavy and clumsy indeed. Rather, bone has a spongy, porous texture, with many open spaces. In fact, you could describe bone as somewhat like a miniature house: complete with frames, walls, corridors, and many tiny compartments or rooms.

This design makes bone perfect for locomotion in that it provides strength without adding excess weight. Also, with building materials conveniently made of retrievable minerals, bone tissue functions ideally as a storage facility too. In fact, over 98% of the 1–2 kg of calcium and also most of the phosphorus each of our bodies contain resides in the bone. Since the function of every cell in the body depends on precise blood levels of these and other minerals, a ready storage and retrieval system (enter our stars, the osteoblasts and osteoclasts!) is crucial. Thus, bone provides an accessible inventory of our vital minerals.

Bone uses two broad categories of ingredients with which to build our skeleton. We call these the *matrix* and the *mineral* portions of bone. The matrix, likened to the steel reinforcement that shapes a concrete structure, is comprised of collagen and protein as raw materials. Collagen is the strong, rubbery component most abundant in cartilage. In bone, it acts like "superglue" that keeps bone flexible and resistant to shearing forces. Our famous osteoblasts formulate collagen and protein, and lay down this strong matrix to kick off the process of bone building.

One of the most important proteins in this bone matrix is called *osteocalcin*. Osteocalcin, and other proteins like it give proper shape to the matrix. We will see how important the maintenance of proper shape becomes later, when we talk about the process of osteoporosis. We will also learn how a certain vitamin affects osteocalcin.

After weaving the matrix (putting up the framework), osteoblasts begin the process of *mineralization* (pouring the cement). They attract the calcium, phosphorus, and other minerals that will line and support the strands of collagen and protein, and later fill in, or calcify, part of the space between these strands. This microscopic process occurs in bone everywhere throughout the body.

Bone building occurs most rapidly on the insides of bones, where lots of bone cells live and work in the cavernous, spongy open tissue known as *trabecular* bone. (See Figure 7.2.) Changes in our internal environment, such as hormonal changes at menopause, can in fact, affect the density of trabecular bone in a relatively short period of time. Watching changes in trabecular bone can help us determine whether or not a certain therapy is working. By contrast, the denser layers on the outside of bone, known as *cortical* bone, sees less action and therefore responds more slowly to therapies.

During our adult years, we optimally want an equal balance between the breakdown and rebuilding of bone. This means that we experience neither a net gain nor a loss of bone mass. Understandably, the bones of growing children shift toward bone-building. At menopause, and other

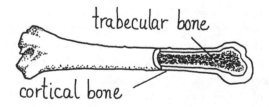

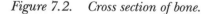

Figure 7.2.   Cross section of bone.

times as we'll discuss later, this balance shifts toward bone breakdown. Basically, if the osteoclasts outpace the osteoblasts—we're losing bone.

A decrease in normal bone density is called *osteopenia,* or "low bone density." If this process goes beyond a certain point, *osteoporosis* occurs. Osteoporosis means literally, "porous bone," and is defined as bone below a certain level of mineralization (see page 129). In osteoporotic bone, one can see actual holes in the "cement" that our osteoblasts laid down. Sometimes, threads in the tapestry of our bone tissue actually break or disappear altogether. When this happens, we have an increased possibility that our bones will fracture, sometimes even from minimal stress.

It's About Form as Well as Content

Information about osteoporosis has focused mainly on bone deminer-alization (loss of its calcium content), as the main predictor of fractures. But as we saw above, calcium alone does not a healthy bone make. If cal-cium were enough, it wouldn't be so easy to snap a piece of drawing-board chalk (which is pure calcium carbonate) in two. Rather, bone strength de-pends also upon that carefully woven matrix of collagen and protein around which calcium and other minerals lie down. Its microscopic shape, resembling cylinders more closely than rods, also adds strength through a superior structure.

The *organization* of its matrix contributes to another important quality of bone—that of elasticity. To illustrate, let's do a little experiment. Locate one of your ribs right now, and push on it. You will notice that it gives way and bends. Bone is not stiff. Healthy bone is flexible as well as strong, and flexible bones don't break as easily as brittle ones.

In some studies, degree of osteoporosis does not correlate to incidence of hip fractures.[1] For example, Chinese women have lower bone densities than white women in the United States, but also a lower rate of both ver-tebral and spinal fractures.[2] In her book *Better Bones, Better Body,* Susan E. Brown, Ph.D., eloquently makes the case that bone thinning, and "osteo-porosis itself does not cause bone fractures." Brown explains that "bone which fractures isn't only thin, but also of poor quality with diminished self-repair capabilities."[3] She is referring to the normal ability of os-teoblasts to rebuild resilient adult bone by laying down collagen in an or-ganized pattern.

Bone which breaks due to osteoporosis has less calcium than normal bone, but important to note, often a *disorganized* microscopic structure as well. This important quality has little to do with calcium and more to do with vitamins D and K, as we will soon learn in more detail. Societies, such as the Mayan culture, which have abundant access to these vitamins in particular via sunshine and fresh vegetables, have an advantage in this regard. It is quite possible that women in cultures where bones undergo considerable decalcification without breaking are benefiting from superior bone architecture.

Macroscopic structure undoubtedly influences bone strength too. Men generally have bigger bones than women, and hence fewer fractures, even if the density of their bones is equivalent. As we'll see in the next section, genetic differences in bone shape also play a role in whether or not someone will fracture a bone.

What Determines Bone Health?

Today, we have an enormous amount of information about the various factors that determine the strength, function, and longevity of our bones. In fact, we hear so much that it's easy to get confused about which factors play big roles and which play relatively small ones. To sort this out, we'll discuss the key physiologic and nutritional factors and the supporting factors.

Key Players in Bone Health

A lot of what determines bone health we inherit. Even some of these inherited traits, however, we have the power to influence. Here's the scoop.

Genetics

Family history profoundly affects our risk for osteoporosis. Bone density studies of families and twins have found that this quality is somewhere between 46% and 80% dependent on heredity.[4] This is a lot.

Most probably, what we inherit regarding bone strength comes largely from our mother's side of the family. Knowing about your mom's bones, her mother's bones, and to some extent her father's bones can give you valuable information when assessing your risk for osteoporosis. Note whether or not any of these people broke any bones as an adult, and if so, what bones fractured. Hip, forearm, and spinal fractures after age 30 may indeed signal osteoporosis. Other bones that have broken from minimal trauma are

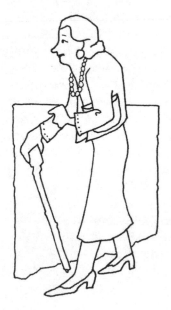

also worth noting. The presence of a dowager's hump also points to osteo-porosis.

Race has a bearing on bone health. Dark skin and an ethnic back-ground that originates in warmer, Southern climates usually translate into stronger bones. Black women have denser bones and fewer osteoporotic fractures than white women.[5] Northern European heritage is associated with higher incidence of osteoporosis. Asian women have bone thinning akin to Northern Europeans, yet have fewer hip fractures.[6] Some re-searchers feel this is due to Asian women having shorter hip bones (called the femoral neck) which makes them less prone to breakage here.[7] How-ever, others feel than lifestyle factors must play a part too. In a disturbing trend, the incidence of hip fractures is climbing in Japan,[8] and some epi-demiologists consider a Westernized lifestyle contributes to this.

Genetic researchers are currently trying to understand exactly how our genes help determine the strength of our bones. One of the most popular theories involves our usage of vitamin D. Vitamin D helps us absorb and use calcium. It does this with the help of vitamin D receptors in our in-testines. Apparently, there are genes that determine how well our vitamin D receptors work.[9,10] Regardless of whether or not this explanation holds up under scrutiny and time, it's bound to be just one of many ways in which we inherit the bones of our ancestors.

Weight

Canadian researchers studying osteoporosis risk factors found that women weighing less than 132 pounds were almost ten times as likely to have low bone density of the spine and hip than women weighing more than 155 pounds.[11] There are a couple of reasons for this. First of all, larger women literally bear more weight on their bones, which will lead to stronger ones. In addition to contributing their own weight, the fat tissues in our bodies, as we also learned in Chapter 5, make estrogen. After menopause, fat can actually produce enough estrogen to help protect our bones.[12] Central abdominal fat is especially good at doing this. Therefore, you can thank your belly for contributing to bone density.

Hormones

Within the realm of reproductive hormones, estrogen is undoubtedly the most important in influencing bone density for women. We'll discuss it, as well as the roles of progesterone and other hormones.

ESTROGEN

Estrogen influences bone both directly and indirectly. First of all, this hormone affects our proficiency at absorbing calcium from food and supplements.[13] The vitamin D receptors in the gut, which grab calcium on its way through, are either turned on or off by the presence or absence of estrogen.[14] Similarly, estrogen levels help determine how much calcium we can salvage from circulation in the kidneys, where calcium would otherwise be on the way out of the body via the urine.[15] By helping pull calcium into the body, estrogen has an *indirect*, although extremely important, action on bones.

We know that estrogen also has a *direct* impact on bone tissue because both osteoblasts and osteoclasts have receptors for estrogen on their surfaces.[16] Science has yet to uncover exactly what these bone cells do once the hormone docks there, however. One theory states that estrogen turns on certain enzymes in osteoblasts that help make proteins for bone. Another asserts that chemicals, which aid osteoclasts in resorption, are produced when there's no estrogen around. Some bone researchers have an even simpler way of understanding the impact of hormones on bone: estrogen speeds up the death of osteoclasts, while prolonging the life of osteoblasts.[17,18]

One way we can actually see the impact of our reproductive hormones on bone is by comparing estrogen levels with bone density levels over a lifetime. Figure 7.3 overlays these two measurements.

Let's follow the dark line, which represents the density of our bones over much of our lives. Clearly we build our bones maximally during our youth. As you can see, bone mass increases steadily from birth and peaks somewhere between ages 18 and 25. We maintain this peak density until sometime in our thirties. From then on, it's downhill, albeit slowly, until we reach menopause.

For most women, something very interesting happens to our bones at menopause (shown at age 50 in this figure). For a period of time corresponding to the initial 3–5 years of menopause, bone density decreases at an accelerated pace. If you look at the thinner line that represents our estrogen levels, you'll see that estrogen plummets right at the time that bone declines more quickly. We believe that much of the (mainly trabecular) bone that was dependent on estrogen actually dies at menopause, if it doesn't receive estrogen from another source. The bone that remains depends less on estrogen. It continues its slower pace of decline. This correlation between plummeting estrogen levels and the steep drop in bone density at menopause, tells us just how much some bone tissue depends on estrogen.

We can also look to the other end of our reproductive years (puberty)

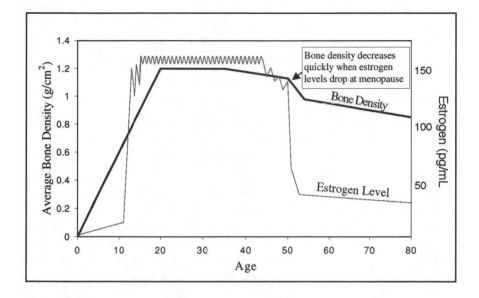

Figure 7.3. Estrogen levels and bone density over a woman's lifetime.

for evidence about this relationship between bones and hormones. We know that heavier girls menstruate earlier than thin ones, and that thinner girls who begin menstruating late have been shown to have an increased risk of osteoporosis later in life.[19] Estrogen derived from fat cells—or lack thereof—is generally accepted as the explanation for this phenomenon. The longer time women spend in their reproductive years, the denser are their bones. Conversely, the shorter time women spend here, the thinner their bones become.

Lack of body fat due to either overtraining or eating disorders can also lead to decreased bone density and have important ramifications later in life. Athletic girls and women who stop having periods for a year or more lose bone density during that time.[20,21] By the same mechanism, anorexia nervosa and bulimia can set up a future problem with bone density.[22,23] In all of these cases, there's the issue of not having much weight to bear in the first place. However, having very little fat tissue does deprive the body of estrogen, which most likely causes loss of bone. Loss of fat from over-exercise or from eating disorders can translate into estrogen levels as low as any postmenopausal woman and cause *amenorrhea,* or an absence of menses.

Estrogen deficiency in girls or young women leads to bone loss similar to that which occurs in menopause—only it's happening when young women are supposed to be *building*, not losing bone. If periods stop for less than six months, a woman can usually gain back lost bone. Two or more years of amenorrhea may result in permanent bone loss that prevents a woman from ever achieving a desirable peak bone mass.

PROGESTERONE

Some scientists suggest progesterone plays a role in bone formation. The most significant researcher in this regard is J. C. Prior, M.D., whose 1990 research at the University of British Columbia started a small amount of laboratory research on the subject. Some research supported Prior's assertion that progesterone is important in preventing postmenopausal osteoporosis.[24] Other research did not.[25] Prior felt that the existing information on progesterone and bone, derived largely from animal studies, provided "the preliminary basis for further molecular, genetic, experimental, and clinical investigation of the role(s) of progesterone in bone remodeling," and added that much further data are needed.[26]

Proponents of natural progesterone are quick to overemphasize the positive findings regarding this hormone for bone health, while minimizing its risks. Popular literature extolling the miracle of natural progesterone cream has influenced many women to forego proven treatments for bone in favor of what they erroneously believe is a risk-free, proven method. There is clearly not enough evidence today to suggest that progesterone, in any form, can prevent or reverse osteoporosis. While progesterone probably does exert an influence on bone, we are very far from knowing what it is. Any woman who chooses to follow a progesterone-only protocol for bone health should do so knowing she is using an experimental treatment—and she should be monitored regularly for its actual effect on her bone. In the section on "evaluating bone health," we will discuss several methods for doing this.

ANDROGENS

Male hormones, or androgens, such as testosterone, seem to have some effect on determining women's peak bone density.[27] As with progesterone, science has a poor understanding of the affect of androgens on women's bones. Currently, there exists no reliable protocol for androgens in the treatment or prevention of osteoporosis for women.

Peak Bone Density

The importance of achieving a high peak bone mass or density early in life is gaining prominence as a fairly accurate predictor of osteoporosis risk over a lifetime. Optimally, we want to do everything possible to ensure that we stockpile very dense bones by age 25, so that we can afford to lose the bone we inevitably shall lose.

Figure 7.4 shows how peak bone mass early in life can be critical in determining whether or not we ever fall below a "fracture threshold." It shows the bone densities of three different women over their lifetimes. Each achieved a different peak bone mass, influenced by genetics, diet, lifestyle, hormonal, and other factors.

Each went through a "natural menopause" without HRT. As their bone density normally declined over the years, one approached, and another fell well below 70% of peak bone density in healthy young adults. Another stayed well above this mark. Levels below 70% of peak bone mass have over 5 times as great a risk of fracture than average. The denser your bones were at 18, the better chances you have of staying well above this hypothetical threshold, naturally.

Activity Level

Astronauts lose bone density in space.[28] Likewise, people confined to bed after illness or injury begin to lose calcium from their bones after only a few days and have detectable decreases in bone density in a few weeks.[29]

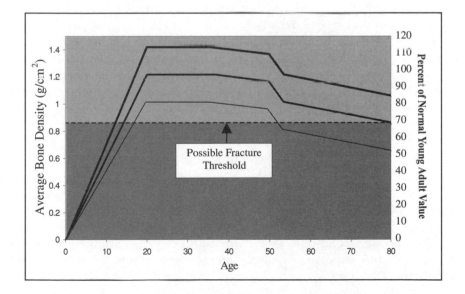

Figure 7.4. Spinal bone densities over three women's lifetimes.

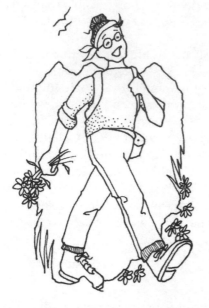

These findings underscore the importance of weight-bearing activity for bone density.

Timing of weight-bearing activity matters. Exercise during the teens contributes to bone density more than at any other period in a woman's life. In a study of nearly 1,500 women in Toronto, Canada, a history of past exercise activity around age 16 prevented more hip fractures than exercise at any other age.[30] Activity in midlife also decreased hip fracture risk, although less so.

A report from the United Kingdom evaluating 2,631 women between ages 45 and 74, found that those engaging in regular high impact physical activity had greater heel density—a finding which correlates to decreased hip fractures. Specifically, these activities, such as running, high impact or step aerobics, tennis, squash, rugby, volleyball, and basketball, all involved some degree of impact, plus an element of being airborne. Likewise, the study found that the number of flights of stairs regularly climbed increased heel density. Not surprisingly, number of hours spent watching television or videos had a negative impact on heel density.[31]

In addition to adding bone density, exercise can give us more muscle mass and coordination. Yoga, martial arts, dance, skating, roller-blading, swimming, and other activities can actually increase our balance and prevent falls. Some osteoporosis experts feel that extra muscle mass in elderly women may in fact cushion and protect the hip from breaking if a fall occurs.

As adults, we must teach young people about the importance of physical activity for bone health. Some international foundations have begun this work. The Finnish Osteoporosis Society has put together a school project called "Rolling Bones" to promote bone health in growing kids. In a similar effort, the Jordanian Osteoporosis Prevention Society has produced a television spot aimed at girls from ages 7–12, teaching them how they can create strong bones—for life. Targeting this population makes sense: *Over 50% of the bone's mineral content in the lumbar spine is accumulated in puberty.*[32] Pass it on.

Key Dietary Players in Bone Health

With regards to diet, you may have heard many, and perhaps conflicting, reports about what to focus on to keep our bones healthy. Let's start with the universal, all-important dietary factors that *everybody* needs to know about—calcium and vitamin D.

Calcium

Intake of dietary calcium over a lifetime, and particularly again in youth when bones grow quickly, has a huge impact on long-term bone health. Calcium intake during the perimenopause and menopause also shows a similar, although less dramatic, impact on bone. In a review of 43 studies done on calcium intake for postmenopausal women, 26 showed a positive effect on bone mass—and 17 did not.[33] *Timing,* again, may account for the fact that over one-third of the studies did not find calcium alone to affect bone mass. During the first 3–5 years after women stop having periods (when bone mass decreases fastest), calcium supplements have a hard time counteracting the effect of estrogen loss. We can see a greater influence of calcium supplementation in women who are at least five years into menopause.[34] At this time, women's bones have adjusted to the new (lower) levels of estrogen in the body, and aren't continuing to lose density at the accelerated pace of the transition period.

You are unique, and so are your bones. Understanding your individual situation will help you sort through all the various opinions about what you should do to protect your bones. If you had a high peak bone density, you'll probably be fine taking basic preventive measures all throughout your later years. However, if you had below-average bone density as a young adult, you will need to make an extraordinary effort to counteract the gradual bone loss that naturally occurs after thirty, and which temporarily accelerates at menopause. Calcium supplements and exercise at menopause then, may not be enough. Later in this chapter, we will describe how you can learn your bone density now, and decide how much intervention you'll need.

The pronounced effect of calcium on bone density early in life vividly illustrates the phrase "an ounce of prevention is worth a pound of cure." Meanwhile, here we are—most of us—already on the gradual downhill slide. Should we even bother with calcium? Of course! Any osteoporosis expert you ask will tell you that optimal calcium intake is a "given" essential for women in or approaching menopause. Calcium supplements have an important role, because it is actually hard to obtain the recommended daily allowance (RDA) of calcium entirely from food sources. Without

enough raw materials absorbed from food and supplements, our osteoblasts won't have enough to work with. And remember, if we don't
keep our blood levels of calcium up from consuming it, our osteoclasts will
certainly mine it out of our bones. This chapter's final section on treatment will detail how much, what form, and when best to take calcium.

Vitamin D

Vitamin D, like estrogen, actually affects bone health in a number of
ways. First, we need this vitamin to absorb calcium from our diet. This is
why milk gets fortified with vitamin D. Second, we need vitamin D to produce *osteocalcin*, the protein that allows our bone to maintain the best microscopic architecture, lending them strength and resiliency.

Studies have verified vitamin D's importance in preventing fractures.
Elderly women whose diets were supplemented with vitamin D were
shown to have a slower rate of bone loss and actually a reduction in hip
fractures.[35] Inadequate levels of vitamin D can have, by contrast, a devastating effect on the bone. Hip fractures are more common in vitamin D–
depleted women. Despite the fortification of milk with vitamin D in
Western nations, deficiency of this nutrient is actually more common than
previously thought—and it is on the rise.[36] This fact has motivated some
forward-thinking researchers to suggest the routine testing of vitamin D
levels in people at risk of deficiency.

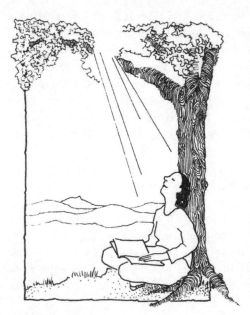

The sun remains the most important source of vitamin D.
People who get little exposure to
sun have the highest risk of deficiency. The elderly, who tend to
spend less time outdoors, often
fall prey to this problem, and in
fact, 25% of elderly women in
northern climates are deficient
in vitamin D. However, people at
any age who don't get regular sun
exposure are also at risk.

A Danish study in which blood
levels of Vitamin D were measured in Moslem women who
wore veils illustrates this point.
Despite their average consumption of over 600 IU of vitamin D
in their diets (three times the
RDA value), these sun-deprived

individuals were *still* deficient in vitamin D. This finding suggests that the RDA of 200 IU is inadequate for women who have little or no sun exposure. Even the 400 IU commonly recommended to women in menopause probably falls short for elderly women or for any woman living in northern climates. The Danish researchers recommended that the daily intake be increased to 1,000 IU for women who get little or no sun.[37] The same advice may then hold true for women who continuously wear sunscreen outdoors.

A small but provocative study from New Mexico found that where a woman grew up may actually affect her current rate of bone loss. Forty women who lived in a retirement community were divided into four groups, depending at which north to south latitude they had lived most of their lives. Each woman was measured for a urinary marker, which correlates to the current rate of bone loss. (We'll say more about this test later.) The study found that relatively few women who had grown up in southern regions were losing bone. By contrast, almost half of those who grew up north of the 40 degree latitude line had results suggesting osteoporosis.[38] This study begs the question of whether previous years of sun exposure (and therefore vitamin D) can possibly affect present rate of bone loss. Whether or not this finding holds up over time, there's no argument about the essential nature of vitamin D for bone health.

Additional Factors Affecting Bone Health

Depending on your personal health history, the following factors will be more or less important for you.

Medications

Several important classes of drugs, including corticosteroids, long-acting benzodiazepines, and anti-seizure medications can have seriously detrimental effects on bone health. Although long term usage of high dose corticosteroids (such as prednisone) are most notorious for causing osteoporosis, even low-dose, chronic use of steroids can dissolve bone.[39] Most of the bone loss with chronic corticosteroid use occurs within the first 1–2 years of use. Calcium supplementation alone or with vitamin D does not sufficiently prevent damage from these drugs.[40] Therapies now being tested to prevent corticosteroid-induced osteoporosis include HRT and the *bisphosphonates,* which we will cover in our section on treatment.

Long-term anticonvulsant drugs, like Carbamazepine (Tegretol®) and phenytoin (Dilantin®) reduce bone density in the hip, increase urinary markers of bone loss, reduce blood vitamin D levels, and even decrease calcium blood levels.[41] Other anti-seizure drugs, which double as antianxiety remedies (from a class called benzodiazepines), may increase hip fracture risk.[42] Clonazepam (Klonapin®) is one such drug. Unfortunately, doctors prescribing them don't always know about, or inform patients of possible risks to bone health with these drugs.

Smoking

Smoking can contribute to poor bone health in at least four ways. First, smoking can cause an early menopause,[43] which will, in turn, increase osteoporosis risk. Second, smokers have lower estrogen levels because they clear it from their bodies faster than nonsmokers. The overall lower estrogen levels in the blood of women who smoke can lead to lower bone density.[44] Third, smoking has been demonstrated to interfere with calcium absorption.[45] And fourth, smoking can keep body weight down, which we've seen is associated with lower bone density. Smokers have lower bone densities, and more hip, forearm, and spinal fractures than non-smokers.[46,47]

Number of Pregnancies

Women who give birth to more babies have stronger bones. A new report in the *American Journal of Obstetrics and Gynecology* found that women who have never delivered a child had the highest risk for osteoporotic fracture, and those with over two deliveries had the lowest. These results were sustained well into women's advancing years (60s and 70s).[48]

Alcohol

While chronic alcoholism is associated with low bone density at present, the effect of moderate alcohol consumption on bone density remains unclear. Conflicting studies do not allow us to make a judgment call about alcohol and bone health at this time. Some studies even suggest that moderate alcohol intake may actually increase bone density by enhancing the conversion of androgens to estrogen[49]—but you won't find any practitioners advising their patients to drink for this reason!

Caffeine

Ingestion of caffeine leads to calcium loss through the urine.[50] There is good evidence to suggest that heavy consumption of caffeine can increase hip fracture risk.[51] Not all studies agree on the dangers of coffee, however. The current wisdom indicates that caffeine ingested without some calcium source might rob calcium from the body. If you can't entertain the idea of giving up your morning coffee or black tea, you can likely mini-mize this effect by making sure you have plenty of calcium on board (from food or supplements) when you ingest caffeine. (Hence, the wisdom of cream in tea or coffee, perhaps?)

Salt

Salt increases calcium loss. Postmenopausal bone loss can be curbed, in part, by reducing salt intake. Every 100 units of salt ingested takes 1 unit of calcium out of the body.[52] In a Japanese study, women age 50–79 who had higher sodium intake had higher bone loss as measured through urine output of bone breakdown products.[53] A similar Chinese study found salt to be the most important dietary factor influencing urinary calcium out-put.[54]

Protein

The exact impact of protein on bone is incompletely understood, and somewhat controversial. No one disagrees that protein comprises an es-sential part of the matrix of bone. Protein malnutrition can certainly lead to a weakening of this structure, and to poor bone formation. In a study of 44 postmenopausal women, dietary protein, and especially animal pro-tein, reduced incidence of hip fractures.[55] Another study of protein intake in elderly women and men echoed these findings.[56]

However, an opposing view is generating a good deal of talk these days. Some researchers have found that dietary protein—and particularly from animals, can actually hurt bone. They even hypothesize that rela-tively low animal protein intake in Third World countries partially ex-plains the lower rates of osteoporosis there. In one study, doubling women's intake of animal protein from 40 to 80 grams daily increased the excre-tion of calcium from the urine by about 1 millimole (mmol) per day.[57] (The millimole is a standard unit of measurement for minerals.) In an-other, ovo-lacto-vegetarian women from ages 50–89 had half the amount of long-term bone loss as meat eaters: 18% as compared to 35%.[58]

The explanation put forth by those finding meat to be potentially detri-mental to bone has to do with the maintenance of pH in the blood. Meat contains high amounts of organic acids (from phosphorus and sulfur) which need to be buffered by a nonacidic, or alkalinizing agent. Cal-cium is one such equalizer. The kidneys couple calcium with the acidic by-products of meat to excrete them. If blood calcium is low—you know where the body goes to mine for calcium. Dr. Susan Brown's *Better Bones, Better Body* contains an interesting and detailed argument for the impor-tance of acid/base equilibrium in preventing osteoporosis.

The issue of calcium excretion and protein (like most things in life) may turn out to be one of balance. Weighing the available evidence, we know that protein deficiency leads to poor bone. It also looks like excess animal protein in the absence of adequate calcium is a problem. Until the evidence becomes a little more one-sided, it's probably wise to eat in the center of either extreme. The section on treatments will provide you with dietary strategies for taking the middle path.

In contrast to protein from animal sources, soy protein seems to have a positive effect on bone density. In a three-year study of 130 Chinese women age 30–40, those consuming the largest amount of soy lost only 1.1% of bone mass, compared to 3.5% for those who ate the least soy. Lead researcher, Dr. Suzanne Ho, believes that soy consumption positively effects peak bone mass as well.[59]

Colas

The Pepsi Generation is about to receive some bone-breaking news. Phosphoric acid in cola drinks causes calcium to be pulled from bone—

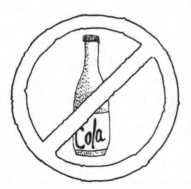

again to balance our body's pH.[60] Harvard researcher Grace Wyshak reported in her recent study of 9th and 10th grade girls that cola drinkers fractured bones during heavy sporting activity five times as often as equally athletic girls who didn't drink colas. "The bone mass girls acquire during adolescence is directly related to their bone mass in postmenopausal years," Wyshak commented.[61] Particularly at a time when a young girl needs to be building bone, shunning milk and downing diet cola is a dietary strategy that may cause not only fractures in her teens, but also frighteningly severe problems with broken bones in later life.

Other Vitamins and Minerals

A study of 62 healthy women aged 45–55 found that women who had eaten higher amounts of fruits and vegetables in childhood had greater density in the hip.[62] The reason for this may have to do with pH again. Fruits and vegetables produce an alkaline environment in the body, as opposed to animal products, which leave an acid residue and require calcium to balance it out.

Then again, fruits and veggies might add to bone density by delivering to us dozens of macro- and micronutrients that assist in bone maintenance. Magnesium, zinc, potassium, boron, vitamin K, manganese, silicon, and others vie for inclusion in anyone's "Top Ten" list of nutrients for bone health. Nutritional medicine expert Alan Gaby, M.D., in his book *Osteoporosis Prevention and Treatment,* details the cases made for nutrients in addition to calcium and vitamin D that may be critical to our bones.

One of the nutrients we know something about is magnesium. In a four-year follow-up of the Framingham Heart Study, a large Massachusetts-based study that advanced our knowledge of how to prevent heart and other diseases related to aging, women who consumed more magnesium from dietary or supplemental sources maintained greater bone density.[63] The researchers speculated that blood chemistry, once again, produced this result. Magnesium (and potassium as well) produce a more alkaline environment in the body which spares calcium from being recruited from bone as a buffer.

A couple of micronutrients attracting attention these days are vitamin K and boron. Vitamin K, like vitamin D, is important to healthy osteocalcin formation. It has been shown in animal studies to prevent bone loss.[64] More impressive, an analysis of 72,327 women from the famed Nurses' Health Study found an actual reduction in risk of hip fracture among women who consumed higher amounts of vitamin K in their diets.[65] Boron is a unique mineral because it seems to have a direct effect on actual levels of estrogen and testosterone. Because boron has been shown to increase estrogen levels, it may be contraindicated for women who have a history of breast cancer. Boron additionally improves the utilization of calcium and vitamin D.

We've spotlighted here just a few of the nutrients that may be important to bone health. Authors Gaby and Brown are good resources for those wishing to delve more deeply into this area. No matter how much we've discovered to date, though, it is likely to be just a fraction compared to what we don't know. Scientists are just beginning to understand the complex interactions between nutrients, hormones and the mechanics of our skeleton. Our magnificent bodies, with their interweaving of chemistry, structure, and life force, continue to inspire our exploration and provide the frontier upon which to do it as well.

Evaluating Your Bone Health

Now that we know how many individual factors influence the dynamic life of our bones, let's see how several of these combine in *you* to provide a rough assessment of your own risk of encountering osteoporosis. The information you learn by taking the following quiz can help guide you and your clinician in deciding whether or not to go ahead with further laboratory or image-testing, which we will discuss shortly.

To take the quiz, read each statement and determine if it is true or false for you. If it is true, give yourself the number of points indicated at the end of the statement. If it is false, give yourself zero points.

Osteoporosis Risk Assessment Quiz

1. My mother has/had osteoporosis. (Including a hip or any other fracture after age 50 or a dowager's hump.) **3 points**

2. My father has/had osteoporosis, or any fracture after age 50. **2 points**

3. My maternal grandmother and/or grandfather have/had osteoporosis. (If you are unsure, but either of these people broke a hip or had a severe dowager's hump, give yourself 1 point.) **1 point**

4. I went into menopause by age 43 and didn't take hormones. **1 point**

5. I weigh less than 132 lbs, *or,* I am tall and thin. **1 point**

6. I have been on low-dose steroid medication (=< 20 mg prednisone for 3–6 months; =< 15 mg for 6–12 months or =< 5 mg over 1 year). **1 point**

7. I have been on high-dose steroid medication (prednisone 20 mg for over 6 months). **2 points**

8. I take anti-seizure medicines or long-acting benzodiazepines (1 point for each). **1 point**

9. I currently smoke. **1 point**

10. I am on my feet less than 4 hours per day. **1 point**

11. I personally have had a fracture (of any bone) after age 50. **1 point**

12. I have had a bone density test, and my T score is between –1 and –2.5. **1 point**

13. I have had a bone density test, and my T score is less than –2.5. (These are negative numbers, remember! *Less* than –2.5 are numbers like –2.7, –3, etc.) **2 points**

14. I do weight-bearing exercise more than 4 hours per week. ***Subtract* 1 point**

When you have finished reading all the statements, total your points. A score of one to three indicates that your risk of developing osteoporosis in your lifetime is low. A score of four to six indicates that your risk is moderate. A score of seven to nine indicates that your risk is high. (Note that this quiz is intended only to help you work with your clinician regarding your osteoporosis risk. It is not a substitution for standard bone density testing and has not been verified for accuracy by large scale study.)

Bone Density Testing

Routine bone mineral density testing has revolutionized our understanding of osteoporosis. We now have the ability to somewhat predict the future in terms of your bone strength. Bone density testing provides the most accurate, objective information about your actual risk of osteoporotic fracture.

Dual Energy X-Ray Absorptiometry

Dual energy X-ray absorptiometry (DEXA) is a low-dose radiation technique that uses either a pencil-thin, or in the case of newer scanners, a fan-shaped X-ray beam to scan for bone density. The radiation is so low, and so specific, that technicians rarely even wear protective clothing for themselves. Specifically, the DEXA scan determines the calcium content of bone. Don't confuse this with a "bone scan," a tool used by doctors for detecting fractures and cancers.

DEXA bone density tests can theoretically be taken over any part of the body. Some less expensive machines measure bone density in the hand, or in the heel, for example. Central DEXAs—those measuring density of the hip and spine—provide a much more accurate estimate of fracture risk in these areas. Importantly, central DEXAs of the spine measure density in the highly metabolic trabecular bone, which changes much faster than cortical bone. When monitoring a new therapy, a central DEXA can detect a change better than any other form of bone density testing.

Today, most large hospitals offer central DEXA testing, which runs about $250, and many smaller hospitals or large clinics offer less expensive peripheral testing. Insurance companies are now catching on to the long-term cost-benefit of bone density testing, and most, though not all, provide coverage. If you don't have insurance or aren't covered for this test, you might consider making the investment out-of-pocket. It could be the most important money you've ever spent on yourself.

Heel Ultrasound

Ultrasound of the heel is a newer, more cost-effective way to evaluate bone mineral density than with DEXA. Some researchers feel it now rivals DEXA's ability to predict one's lifetime risk of having any osteoporotic fracture. In the future, this emerging technique may allow us to discern more important information about actual bone architecture, which would be a real advantage over the DEXA's ability to assess density alone.

The World Health Organization recognizes the importance of ultrasound for bone density testing, but cautions that no standard exists yet for precise interpretation of the results. In other words, we know that a heel ultrasound produces an accurate measurement, but don't know what values translate into fractures. Some experts say many women who get heel measurements are being told they're osteoporotic when they're actually not.[66]

Central DEXA can serve as the "final arbiter" in equivocal cases. That means that if you have a borderline heel ultrasound, you may want to consider getting a central DEXA, to clinch whether or not you truly have osteoporosis. Also, if you obtain a heel ultrasound, are told you are osteoporotic and therefore should go on a therapy you are not completely sold on, talk to your practitioner about obtaining a central DEXA test. It's possible that you're in better shape than the ultrasound indicated. Also, while some newer types of these machines seem to be approaching the DEXA's ability to determine risk of an actual hip fracture,[67] people who want to know their spinal density are still better off with a DEXA, which takes a picture of the area in question.

Who Needs Bone Density Testing?

Not everyone needs bone density testing. Black women, for instance, have a very low rate of osteoporosis, and rarely need testing. Healthy premenopausal, Caucasian women who don't have much in the way of risk factors can similarly forego this test. If you fall into any one of the following categories, you can probably save yourself money and time and forego testing and just stick to a reasonable prevention plan:

- Premenopausal women without significant risk factors
- Postmenopausal women on HRT who have no extraordinary risk factors
- Women for whom bone density results will not affect treatment.

Additionally, if your score on our osteoporosis risk assessment quiz on page 146 placed you in the mild risk category, you are likely to not need further bone testing. Because there are always limitations of any assessment quiz, you should verify this by talking with your practitioner.

If you are a postmenopausal woman, the National Osteoporosis Foundation recommends you do obtain a bone density test if you fall into any *one* of the following categories[68]:

- Women 65 or older
- Postmenopausal women who've had a fracture
- Those with a parent or sibling who fractured a hip, wrist or vertebra
- Women under 127 pounds
- Current smokers

We would like to expand on this list. If learning your bone density would affect your decision-making about therapies in menopause, go ahead and get tested. Even if you are pretty sure you want to have a "natural" menopause (without hormones or other pharmaceuticals), if your scored is moderate to high on the ostcoporosis risk assessment quiz, it's prudent to have bone density tested. With a baseline central DEXA (the type which measures trabecular bone and shows up changes fastest), you can obtain another for comparison after a few years to evaluate the effectiveness of any natural (and usually less well-proven) therapies.

Finally, any woman who scored in the "high" range on our quiz should obtain bone density testing. In our next section, we'll help steer you in the direction to the testing method that will give you the most pertinent information for your situation.

When to Do Bone Density Testing

There are situations that call for bone density testing well before menopause. These include cases in which a woman with risk factors for low bone density fractures any bone, at any age, following minimal trauma. Women of reproductive age whose periods disappear (a condition called secondary amenorrhea) for over two years should also talk to their practitioners about this evaluation (and in some cases, advocate for themselves if practitioners are reluctant to order the test). Early bone density testing in cases like these can alert a woman to a potential future problem, and allow her to begin addressing bone health sooner rather than later.

For most women who have an indication for bone density testing, perimenopause provides the perfect opportunity to do so. If you refer back to Figure 7.3, you will see that a steep drop in bone density occurs for the first 3–5 years after a woman's last menstrual period. *Obtaining your bone density just before this drop happens can show you whether you have bone to spare—or alternatively, if you can't afford the drop.* This information can play a critical role in your decision about which therapies to choose.

Repeat, or follow-up DEXAs should be spaced about two years from the last one if monitoring a new prescription medication for osteoporosis prevention. The reason for this timing has to do with the sensitivity of the testing method. Repeating a DEXA before these time periods does not guarantee accurate testing. In some cases, such as with women on steroids, repeat testing earlier than 2 years is warranted.

Janice

At 52, Janice was unsure about whether or not to take hormones in menopause. Her periods had tapered off last summer, and she hadn't had one for three months. She still had 1–2 hot flashes a day, plus minor sleep disturbances, but these weren't a problem, and she usually could control them if she remembered to take her black cohosh.

Yet, Janice's mother, a smoker of 25 years, had just been prescribed a medication for osteoporosis, and her maternal grandmother (also a smoker) had suffered a hip fracture in a nursing home at age 75. In addition, Janice had grown up in Minnesota, a descendant of Norwegian and Irish parents. After doing some reading, Janice figured she had a moderate to high risk of osteoporosis because of her genetic heritage and from living in a Northern climate. She wondered if being more physically active, not smoking, and taking calcium supplements was protecting her bones adequately.

She scheduled a visit with her nurse practitioner to talk about this. Janice's practitioner agreed that bone density testing would help them know whether or not she should be thinking about hormonal or some other kind of preventive medicine for osteoporosis. Together they scheduled a bone density test at the nearest facility.

Choosing Bone Density Testing Methods

Perimenopausal women who would likely opt to take HRT if bone density is low can usually get by with the less expensive heel ultrasound bone density test. Likewise, women for whom the high cost or lack of availability makes the DEXA inaccessible, heel ultrasound, or another peripheral study such as DEXA of the heel, are reasonable alternatives.

A woman entering menopause who's leaning toward a natural meno-pause (without hormones), on the other hand, should opt for a central DEXA, which will give her a measurement of the spine. Because the spine shows changes first, prudent monitoring of a central DEXA can help her know if she's on the right path. In fact, any woman who wishes to monitor progress over time should utilize central DEXA testing for the same rea-son. Aside from the cases listed above, central DEXA is usually the pre-ferred form of bone density testing.

What Does Bone Density Tell Us?

DEXA bone density tests give us a picture of the calcium content, or density, of the bones. Measurements of the hip correlate well to actual hip fracture rate. Spinal measurements, however, don't correlate quite as well with spinal fractures.[69] This is particularly true in women over 65, who often have age-related bone change in the spine.

Janice (see page 150) and her nurse practitioner decided that she could use the peripheral heel ultrasound testing offered by the small nearby hospital, because Janice was willing to be on HRT if her bone den-sity was too low. After her test showed her to be in the low risk category for fracture, Janice and her nurse practitioner decided that she could forego any prescription medication for bone at this time, as long as she keeps up with her calcium and weight-bearing exercise. They decided to have a re-peat bone density measurement in two years, and at that time, will revisit the question of medication.

The T-score is the most important measurement obtained in a bone density test. Expressed either in positive or negative numbers, the T-score tells us how much our bones deviate in density from normal, healthy bones. Positive T-score numbers mean we have dense bones. Negative T-score numbers indicate we have a risk of fracture. Specifically, a T-score of –1.0 indicates twice the average fracture risk, a score of –2.0 indicates four times the average fracture risk, and a score of –3.0 indicates eight times the average fracture risk.

The World Health Organization (WHO) has established criteria for di-agnosing osteoporosis using the T-score. These criteria are summarized in Table 7.1.

Limitations of Bone Density Testing

Although bone density tests are the best tools available today in esti-mating an individual's risk of fracture, they are still far from perfect. Because it only measures calcium content, a DEXA indicates the *quan-*

Table 7.1. WHO's Criteria for Diagnosing Osteoporosis[70]

T Score	Risk for Osteoporosis	Recommended Measures
Below -1	Below average	Adequate diet and lifestyle measures.
Between -1 and -2.5	Above average	Hormone replacement [or natural alternative, we'll add]. Repeat bone density tests in 2–3 years.
Below -2.5	High	Therapeutic intervention (for B most patients).
Below -2.5 plus one or more osteoporosis-related fracture	Very High	Therapeutic intervention and further diagnostics.

tity—but not the *quality* of bone tissue. Bone's microscopic structure is invisible to the DEXA's eye. Bone density testing can't measure microscopic architecture, and therefore the qualities that determine bone's resiliency.

Patients and practitioners can sometimes overinterpret the meaning of a DEXA test. DEXA gives us a relative percentage of bone density, and from it, extrapolates a person's chance of having a fracture. It cannot absolutely predict whether or not you will break a bone. Any bone density result needs to be interpreted in the context of the whole person. One's age, lifetime calcium intake, family history, and other factors that affect bone health can effectively adjust the risk stated on a DEXA value either up or down. According to Dr. Edward Leib, director of the Osteoporosis Center at the University of Vermont Medical Center, this means that two women with identical "T" scores can, in fact, have very different fracture risks. "If a woman has a T score of –2 and has no other [risk] factors, I may not treat her beyond recommending calcium, vitamin D and exercise. But if a woman has a T score of –2, a family history [of osteoporosis], and is a smoker, I would probably treat her."

Dr. Leib also points out that a 50-year-old woman and a 70-year-old woman with identical scores on bone density testing have different risks of fracture. Age-related decline in bone strength due to changes in microscopic architecture probably have a role here. Also, over time, a woman's muscle strength, balance, and coordination will help determine whether or not she will actually fall. Daily mechanical stress of poor posture can influence development of a dowager's hump. Finally, a decline in muscle mass, which happens with age, provides less "padding" to cushion any falls that do happen. DEXA or ultrasound bone density tests cannot measure these important factors. Therefore, after receiving your DEXA results—you and your practitioner will both need to factor in your overall health status to arrive at an accurate interpretation of your risks. For example, if you have great posture, practice yoga, and take a good multivitamin, your bones are likely in better shape than someone with the same bone density who drinks diet cola and watches TV all day.

Cross-Fiber Testing

DEXA and heel ultrasound bone density tests give a snapshot image of our bone density at the moment of the test. They cannot, however, tell us if we are currently gaining or losing bone. A different type of testing may help in this regard. As you recall, bone is comprised of protein and collagen fibers, upon which osteoblasts lay calcium. Our busy bone cells actively break down bone and build it back up all the time. We can actually measure this process, by measuring how much of the protein and collagen fibers from bone are leaving the body via the urine.

In the past decade, tests that measure the urinary excretion of bone breakdown products have become commercially available. Naturopathic physicians and other holistically oriented practitioners have been employing these tests for several years to gain more insight into the dynamic processes that are taking place within a patient's bone tissue. As the technology improves and knowledge of these tests increases, some conventional providers are beginning to use these urinary cross-fiber tests in patient care. Some preliminary studies have gone so far as to conclude that these studies can, like bone density tests, predict bone loss and fracture risk.[71,72] Others have found only a weak correlation between levels of these cross-fibers in the urine and hip fractures in women.[73]

While the jury is still out and the technology advancing, we feel that urine cross-fiber studies can be a helpful addition to—but not a replacement for—bone mineral density testing using DEXA or heel ultrasound. Cross-fiber studies actually provide a type of information different from bone density testing. While bone density testing provides us with the static picture of how much calcium resides in the bone, urine cross-fiber testing tells us whether or not we're hanging on to that bone.

Gathering information about both the static and dynamic state of our bones can help us make clinical decisions. For instance, suppose you have some bone loss, and are deciding on whether or not to take HRT, another bone-sparing remedy. If a baseline urine cross-fiber test indicated that you were losing bone at a significant rate right now, you might choose a differ-ent course of action than if it looked like the bones were remaining stable. Likewise, re-testing the urine after being on a therapy for three to six months may tell you if the therapy is working to protect bone.

This kind of "before and after" test is particularly helpful if you are choosing a therapy that has not yet been proven to prevent osteoporosis. Make sure you obtain a baseline test before beginning on the therapy, to get an accurate picture of how the therapy affects the bone. Again, you are much more likely to find this type of testing offered by a naturopathic physician or other holistically oriented practitioner until it becomes more mainstream. Used in this complementary fashion, cross-fiber testing via the urine may give you helpful information long ahead of a repeat bone density test, and allow you to change the course of therapy if it looks like something else is needed.

Why Calcium Blood Levels Aren't Helpful

Many patients ask if there is a blood test for calcium that can check their bone status. The answer is "no," and here's why. Calcium is one of the most important elements in the body—and not just for making bone. Every muscle in the body—from our skeletal muscles to those that line our blood vessels to our all-important heart muscle—needs calcium to con-tract. Nerves use calcium to transmit their impulses. Even functions like insulin release and blood clotting depend on calcium.

Because so many systems depend on calcium, our body must carefully maintain a very steady level of it in our bloodstream. As soon as our bodies perform a function that requires calcium and takes it from the bloodstream, we pull calcium out of bone, and also salvage some from excretion by the kidneys. (Since our bones are viewed as a large storehouse of calcium, the body would much rather deplete bone storage than allow blood levels to dip.) At the same time, vitamin D gets activated, and increases its absorption of calcium from the bowel. These functions together bring our blood cal-cium back up to the normal range. The body's sensitivity to, and correction of, blood calcium levels happens in the blink of an eye. We can never, then, measure blood levels to get an accurate sense of our calcium nutriture.

Keeping Our Bones Healthy

In the beginning of this chapter, we saw how modifiable factors of diet, exercise, and lifestyle choices can influence bone health. In this section, we will discuss the practicalities of implementing such choices. We will also detail the natural and conventional medicines that work the best for pre-venting and treating osteoporosis.

Whether you have a mild, moderate or high risk of osteoporosis, the information on nutrients and exercise certainly apply to you. Optimal diet, calcium, and supportive mineral intake, along with weight-bearing exercise, are essential for every woman.

If you have a moderate or high risk of osteoporosis, or already have been diagnosed with osteopenia (low bone density) or osteoporosis, you will want to pay special attention to the natural and conventional medicine options. In each section, you will learn the indications, expected results, and side effects known for the remedy in question.

Diet

We've seen how salt, caffeine, and cola drinks influence calcium excretion through the urine, stealing calcium from our bones. It won't come as a surprise, then, that our first dietary recommendation will be to minimize salt, caffeine, and colas.

Regarding protein from animal sources, balance is key. Nonvegetarian women who have low bone density may want to move in the direction of a vegetarian diet, receiving protein from dairy products or vegetable sources when possible. Vegetarian and vegan women, on the other hand, need to look for food combinations that provide complete proteins so they don't develop protein deficiencies. Books like *Laurel's Kitchen*, and Francis Moore Lappé's classic *Diet for a Small Planet* instruct those new to vegetarian cooking how to derive a protein-rich diet from plant sources.

Milk

In some natural medicine circles, milk and dairy products have received harsh condemnation, while most conventional sources tout milk as a perfect food. Research landing on both sides of the fence has fueled the controversy. Studies like that done at the Channing Laboratory in Boston, where increased dairy intake actually led to a slight increase in osteoporotic fractures in 77,761 women ages 24–59 over 12 years[74] have lent support and some validity to those who crusade against dairy products.

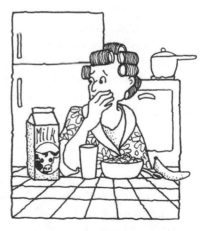

On the other hand, dairy proponents retort with studies of their own, which show slowing of bone breakdown and greater bone density among milk-drinkers. For instance, a study of Taiwanese vegan nuns found their bone density at the hip to be markedly reduced, and their spine even worse, near fracture threshold.[75] (Vegans do not consume any dairy or animal products.)

In one review's attempt to answer the "dairy dilemma," Creighton University professor R. P. Heaney analyzed all published research from 1975 to 2000 concerning dietary intake of calcium through dairy and calcium supplements and its effect on osteoporosis. He looked at the strengths and weaknesses of the methods used and sorted through the problems associated interpreting results in an issue with many factors, such as osteoporosis. Heaney reported that the vast majority of well-designed studies supported the positive effect of dairy calcium and bone health.[76] In a study conducted by his own research group, Heaney found calcium from dairy and supplements to affect bone density equally. He made a comment that seems comical in its self-evidence, but in this day and age where we focus on pills, it nonetheless bears repeating: "Dietitians can be confident that food works."[77]

The debate over dairy is fueled partly by separate health issues that some individuals have with milk products. Lactose intolerance (due to the deficiency of an enzyme that digests milk), dairy allergy, and many other chronic health conditions present some women with good reasons to avoid milk products. Confusion arises when either the problems or the virtues concerning dairy products for certain groups of people become overgeneralized. In truth, milk is a perfect food for some women, highly problematic for others, and somewhere in between for most.

For people who eat meat, animal sources actually offer up better-absorbed calcium than do vegetables. Omnivores absorb about 45% of milk's calcium, whereas vegetarian sources of calcium (like spinach, sesame seeds, and watercress) yield about 27% absorption. People who do not eat meat develop a natural strategy for increasing the amount of calcium they can actually absorb from food. Vegetarians have been shown to have a slightly altered gut ecology when compared to omnivores. The normal bacteria that inhabit the intestines in vegetarians produces chemicals called *phytases*, which result in an increased absorption of calcium. What a beautiful example of the body's extraordinary adaptive powers!

The question of whether or not to eat dairy products gives us yet another opportunity to resound our ongoing theme—that every woman's situation is unique to her. If you digest dairy well, and have no other health detriment from eating it—rest assured that dairy provides a good source of calcium for you. If you have an intolerance to dairy for any reason, by all means, choose vegetable or supplemental sources of calcium.

Most women consume far below the recommended daily allowance of calcium. Even health-conscious people, like 45-year-old Theresa, who attest to eating excellent sources of plant and/or dairy calcium, find themselves shocked when they actually do the math to calculate their daily calcium intake. To find out how much calcium you're getting in your food, use the following to help you tally up what you might eat on a typical day.[78] Note that each of the calculations is based on a 3.5-ounce serving of the food.

- **Dairy products**
Cheddar cheese	750 mg
Goat's milk	129 mg
Whole milk	119 mg
Yogurt	120 mg
- **Nuts and Seeds**
Almonds	234 mg
Sunflower seeds	120 mg
Sesame seeds, hulled	110 mg
Walnuts	99 mg
Pumpkin seeds	51 mg
Cashews	38 mg
- **Vegetables**
Kelp	1,093 mg
Collard leaves	250 mg
Kale	249 mg
Parsley	203 mg
Dandelion greens	187 mg
Watercress	151 mg
Olives, ripe	106 mg
Broccoli	103 mg
Lettuce, romaine	68 mg
Green beans	59 mg
Artichoke	56 mg
Cabbage	49 mg
Sweet potato	32 mg
- **Grains**
Wheat	46 mg
Rye	38 mg
Barley	34 mg
Brown rice	32 mg
- **Legumes**
Tofu	128 mg
Soybeans, cooked	73 mg
- **Dried Fruits**
Apricots	67 mg
Raisins	62 mg
Prunes	51 mg

Soy

Again, soy scores high marks here for bone-building. Japanese researchers found postmenopausal women who consumed more soy had higher bone densities.[79,80,81]

Soy's bone-building action comes both from its calcium content and also from the same isoflavones that act as phytoestrogens for perimenopausal symptoms. All soy is not alike, however. Soy products rich in isoflavones exert a more potent protection on perimenopausal bone loss in the spine than soy without high isoflavone content.[82] Refer back to Chapter 4 for a list of the isoflavone content of various soy foods.

Nutritional Supplements

Some type of supplement to insure bone health is about the only remedy that we recommend for nearly every woman, beginning at the approach of her menopausal years. Here's our take on what's important to know about a good one.

Calcium

The body absorbs calcium best at night, during sleep. Optimally, then, you should take at least part of your daily dose of calcium before bed. The

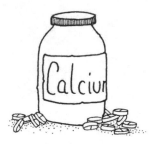

National Institutes of Health recommends 1,000 mg of calcium daily for postmenopausal women on estrogen, and 1,500 mg for those not on estrogen. We recommend that women in perimenopause begin consuming this amount as well, simply because menopause could happen at any time. After age 65, the recommendation of 1,500 mg applies to everyone.

Women with osteopenia or osteoporosis who, for whatever reason, are not on additional bone-building medicines, can—and probably should—consume 2,000 mg of calcium daily. Only very rarely (such as for women who have a history of easily forming calcium-based kidney stones) is calcium supplementation a problem. The Food and Nutrition Board of the National Academy of Science has set a tolerable limit for calcium at 2,500 mg/day.[83] To know how much calcium you will need to supplement, subtract the average daily intake from food, as calculated above, from your recommended daily intake.

CALCIUM CARBONATE

Calcium carbonate, commonly known as "oyster shell calcium" is the most popular and least expensive form of calcium available. It has an added benefit for those who don't particularly enjoy taking pills: calcium carbonate is very dense. This means that one can consume more calcium in a smaller pill size than with any other form of calcium. Perhaps the most important benefit of this form of calcium, however, is that the vast majority of studies regarding supplemental calcium and bone density are done on calcium carbonate. Calcium carbonate therefore, sets the standard for RDAs. It is the only form of calcium that we can say with assurance what dosage works.

Calcium carbonate has some disadvantages too. First, some studies of major supplement brands have found unacceptable levels of lead in their calcium carbonate products.[84] This problem also surfaces in *hydroxyappatite* forms of calcium. Second, calcium carbonate poorly absorbed compared to other forms. Calcium requires stomach (hydrochloric) acid for optimal absorption, and calcium carbonate inactivates acid. This presents a problem for people who have low stomach acidity.

CALCIUM IN ANTACIDS

Many practitioners recommend Tums® antacid as a calcium source for their patients. While convenient and fine for most people, this form of calcium is inadequate for some. Low stomach acidity, which affects about 10% of elderly women, can prevent adequate absorption of Tums®, or any form of calcium carbonate, particularly if taken on an empty stomach. Antacid calcium supplements obviously neutralize stomach acid. (As an important aside, they may also contain aluminum, a potentially detrimental metal, which has itself been implicated in adversely affecting bone density.) Women who always take their supplements with meals can usually get away with using the antacid or other calcium carbonate sources, as food gets the stomach to pump out more acid.

CALCIUM CITRATE

Other forms of calcium, such as *citrate, malate,* and *aspartate,* provide more absorbable calcium than the carbonate form. People with low stomach acidity are better off using this form. One study found that these people absorbed 45% of the calcium from calcium citrate, and only 4% of that from calcium carbonate under fasting conditions. (If taken with a meal, they were able to absorb both forms comparably.)[85] Additionally, calcium citrate has not been implicated in kidney stone formation.[86] In one study comparing two popular forms of calcium supplementation, calcium citrate had a 75% greater rise in blood calcium levels than did calcium carbonate.[87]

The main drawbacks of calcium citrate and the other forms mentioned are cost, bulk, and lack of studies. Where you might be able to get 1,000 mg of calcium in carbonate form with two pills, you would likely need to take four to six calcium citrate pills to deliver 1,000 mg of calcium. Some women wonder if they can take less calcium citrate, because more of it makes it into the system. The answer here is "*probably*—but we don't have the studies to prove this." As you can see, lack of data here produces a dilemma for clinicians and their patients. We desperately need more studies on calcium sources other than carbonate form.

Different women solve this dilemma in different ways. For people on a budget, calcium carbonate affords the cheapest and easiest option. Women who are more concerned about lead levels will want to stick to calcium citrate. Yet others find that mixing and matching, using some combination between calcium citrate and calcium carbonate keeps costs and number of pills at reasonable levels, while ensuring that the best form of calcium also gets included in a woman's regimen. For any woman who finds that her calcium supplement causes constipation, gas or bloating, experimenting to find which mix works with her digestive system may determine what form of calcium she ultimately chooses. One thing we know: consistent supplementation with *any* form of calcium will benefit women more than inconsistent use of even the most bio-available forms.

Vitamin D

Native cultures in northern climates may have avoided vitamin D deficiency by eating a traditional fish-based diet. Dishes with fishes—in particular, fatty fish (for example, salmon, mackerel, herring, halibut, sardines, and fresh tuna) provide excellent sources of vitamin D. Egg yolks, butter, fortified milk, wheat germ, and liver also provide us with significant vitamin D.

Women of all ages should get at least 400 IU of vitamin D per day. If you are middle-aged or younger and live in a sunny climate all year, thirty minutes in the sun with a short-sleeved shirt or shorts 2–3 times per week will provide you this level or more. As we age, our skin loses some ability to convert sunlight to vitamin D. Hence, we may need to supplement even if we do get adequate sun exposure. Also, sunscreen blocks vitamin D production. Therefore, if you usually wear sunscreen, you need to treat your vitamin D supplementation as if you lived in the north.

To adequately prevent vitamin D deficiency and to protect bones, women who live in northern climates should supplement with 800 IU of vitamin D daily. Many good calcium supplements will come with 200–400 IU of vitamin D already in them. Topping this level off with some sun exposure, vitamin D from a multivitamin you may be already taking, or from a dietary source of vitamin D, is a manageable way to ensure you're getting an adequate supply.

Micronutrients

Fresh fruits and vegetables provide us with most of the additional nutrients good for bone health. Particularly if you eat plenty of local and/or organic produce, along with whole grains and unprocessed foods, you'll find most of what you need right on your plate. Following are the best food sources of five vitamins and minerals particularly important for bone health:

- **Vitamin D**
  Tuna
  Egg yolks
  Salmon
  Wheat germ
  Liver
  Sardines

- **Vitamin K**
  Spinach
  Green cabbage
  Tomatoes
  Liver
  Meat
  Egg yolks
  Whole wheat
  Strawberries

- **Silicon**
  Oatmeal
  Brown rice
  Root vegetables

- **Manganese**
  Whole grains
  Nuts
  Dried fruits
  Green, leafy vegetables

- **Zinc**
  Oysters
  Pumpkin seeds
  Ginger root
  Pecans
  Split peas

Also important is boron, available in fruits and vegetables grown in boron-rich soil.

If, for whatever reason, you can't move in the direction of more nutritional foods, getting a "state of the art" calcium supplement is your next best option. The best nutritional supplement companies will have done their homework and included several of the nutrients important in bone health in their top calcium supplements. If you shop around you can find several micronutrients, including magnesium, boron, vitamin K, zinc, phosphorus, potassium, manganese, silicon, and even hydrochloric acid on the label, right beside calcium.

Ipriflavone

Scientists are actively investigating ipriflavone, a soy derivative, as a viable treatment for osteoporosis prevention. Ipriflavone has received favorable reviews from early research done mainly in Japan, and a recent unfavorable one from Europe. Let's look at the positive research first.

Ipriflavone, at doses of 200 mg three times per day, has been helpful in treating existing osteoporosis in postmenopausal women.[88] A Japanese study of 60 postmenopausal patients who were randomly assigned to receive either 600 mg/d of ipriflavone (IP) or 800 mg of calcium lactate found that the IP group maintained bone density after one year, while the calcium group lost bone. Additionally, urinary markers of bone loss decreased in the IP group, suggesting that bone resorption had slowed.[89] A small study of seven women showed that ipriflavone slowed down the progression of bone loss via urinary metabolite assessment.[90]

One of ipriflavone's actions is to enhance calcium uptake in the gut, in a similar, although less potent way than estrogen does.[91] However, animal studies have suggested that ipriflavone acts differently from estrogen directly on bone tissue.[92] The current evidence suggests that ipriflavone does not increase risk for breast cancer.

Researchers have just begun comparing ipriflavone's effect on bone density with other therapies. A Japanese group compared 600 mg ipriflavone with weekly intramuscular injections of 10 units of eel calcitonin (see page 168) in 30 postmenopausal women. Ipriflavone had a more pronounced effect on the density of the radius, while calcitonin was more effective on the lumbar spine. Calcitonin prevented a decline in osteocalcin levels best, while ipriflavone better slowed down loss of bone metabolites in the urine.[93]

Now for the bad news. The Ipriflavone Multicenter European Fracture Study Group completed the largest study of ipriflavone for postmenopausal women to date. In this study, 234 women were randomly assigned to receive ipriflavone (200 mg three times per day) or placebo. All participants took 500 mg of calcium. After three years, bone density measured at the hip, spine, and forearm did not differ between the ipriflavone group and the control group. Likewise, there was no difference in the urinary markers of bone turnover. Alarmingly, 13% of the women on ipriflavone developed low white blood cell counts, and half of these did not return to normal after one year.[94]

Where does this leave us with regard to ipriflavone? The recent findings have somewhat dampened the initial enthusiasm regarding this as an alternative to HRT for bone health. For some women, ipriflavone does work and should not be discarded as an important therapy. For others, it does not work or could be potentially harmful.

Fortunately, there are ways to tell which category you fall into. Monitoring this therapy with bone density and urine cross-fiber testing can tell you whether or not it's working for you. Obtaining a baseline bone density, and a baseline urine cross-fiber testing, if available, is important. Repeating the urine test after 3–6 months and the bone density after two years will give you an indication of whether or not ipriflavone is working for you. Checking white blood cell levels before and after initiating ipriflavone will also be important.

Exercise

Bone depends on weight-bearing for maintenance. In other words, "use it, or lose it." If we don't use our bones, they (understandably) react as though we don't need them. It makes sense that we can best maintain the health of our bones by putting them to task.

Walking places the weight of our upper body on our low spine, hips, and legs, and so activates bone formation there. Running, dancing, skiing, and snow-shoeing also increase hip and leg bone density. Lifting exercises with hand-held weights helps build bone in the wrist and arms. So does tennis, golf, volleyball, or rock-climbing. For women concerned about spinal bone density, activities like canoeing, shoveling, horseback riding, weight-lifting, and certain forms of yoga can help build bone.

Repetition helps too. "Any exercise activity that produces repetitive stress loading to a part of the skeleton will tend to increase bone density at that site," says Roger Wolman in the *British Medical Journal*. He points out

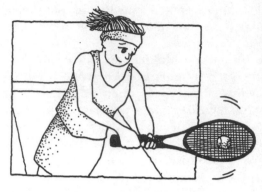

that professional tennis players develop the bones in their playing arm up to 30% larger and denser than their nonplaying arm.

As we've discussed in previous chapters, finding an activity that you enjoy is often the key to maintaining it. Be sure to include activities for all seasons. Great weight-bearing activity that only happens one or two seasons out of the year, unfortunately, isn't doing anything for you during the rest of the time. If all else fails, buy a jump rope! The repetitive, weight-bearing exercise received from jumping rope will activate bone growth in the entire spine, hip, legs, and arms.

Hormone Replacement Therapy

On June 17, 2000, at a concluding session of the World Congress on Osteoporosis 2000, Dr. Lawrence Riggs reviewed what we currently know about hormone replacement for osteoporosis prevention and treatment. He pointed out that despite all the evidence, we still lack the kind of proof that researchers like best; the large, long-term, randomized, double-blind, clinical trials that have not yet been conducted on HRT and osteoporosis.

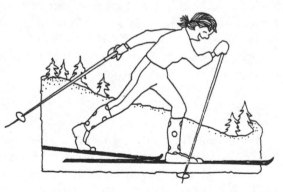

In several smaller studies, estrogen replacement therapy (ERT) has shown consistent ability to reduce bone loss and also increase density in the spine and hip (affecting trabecular bone most). This effect does indeed translate into reducing the risk of fractures in these important places for postmenopausal women. The United States Food and Drug Administration has been impressed enough with the available studies on ERT to approve it for both the prevention and the management of osteoporosis. Currently, HRT is considered the front-line conventional therapy for these purposes.

Larger studies are coming down the pike. The Women's Health

Initiative study, a large, multi-center trial of HRT, is currently underway. Most people expected its results to support those of the current smaller studies, and further illuminate what forms and doses of HRT best can prevent or reverse bone loss. If they're right, you can expect an even greater push for the use of HRT in treating and preventing osteoporosis than we see currently.

How Estrogen Works on Bone

Estrogen affects bone in many different ways. First of all, we know that estrogen indirectly influences bone by affecting the absorption of calcium in our diets. It does this by improving the performance of vitamin D receptors in the gut, which in turn influence how well we absorb calcium.

Secondly, estrogen acts directly on bone. We know this because osteoblasts, osteocytes, and osteoclasts all have estrogen receptors on their surfaces.[95] What these receptors are doing there is keeping a lot of researchers up nights trying to figure out. One research group has found that estrogen seems to be involved with the actual growth of our bone-building osteoblasts.[96]

Estrogen also directly affects bone density by influencing how osteoblasts build bone in response to mechanical stress. One group of researchers found that the more estrogen receptors a bone cell has, the more prolific it is when either estrogen or strain initiate bone growth. Furthermore, when the estrogen receptors were inactivated (by tamoxifen), weight-bearing itself did not result in bone cell proliferation.[97] These findings were supported in another study, which found that estrogen receptors mediated the bone proliferation that occurs with strain, or weight-bearing.[98]

Although still speculative, the implications of these findings are large. These studies suggest that exercise and estrogen may be intricately intertwined, rather than separate determinants of bone density. If bone growth induced by strain depends on the presence of estrogen, it may mean that some women need certain levels of estrogen for their exercise to successfully build bone.

Swedish health officials are looking into a novel hormone-like medication called tibolone for bone health.[99] Tibolone has qualities like estrogen, progesterone, and testosterone, with far fewer side effects. You may be hearing more about this agent in the future.

How Much and Which Form of HRT Is Best

Again at the World Congress on Osteoporosis 2000, Dr. Lawrence Riggs pointed to an important study in which women given about half the standard dose of conjugated estrogens (0.3 mg) plus 1,000 mg calcium a day increased their lumbar bone density and did not increase endometrial thickness.[100] At this low dose of estrogen, a form of progesterone was not needed to protect the uterine lining for participants in this study—although we should point out that no long-term studies yet exist to prove the safety of low-dose estrogen without progesterone. Dr. Riggs emphasized that natural micronized progesterone was a better choice than synthetic progestins if a woman takes progesterone.

Doctors at the University of Connecticut found that as little as one-fourth the usual dose of estrogen effectively prevented bone loss. When 107 older women living in nursing homes randomly received either 1.0, 0.5, or 0.25 mg per day of estradiol, loss of collagen cross-fibers in the urine slowed equally in all groups.[101] Side effects of estrogen differed significantly between the groups, with those on less estrogen experiencing less breast tenderness, vaginal bleeding, and endometrial growth. Results like these are encouraging for practitioners and patients who want to enjoy the benefits of estrogen on bone minus its side effects and risks.

Estriol

Dr. Riggs's statements reflect an evolution in the thinking about doses and forms of HRT. Women and many clinicians are interested in taking the least amount, and the most natural forms of hormones that will work. This interest has spawned study into the use of a weak and possibly safer form of estrogen called estriol, for bone health. In Chapter 10, we will discuss estriol, as well as all the available forms of HRT in detail. For now, let's see what we know about this weaker form of estrogen and bone.

About half a dozen studies to date on estriol and bone density have yielded mixed results. Most of the reports suggesting that 2 mg of estriol daily slowed or even reversed bone loss resulted from studies done in Japan, one even suggesting that 2 mg estriol was equally effective to 0.625 mg conjugated estrogens in preventing bone loss.[102] Other studies, like one in Scotland, found that doses as high as 12 mg/day did not offer sufficient protection from bone loss.[103] One reviewer has speculated that the soy phytoestrogens in the traditional Asian diets may have somehow increased the effect of estriol in the Japanese women.[104]

Although estriol for bone protection has shown some promise, we can't guarantee its effect in all women. If after researching your options, you choose to try estriol or some product mostly comprised of estriol (again, you will learn more about these options in Chapter 10) for bone protection, we advise working with a practitioner who agrees to monitor your bone density closely, via DEXA and perhaps urine cross-fiber testing as well, to see if it's working for you. With close supervision, you can change to a different therapy early on if it looks like estriol doesn't offer enough bone protection.

Additional Medications

Our aging population has created a high demand for the creation of new therapies aimed at maintaining bone health. We've presented the most common of these currently available. We can expect that variations on these drugs, and others, will surface in the years ahead.

Raloxifene

Raloxifene (Evista®) acts both like an estrogen and unlike an estrogen. It belongs to the hot, new class of so-called "designer estrogens," known as selective estrogen receptor modulators, or SERMS, for short. Raloxifene acts like an estrogen, in that it activates to estrogen receptors in some parts of the body—notably bone, in this context. It has been shown that 60 milligrams of raloxifene reduces risk of spine fractures by 50%, if taken for three years. Raloxifene per day. is unlike estrogen, in that when it binds to estrogen receptors in the uterus or breast, it does not activate them. This means that breast or endometrial cancer risks do not increase—and may actually even decrease on raloxifene. We'll discuss raloxifene and other SERMS more in Chapter 10.

Bisphosphonates

Like ERT, alendronate sodium (Fosamax®) and risedronate (Actonel®) are approved by the FDA for both the prevention and treatment of osteoporosis. They belong to a category of drugs known as bisphosphonates, and were first developed to treat metabolic disorders of bone. Also like ERT, the bisphosphonates increase bone density in the spine and hip, reduces bone loss, and—bottom line—decreases risk of both hip and spinal fractures.

Unlike ERT, alendronate and risedronate have nothing to do with estrogen or progesterone-related side effects. They neither increase breast or uterine cancer risk, nor increase risk of blood clots, bloating, mood or other changes that hormones can cause.

The bisphosphonates can have annoying gastrointestinal side effects for some women: most notably gastric reflux or heartburn. They also can be difficult to absorb. The drug's manufacturer therefore recommends taking either drug first thing in the morning, on an empty stomach, chasing it down with 8 ounces of water, plus remaining upright and not eating for a half hour afterwards. If you can handle the acrobatics and don't get the side effects, these drugs can be important medicines for women with real osteoporosis concerns. Future drugs of this class may come with fewer gastrointestinal problems.[105]

Doses of alendronate differ depending on whether or not the goal is prevention, or treatment of established osteoporosis. A dosage of 5 mg/day addresses prevention, and 10 mg/day works for treatment. Weekly dosing has been available now since October 2000, partly as an attempt to make the drug more tolerable to people who have side effects. The FDA has approved doses of 35 milligrams once weekly for prevention, and 70 mg once weekly for treatment.

Calcitonin

Calcitonin is a hormone produced by our parathyroid glands. Along with parathyroid hormone (PTH, which *itself* is under investigation as a treatment for osteoporosis), calcitonin helps us keep the level of calcium in our bloodstream within a narrow, optimal range. When blood levels of calcium fall below normal, our body secretes PTH, which pulls calcium out of storage (bone). Calcitonin does just the opposite. We normally secrete calcitonin when blood levels of calcium are high—and it aids in the transport of calcium into bone for storage.

The pharmaceutical industry has been able to exploit calcitonin for the purpose of pumping calcium into bone for women who are at least 5 years beyond menopause. Injectable or nasal spray forms of calcitonin are derived from eel or salmon sources.

Calcitonin nasal spray reduces risk of spinal fractures. Outside the

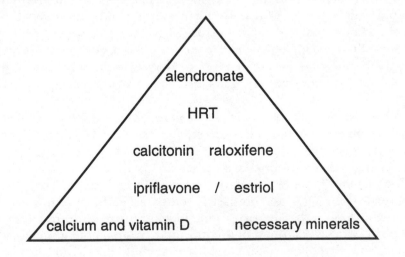

Figure 7.5.   Relative strength of bone-building agents.

spine, calcitonin does not help to increase bone mass. Therefore, if hip fracture is your greatest risk—it's better to find a different remedy. Typically practitioners recommend 200 IU/day of calcitonin nasal spray. Side effects tend to limit themselves to the nose: irritation, runny nose, and the like. These are usually mild.

Simplifying Your Process

Phew! You've just learned more than you probably ever wanted to know about osteoporosis. Before you get overwhelmed, let's step back and look at your situation, individually. You'll be able to eliminate a lot of choices right off the bat.

First of all, let's go back to the risk assessment quiz on page 146. This simple tool can guide you to your next step. If you have a low risk of osteoporosis, it's likely that you only need to concentrate on maintaining a healthy diet, lifestyle, and weight-bearing exercise. If you have moderate or high risk, you should obtain a bone density reading. Talk to your practitioner about getting one. If you have a question about which type of testing to choose, reread "Choosing Bone Density Testing Methods" on page 150 for help in deciding on a method.

If your bone density is good, your process will be easy. A single contact with your practitioner to go over your prevention plan should be sufficient. You will probably do fine using minimal intervention, such as calcium, vitamin D, and exercise. If your bone density is low, however, you should embark on some type of treatment. Schedule a separate visit with your practitioner to talk about your therapeutic choices. Plan it with enough time so that you're able to do your homework on your options. For a visual reference, see Figure 7.5, which presents the bone-building agents in ascending order of strength.

If you're willing to jump through these few hoops now, you can extend the health of your bones for several years. Remember, seven years from now, you'll have made an entirely new skeleton. Medical advances have made it possible to gauge where our bones stand, where they're going, and what's likely to affect that journey. To a large degree, you are the architect and builder. The choices you make now will literally shape your future. What's it going to look like?

8 Sexuality and Bladder Health

Contrary to any other time in history, women today live one third of their lives beyond reproductivity. But while our reproductive organs may themselves be ready to take a back seat, many of us aren't quite ready to let them retire. Most women of the baby boom generation, in particular, regard sexual health important to overall health,[1] yet up to 50% admit to some difficulty with sexual function.[2] As with every other area of menopause, these women also refuse to let medicine dismiss their concerns about sex. As a result, clinicians and researchers have stepped up efforts to both understand sexuality at midlife and beyond, and find solutions for women who encounter challenges.

Changes in Sexuality in Midlife

Sex researchers have divided woman's experience of sex into several distinct parts: desire, physical sensation, arousal, enjoyment, ability to reach orgasm, satisfaction, and frequency of sexual activity. What's useful about this approach is the finding that menopause affects some of these areas, but not others. According to an analysis of 200 women from the Massachusetts Women's Health Study,[3] a large, community-based study of women as they transitioned into menopause, frequency of sexual activity, satisfaction with sex, and ability to reach orgasm had nothing to do with menopausal status, while desire for sex and arousal did. In this study, the only part of a woman's experience of sex that specifically had to do with her *estrogen* status was physical sensation—namely the pain of vaginal dryness. *Lifestyle factors,* such as smoking and marital situation, as well as general health affected overall sexual function more than menopause did.[4]

However, as they say, "your mileage may vary." Certainly it's important to dispel the myth that older people don't have or enjoy sex. At the same time, we shouldn't pretend that *normal* women and men don't evolve in their sexual behaviors and desires. The subtle and not-so-subtle pressure for women to stay "sexy" throughout menopause puts an unnecessary burden on those who have a natural inclination to relax and enjoy a different approach to physical intimacy. This pressure leads women, more than men, to seek remedies for what they feel is their "problem," rather than asking for a change in their partner's behaviors.[5]

For example, Sally brought her concerns to her naturopathic physician. "I could take it or leave it, really," she said. "If I had sex once a month I wouldn't miss it at all. It's my husband I'm worried about. I feel bad because I'm not 'there' for him like I used to be. He say's its OK, but I know he would like to have sex more often."

While there are sometimes medical causes of decreased sex drive (which we'll discuss later in this chapter), in all probability, Sally is experiencing a perfectly normal decline in sexual desire. Before seeking a "solution," Sally might first reframe her experience as something normal. A quick judgment that Sally, and women like her, have a "problem," invalidates a normal process, and can heap yet more distortion onto our culture's overemphasis on sex. Conversely, embracing the diverse, realistic, and mature sexual experiences of menopausal women can move our culture toward a more meaningful take on sex—and one which could heal society in countless ways.

Rewriting the Sex Scene

"Look—my husband and I have been married for 25 years," says Gillian, in a matter-of-fact tone. "We're not newlyweds. Sex is different now. It's mellow, and it's just fine for us. Neither one of us wants sex as often anymore. Once every two or three weeks does it. It also takes longer, and I feel like we're just being together in a relaxed, intimate way. I think all those magazine articles that say you're supposed to have 'hot sex' forever must be by someone who's too young to know better."

While some aspects of sex decline for menopausal women, some in fact *increase.* Many midlife women (as well as men) report an increase in their desire for nongenital forms of loving: hugging, kissing, caressing, and holding.[6] So rather than taking the medical view that many women "suffer from sexual dysfunction," at menopause, we might reframe the experience as one of *sexual evolution.* Mature sex is often less performance-driven and more about relating. If we can release the image of sex created by a youth, male, and commercially oriented culture, we might allow mature sexual intimacy to find its natural expression.

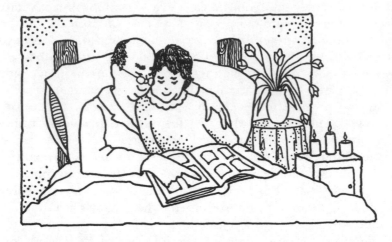

"Sexual evolution" at menopause can lead some women to funnel their sexual energy into artistic endeavors. Some eastern religions, in fact, believe that the same energy that fuels sex also fuels creative endeavors like art, dance, writing, and imagination. Hindu and Buddhist practitioners believe that all of these "creative" energies reside in the second chakra, or "wheel of energy" located in the pelvic region, and that sexual energy can transform, finding outlets through artistic or spiritual pursuits. This belief finds alliance with that of many Western feminist writers, who point out that sexual energy often emerges in other creative forms as a woman matures into menopause.

What Affects a Woman's Sexual Functioning at Menopause?

Need we say it? Sex is complex. How our sexual being expresses itself depends on many factors. Menopause affects some, but not all of these qualities. The comfort we have with our own changing bodies, our love relationship, our overall health and energy, our hormones, and many other factors blend together to form this amorphous thing known as our *libido*, or sex drive. Let's get acquainted with the factors that determine our sexual function at this time.

Vaginal Dryness

There's nothing less sexy than painful sexual activity. Vaginal dryness and thinning of the tissues, due to the drop in estrogen, can make sexual activity (and sometimes even sitting or walking) an uncomfortable experience. The durable cells that line the vagina, known as the *cornified epithelium*, depend on estrogen to, in fact, survive.

After several years of less estrogen in our systems, we actually lose several layers of these cells, which normally allow our vaginas to withstand friction. If this gets severe, we can develop *atrophy*, or a significant thinning of the outer layer of vaginal tissue. Figure 8.1 demonstrates what the inside of the vagina would look like depending upon whether or not there was estrogen around.

Although estrogen seems to have the biggest impact on vaginal cells, other factors can also contribute to their health. Cigarette smoking, for example, has been shown to hasten vaginal atrophy.[7] This occurs because when the liver detoxifies the body of chemicals in cigarettes, it also speeds up the removal of estrogen from the bloodstream. In other words, smokers deplete their bodies of estrogen.

Vaginal pH is also important in tissue maintenance. When estrogen levels go down, pH goes up, and this causes the first layers of cells to die off. Instead of the resilient epithelium lining the vagina, the more fragile

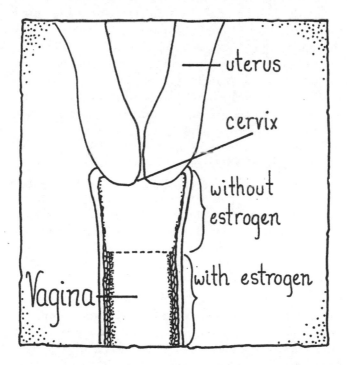

Figure 8.1.   Several years of reduced estrogen cause the normally thick outer layer of vaginal tissue to significantly thin.

"middle skin" which lies underneath the epithelium appears on the surface of the vagina in women who have an elevated pH.[8] We'll discuss more about pH below, when we address infections in the vagina and bladder.

Fortunately, we can easily solve this issue of vaginal dryness and even atrophy, particularly if one doesn't wait decades to address it. At the end of this chapter, you'll learn hormonal and nonhormonal solutions to vaginal dryness and painful sexual activity.

Testosterone

So far in this book we've focused on the "female" hormones estrogen and progesterone. But lately, heightened awareness of libido issues in menopause has prompted discussion about *testosterone*, which is now vying for inclusion in hormone replacement therapy for some menopausal women.

For the first few years after menopause, our primary source of testosterone, the ovary, increases its production of this hormone. At the same time, however, we lose production of testosterone from another source—the adrenal glands. The adrenals, located right above the kidneys, secrete a building block of testosterone known as *androstenedione*, which the body can use to make more testosterone. During the first few years of menopause, the adrenals in most women put out less of this precursor. (Many natural health practitioners refer to this as one sign of "adrenal fatigue," and will offer lifestyle, herbal, and nutritional supports, especially if a woman also experiences overall fatigue.) So despite increased production by the ovaries, women generally have less testosterone around after menopause,[9] although this is certainly not true for everyone.[10]

In some (although not the majority of) women, testosterone can actually begin to fall several years before menopause.[11] This may explain the loss of interest in sex some women feel even before they see the first sign of perimenopause. As levels continue to drop in menopause, a previously hot flame of passion may dwindle into an intermittent flicker, or extinguish itself altogether. For women who are low in testosterone, taking it in supplement form *may* bring back sexual desire, although even this isn't guaranteed.[12]

Some clinicians feel another androgen, dihydroxyepiandrosterone (DHEA) has as much or more to do with libido and overall sense of wellbeing as testosterone. DHEA declines in both men and women gradually as we age. The adrenal glands make DHEA and peripheral tissues convert small amounts of it into both testosterone and estrogen. In Chapter 10 we'll further take up the issue of adding DHEA to a hormonal regimen at menopause.

Estrogen can help with some, but not all aspects of sexual functioning. Estrogen therapy works well in solving problems with vaginal dryness, sleep, emotions, and other things that need to be in place before we're "in the mood." But, estrogen supplementation has been shown to actually *decrease* the amount of free testosterone in the bloodstream.[13] Taking estrogen increases SHGB, the hormone "bus" that carries *both* estrogen and testosterone around in the blood. With more "busses" around, more testosterone is bound up (riding the bus), and there's less free testosterone to act on tissues. While estrogen (with or without progesterone) helps some women regain their lost libido, it doesn't necessarily work for women with low, or borderline low testosterone levels. Therefore, if you are on estrogen and still have no sex drive to speak of, you may want to talk with your clinician about getting a blood test for testosterone.

Testosterone doesn't just affect our sex lives. Low levels can also lead to fatigue or a loss of a sense of well-being for some women. Of course, there are other causes of these problems too, such as thyroid abnormalities, blood sugar problems, anemia, and depression. Be careful not to jump on the "testosterone bandwagon" without ruling out other causes for a lack of energy. However, if you're menopausal and you have a problem with an overall lack of energy, and have ruled out other causes, talk to a practitioner about getting your testosterone levels checked. In women who test low, fatigue and lack of well-being may respond to supplemental testosterone.[14]

Doctors have long offered testosterone to women who have had their ovaries removed, since most of our testosterone is produced in these glands. Although some practitioners who deal with women's health have been using testosterone in regular hormone replacement therapy for over a decade, until recently, most clinicians reserved its use for men who had a serious medical condition involving a deficiency of the hormone. Thus, the mere idea of prescribing it to postmenopausal women is new for many clinicians.

Lack of familiarity may be the biggest reason some clinicians hesitate to prescribe testosterone to women, but there are others as well. First of all, illegal drug use by some athletes for performance enhancement has forced the FDA to categorize testosterone with other drugs of potential abuse and restrict its use. Second, side effects of testosterone, particularly if overdosed, aren't particularly popular: acne, growth of facial hair, and in rare cases, a lowering of the voice. These side effects are almost always reversible if testosterone is stopped. However, chronic and inappropriate overdosing of testosterone can lower a woman's voice permanently, and enlargement of the clitoris has also been noted in some cases. Third, many clinicians believe that testosterone will negatively impact cholesterol levels. Fourth, while data steadily mounts, we don't yet have much in the way of long-term, large studies that most clinicians need to feel comfortable about the safety of using testosterone in postmenopausal HRT.

One important thing to note is that much of the experience, and therefore the fears about testosterone, come from our experience using it for men, and in high doses. The amounts used in postmenopausal women (10 mg per day or less) are very small in comparison to the 100–200 mg daily doses in men. A review of the studies done between 1941 and 1996 on the safety of testosterone showed that the safety issues in its use at higher levels in men "do not apply to the lower doses combined with estrogens for hormone replacement in postmenopausal women."[15]

Although the side effects we mentioned above can occur for some women on 10 mg per day, the more serious problems that many clinicians fear have not been noted. Liver problems are exceedingly rare at these levels,[16] and blood pressure and cardiovascular changes other than cholesterol-lowering are not seen.[17] In contrast, testosterone at these levels, and also in combination with estrogen, seems to provide several benefits, certainly for libido and energy, but also in other areas if added appropriately to a menopausal woman's overall HRT regimen. For instance, while testosterone alone can cause atherosclerosis, given with estrogen it appears to have the reverse effect.[18] It has also been shown to augment the potential benefits of estrogen with regards to heart health by further improving some of the functions of blood vessels.[19] Regarding bone health, testosterone has been shown to augment the beneficial effect of estrogen on bone density in women who had their ovaries removed.[20]

The majority of studies do show that testosterone lowers all major blood fats: total cholesterol, LDLs and triglycerides—but also the good HDL cholesterols. Therefore, testosterone added to HRT may blunt some of the potentially beneficial effects of estrogen on HDL. If you have a good HDL level, this shouldn't be an issue for you. On the other hand, if you have a borderline or low HDL level, note that testosterone may make this worse. For women considering HRT who watch their triglycerides, this benefit might offset the tendency of estrogen to raise triglycerides.[21]

Certainly, testosterone in women does not have the track record of study that estrogen does. Therefore, each woman should proceed with caution before assuming it's the answer for her. Testosterone is not meant for everyone. Also, because it is a new concept for use in postmenopausal women, medicine hasn't worked all of the bugs out of this prescription yet. No one knows exactly what constitutes normal levels for women, and what defines "deficiency" has not yet been clearly established. Furthermore, your access to it may be limited by your practitioner's knowledge and experience.

However, if you are low in testosterone and having significant difficulties with libido or energy, testosterone could make a difference in your life, as it did for Teri (see below). It might be worthwhile for you to search for a practitioner who has experience with this hormone for women.

If you are able to find one willing to explore whether or not this hormone may benefit you, we recommend you follow the guidelines offered in the treatment section of this chapter. There, we'll also discuss the testosterone's forms, doses, and where to find it.

Teri

As a former dancer and now a choreographer, Teri had always felt herself a sensual person. "It's part of my creativity," she told her therapist. "I see my sexuality as part of expressing myself. I think dance and sex ultimately come from the same place. In fact, I notice that if I'm having great sex, my creativity at work, designing dance pieces, is flowing too."

A few years before hitting menopause, however, Teri's libido dropped. After ruling out factors like relationship issues, stress or mood changes, she and her therapist concluded that hormones might be the issue. Teri consulted a doctor in her area known for treating women in menopause, who tested her for testosterone levels. When the results showed Teri's level to be low, he prescribed a low level of testosterone supplementation. After three weeks, Teri noticed the change.

"I'm back," she reported happily to her therapist. "This is who I know myself to be. I thought that testosterone was a male hormone. No way! I'm glad I found this."

Physical Energy

Sexual energy is a subset of total energy. If our body needs extra energy for basic functioning, it may not have enough left over for lovemaking. This is why stress, physical disabilities, insomnia, pain, and chronic illness all can impair one's ability to enjoy sex.

Sometimes, the demands of relatively healthy but busy lives can take their toll on our energy and effect our libido. Middle-aged moms particularly fall prey to this. When menopause coincides with the demands of raising children, sex can go out the window. This is why it's especially important for women with high demands on their time and energy to have regular, significant time for restoration.

State of Mind

"I'm having the best sex in my life," states Joanne. "I think it's where I am in my life now. I'm doing yoga and Pilates three times a week at the gym, I love my job and my relationship is great. I think I'm making up for all the luke-warm sex I endured for 20 years in my former marriage."

Joanne's experience illustrates how both our physical and mental well-being can affect our sex lives. In fact, some experts claim that women's interest in sex has more to do with psychological and social factors than actual physical ones.[22] Either through good fortune or by design, many women find themselves quite pleased with how life is going at menopause. A study of 280 midlife women at Pennsylvania State University found that most of the positive increases in women's sexual experience in midlife resulted from positive life circumstances.[23]

In addition to our external life situation, our internal emotional environment either fans or dampens sexual desire. Depression and anxiety have both been shown to deflate sex lives. In one study, anxiety was the most important influence on reduced frequency of intercourse for menopausal women.[24]

Body image, which we discussed in Chapter 5, plays a major role here too. If a woman feels good about her body, she is more likely to explore her body on her own, and to share it with another. Ask yourself if there are changes in your self-image as you watch your body take on its menopausal shape. Are you loving and kind to yourself? Could your attitude about your desirability be affecting your sex life?

Relationship

Understandably, single people report less satisfaction with their sex lives than coupled people. Outdated, but persistent cultural taboos on masturbation may contribute to this. Self-pleasuring is a normal, natural activity, and actually ought to be encouraged, especially for single menopausal women. Staying "in touch" with ourselves in this way can promote a healthy relationship with our bodies, and also alert us to physical changes that might require medical attention. Also, vaginal secretions produced during masturbation as well as coupled sexual activity can keep tissues healthy.

For those in partnerships, the health of the relationship can influence our sexual function. Communication and the ability to resolve relationship issues can make or break a couple's sex life. By the time we reach menopause, we've usually had plenty of time to harbor resentments or bury grief, if we haven't kept up with routine relationship maintenance. Then again, if we have nurtured our relationship with healthy dialogue, we've had the time to build trust, deep understanding, and love. The success of a relationship can show up in the bedroom, sometimes more plainly than in any other arena.

Menopause often corresponds with changes in relationships or partners. Like Joanne, above, women who find themselves in new relationships can be enjoying the novelty of sex with a new partner, or one with sexual compatabilities more in tune with her own. Some women experience a change in sexual orientation at menopause. Several factors might explain this. As women mature, they may feel more in touch with who they are, and more secure about owning those feelings. Particularly if a woman has raised a family, an "empty nest" allows her now to pay attention to her own needs, which may have been surpressed. "Coming out" at menopause can be at once thrilling and terrifying for new lesbians, given our cultural climate. A change in sexual orientation obviously can have an impact on one's sex life in many ways. Lesbian sexuality is a complete subject in and of itself, and is addressed in *The Lesbian Sex Book: A Guide for Women Who Love Women*, by Wendy Caster, and *The Whole Lesbian Sex Book: A Passionate Guide for All of Us*, by Felice Newman.

Heterosexual women still need to be concerned about pregnancy. "Officially menopausal" women (those one year out from their last period) can leave the fear of pregnancy in the dust. For some this is a welcome relief, and enhances sexuality by interjecting the element of spontaneity. For women who were still hoping to have children, loss of reproductivity can be a blow, sometimes requiring emotional support to work through, and frequently affecting sexual desire via depression, if even temporarily.

Partner's Health

Physical health issues impair *men's* ability to engage in sex much more than women's. Common problems like cardiovascular disease, diabetes, prostate enlargement, as well as some types of medications can all cause sexual dysfunction in men. More rarely does chronic disease affect a woman's sexual function, such as in cases of severe kidney, adrenal, or liver disease that effect hormonal levels and libido. In fact, a recent study found that "having a functioning partner is a more important variable" in women's ability to keep having sex into ripe old age than their own physical health.[25]

Medications

For most of us embedded in Western culture and medicine, getting older means we have a fuller medicine chest. Some very popular prescriptions are known to cause decreased orgasm in women and erectile dysfunction in men. These include the SSRI antidepressants and benzodiazepines for anxiety, and thiazide diuretics for high blood pressure if prescribed in too high a dose. Drugs can affect not only sexual desire, but also one's ability to become aroused and the ability to have orgasm as well.

If you're not getting as much juice out of your sex life as you'd like, and either you or a partner are on medication, check with the prescriber to see if the medicine could be causing your problem. Usually, a practitioner can offer an alternative which will not dampen your desire. If you choose to still remain on the medication, we have suggestions at the end of this chapter which can help.

Sex After Breast Cancer

Breast cancer treatment, and mastectomy in particular, presents those who go through it with additional challenges relating to sexual intimacy. Some women who are diagnosed with breast cancer assume their sex life is a thing of the past. Although initial adjustments require care, time, and compassion by both the woman and her partner, it is heartening to learn that the sex life of these women differs little from that of women without breast cancer.

In a study of 865 women surviving breast cancer, done at UCLA School of Medicine (just down the street from Hollywood, in fact—the *most* likely place for women to be affected by appearance), sexual functioning and their partner's ability to adjust was no different than that of the general population.[26] In the same study, neither did tamoxifen (the anti-estrogen drug used after chemotherapy) detract from sexual experience.

Breast cancer survivors who do have difficulties with sex often complain of vaginal dryness. Vitamin E oil and the vaginal lubricants we will discuss on page 185 are very helpful for this problem—and *safe* even if one has a history of breast cancer. Other issues that come up frequently for breast cancer survivors (especially those on tamoxifen) are hot flashes, night sweats, and insomnia. Getting a flush in the middle of arousal doesn't usually heighten the experience! Nor does lack of sleep contribute to our energy stores, including what we need for sex. For dealing with these problems, try the nonestrogen-related remedies at the very end of Chapter 10.

Psychotherapy can help women overcome psychological blocks around sex after a breast cancer diagnosis and treatment. Group therapy helps women confront and change negative distortions in their body image. Couple's therapy can nurture a loving relationship and supports its evolution toward deeper intimacy, as both people confront their issues around cancer. Seek out a good therapist who can guide you in establishing a healing relationship with your body. It's even possible that you could enter an entirely new chapter of being in touch with your body *because of* a brush with breast cancer. It's important to know that while it is often a challenge, women who have had a mastectomy *can* and *do* overcome fears about what their partners think, and accept their bodies.

If there's anything a body that's gone through cancer and cancer treatment needs—it's acceptance and love. Start by giving it to yourself. Treat yourself to an energy work session, a foot massage, and when you feel brave, a whole body massage. Take a dance class. Get to know this body, in its slightly new form. Touch it yourself. Develop a relationship with your own sensuality. (After all, sensuality is inborn—not dependent on someone else.) If you have a partner now or in the future, you may find that developing your own *individual* sensuality can actually enhance that experience with another.

Sex After Hysterectomy or Oophorectomy

Most women who have a hysterectomy do so because of some kind of pelvic discomfort. Uterine problems leading to hysterectomy (like uterine fibroids) sometimes cause discomfort, or even bleeding with intercourse. In light of this, it's not surprising that most women feel an improvement in their sexual functioning after a hysterectomy.[27]

There are occasions when this isn't the case, however, and it behooves women to know about how some types of hysterectomy *can* disturb their sex life, preferably in advance of making decisions about the surgery. This relates to which organs a surgeon removes—and how much of them. In days gone by, surgeons who set out to remove the uterus frequently ended up taking the ovaries too—whether the ovaries were diseased or not. Today, fortunately, surgeons are much more discriminating about leaving good body parts in place. (But not always! It pays to discuss this with the surgeon beforehand.) Hysterectomy (removal of the uterus) and oophorectomy (removal of one or both ovaries) introduce completely different issues into one's sex life.

In a simple hysterectomy, a surgeon removes the uterus and leaves the ovaries. In theory, and largely in practice, this allows a premenopausal woman to continue producing her own hormones in the ovaries and enter menopause naturally. Occasionally, if a woman is near menopause, removal of the uterus (or any major surgery or other trauma for that matter) can speed up her transition. Some women report that such a large physical stress can make her reproductive system feel like it just aged a couple of years rather than weeks, and hasten the onset of perimenopausal symptoms. Also, disruption of the blood supply to the ovaries by nearby surgery, can sometimes speed their decline by one to two years.

Simple hysterectomies can either involve the removal of the entire uterus (including the cervix) or can leave the cervix intact. Doing the latter will keep the vagina feeling like it did—both to you and to any partner—before the surgery. Removing the cervix can slightly shorten the length of the vagina—a change that some women find less desirable for themselves or their sexual partners. This occurs more often with postmenopausal women who do not use hormone replacement after hysterectomy. If a woman facing hysterectomy wants to retain her cervix, she should discuss this beforehand with the surgeon. Hysterectomies performed vaginally generally do not include this option.

Sometimes, ovaries need to be removed, either because of cysts, endometriosis, pain, or ovarian cancer. In the case of ovarian cancer, surgeons usually recommend that a woman have her uterus removed as well to minimize the possibility of leaving some cancer cells behind, since these organs share a blood supply. For ovary removal due to cysts, endometriosis or pain, however, the uterus can usually stay, unless it also has a problem. The medical name for removal of ovaries (the actual "surgical menopause") is *oophorectomy*. If a woman does not begin hormone replacement therapy after the operation, oophorectomy usually leads to an abrupt plunge into menopause. Women who have oophorectomies then, often experience more sudden, dramatic, and intense menopausal symptoms than women undergoing natural menopause.

Women who have their ovaries removed often feel the effects not only of estrogen loss, but that of testosterone as well, since this is where testosterone comes from in women. Sudden reduction in testosterone levels can sometimes cause energy loss, or decrease in sexual drive. In a study done at Massachusetts General Hospital in Boston, 75 women age 31–56 who had undergone oophorectomy were given tiny amounts (0.15 and 0.30 mg) of testosterone cream daily for twelve weeks. As a result, frequency of sexual activity, including fantasy, masturbation, and intercourse, all increased. Women who had engaged in sexual intercourse once per week increased two to three times per week on average. They reported heightened enjoyment, also, with an increase in pleasure response and orgasm.[28] Most similar studies echo these findings. Thus, testosterone supplementation is often indicated in women who have no ovaries.

Vaginal Infections

Healthy vaginas are like climate-controlled ecosystems. When the weather is just right and we're in balance, several species of *flora* (bacteria and yeast) live at appropriate population levels in our vaginas. Just like species in a forest, normal vaginal flora keep one another in check.

Also, like that of a forest, it is quite possible to upset the vaginal ecology. Disease organisms, sexual activity, certain medications, sugar, stress, and other factors can change this delicate environment. Estrogen levels also contribute to this ecosystem by influencing pH, a measurement of acidity which greatly influences the "weather in there."

The normal pH inside the vagina of reproductive women ranges from 3.8 to 4.2, which is quite acidic. Friendly bacteria called *acidophilus lactobacilli* make it that way by digesting and fermenting a kind of sugar in our cells known as *glycogen*. (You may also have heard that yogurt often contains this friendly bacteria.) Because bad bacteria and excess yeast can't hang out in this acidic environment, lactobacilli perform a crucial job.

Estrogens increase the amount of glycogen in our vaginal tissues that lactobacilli get to work with.[29] More glycogen means a more acidic environment. With less estrogen, therefore, our vaginal pH gets less acidic, and more hospitable for bad bacteria or yeast. For some women, this translates into an increased susceptibility to vaginal infections.

If you suspect an infection, first get a proper diagnosis and treatment from your health practitioner. After the infection clears, inserting a capsule of acidophilus into the vagina for three nights in a row may help reestablish the normal flora in the vagina, return the pH to normal, and prevent recurrence. If you get repeated infections, you can either talk with your clinician about the appropriateness of some form of estrogen, or discuss dietary and lifestyle modifications with a natural health practitioner, to maintain a normal vaginal pH. We'll present a detailed description of topical options at the end of this chapter.

Bladder Health

"I'm up two or three times a night to use the bathroom, not to mention my numerous daytime trips," complains Gail. She is experiencing a phenomenon called *urinary urgency*, common to menopausal women. Like vaginal tissues, those lining the urinary tract also depend on estrogen. Sometime (usually several years) after estrogen declines at menopause, the lining of our bladder and urethra become thinner and more sensitive. As this process progresses, a woman may lose urine while sneezing, coughing, laughing, or exercising. We call this common problem *stress incontinence.*

Some women, like Gail, wake up one, two, three, or more times per night to urinate. Vasomotor fluctuations, which can cause shallow sleep, combined with bladder sensitivity can contribute to this problem, known as *nocturia.* Prolapse of the uterus or bladder, often caused by childbirth or just plain gravity, stretches out the ligaments holding these organs in place, and can further contribute to the problem. At least 40% of women over 60 complain of minor or major problems with urinary incontinence.[30]

In addition to urinary urgency and nocturia, some women have an increase in bladder infections after menopause. This is due to several factors: thinning of the bladder lining, a change in pH (both affected by menopause), and the proximity of the vaginal opening to that of the bladder (see Figure 8.2).

The health of our vaginas and our bladders are intimately linked. Women who find they have recurrent problems with bladder infections after menopause may indeed be sharing bacteria between these two locations. After all, as you can see in Figure 8.2, the opening to the vagina and to the urethra are less than a centimeter apart. It's little wonder that women themselves often have difficulty knowing which symptom is coming from where in that vicinity! This is also why sexual activity can precede a bladder infection, as bacteria from the vagina can easily be introduced into the bladder through the urethral opening during intercourse.

Besides bacteria, the bladder and the vagina have something else in common: namely, a similar pH.[31] As we saw with vaginal infections, bacteria like to live at a different pH than normal tissues do. If the pH in the area goes up or down in either the bladder or the vagina, the other organ often follows suit. In a less acidic bladder environment, therefore, bacteria can move in.

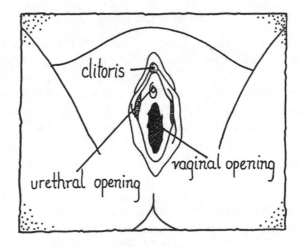

Figure 8.2.   Anatomy of the female genitalia.

Maintaining Pelvic Health and Reclaiming Lost Sexual Desire

Maintaining the health of the vagina and bladder is important for every woman because it will decrease the potential for infections and discomfort and keep those areas in good working order for years to come. Here, we present the best remedies for "routine maintainance," as well as the effective herbal and hormonal approaches for enhancing libido.

Remedies for Vaginal Dryness

Remedies for restoring vaginal health range from topical lubricants to systemic hormones. Lubricants simply moisten the vagina to cut down on friction during sexual activity, protecting delicate tissue. Examples are KY Jelly®, Astroglide®, and Replens®. Transitions for Health® vaginal lubricant contains aloe vera, vitamin E, evening primrose oil, and phytoestrogens, which actually feed vaginal tissues and help restore them back to health. Most naturopathic physicians can direct you in locating this product.

Other products do not provide lubrication per se, but will help the tissues produce their own, as well as encourage the regrowth of cells lining the vagina. These include vitamin E oil and various forms of estrogen. One advantage of vitamin E oil is its safety for women at high risk for breast cancer. To try it, open a vitamin E capsule with 3 or 4 pin-pricks, and insert it vaginally before bed. Wear a pad and your least favorite underwear—because it will stain! Do this nightly for two weeks, then as needed for maintenance: usually once every one or two weeks.

Estriol works well in reversing vaginal atrophy and dryness. In fact, estriol seems to be just as effective as its stronger counterpart, *estradiol* in treating vaginal symptoms.[32] Estriol also effectively treats a problem known as *atrophic vaginitis*,[33] where estrogen loss can lead to significant thinning and inflammation of the tissues.

Vaginal estriol is most commonly supplied in cream form, and is available from specialty compounding pharmacies. A prescription item, it is offered by most naturopathic physicians as well as conventional providers who have made a point to become informed about natural options outside the purview of the pharmaceutical industry. Doses are usually 1 mg of cream nightly applied to the vulva, or inserted vaginally with an applicator, for one to two weeks, then once or twice weekly as maintenance.

Although some does get absorbed into the bloodstream,[34] most clinicians familiar with estriol feel comfortable recommending vaginal estriol to women who have had breast cancer. This is because the vaginal tissues respond in tiny amounts—doses which do not come close to those delivered by oral HRT. Also some practitioners feel that this weaker estrogen may be safer than estradiol in breast cancer. There exist no long-term studies to date which prove this safety, however. For a full discussion on estriol and breast cancer safety, see Chapter 10.

While oral estriol administration requires progesterone to prevent overgrowth of the uterine lining, the vaginal form usually doesn't. Oral, but not vaginal administration of estriol caused endometrial overgrowth in a Swedish study of over 4,000 women.[35] Another study, in which 263 menopausal women with severe vaginal dryness applied 2–4 mg estriol per week, estriol resolved the vaginal problem without increasing the uterine lining.[36] Indeed, it takes five times this normal amount to induce overgrowth of the endometrium.[37]

Estring® is a flexible ring that fits right into the vagina, and usually can't be felt during normal activity. Estring® releases a small amount of estradiol directly into the vaginal skin. A woman inserts and removes the ring herself, and changes it every 90 days. The amount of estrogen provided in the ring is not enough to cause overgrowth of the lining of the uterus, so progesterone supplementation isn't necessary. In addition, very little of the estrogen makes it into the bloodstream. For this reason, Estring® is also a good choice for breast cancer survivors who have vaginal thinning.

Conventional vaginal estrogen creams come under several names, including Premarin®, Estrace®, and Ortho Dinestrol®. These creams all contain certain "active" estrogen compounds, which means that if used regularly, they require intermittent progesterone use to prevent overgrowth of the uterine lining. Exactly how much to use, and how often, depends on your situation. Not surprisingly, the more atrophy a woman has, the more cream she'll need. These creams all come with a vaginal applicator. It's best to insert these before bedtime to allow the cream to remain in the vagina. Even so, daytime use of minipads may be necessary the day after use.

A small vaginal estrogen tablet called Vagifem® has recently become available. This also contains one of the "active" estrogens, albeit a natural one: estradiol, which means that long-term daily use of Vagifem® (sometimes required in severe cases) will require progesterone supplementation. The usual dosage, twice a week, however, does not require progesterone, and is considered safe for women with a history of breast cancer. This small tablet comes packaged on a very thin vaginal applicator and is less messy than the creams for many women.

Remedies for Urinary Symptoms

Estrogen-containing products and muscle-toning exercises form the basis for treatment of menopausal urinary disturbances. If severe prolapse of pelvic organs causes the problem, surgery may be a woman's best option. Let's start with the easiest choices first, for more minor problems.

As we discussed earlier, loss of estrogen can make the bladder and the urethra thinner, and increase sensitivity. If "overactive bladder" is your problem, you can try any of the forms of estrogen above, in addition to the pelvic exercises we'll soon discuss. Danish researchers compared an estradiol-releasing vaginal ring in 134 women with 117 women who wore estriol pessaries (a plastic device inserted into the vagina) for 24 weeks. Urinary urgency, urge incontinence, stress incontinence, nighttime urination were equal in both groups. Patients preferred wearing the ring form over the pessary form.[38]

Increasing the tone of muscles in the area of the bladder and vagina can sometimes help with stress incontinence. A recent Japanese study reported that postmenopausal women with urinary stress incontinence who combined use of 1 mg/day of oral estriol with pelvic floor muscle exercises found significant relief after three months, and improvement continued over the next year.[39] Clinicians recommend Kegel exercises as the simplest way to strengthen this area. To perform a Kegel, contract (pull up) the pelvic floor muscles, as if you were attempting to retain a full bladder. Hold for two or three seconds, then release. Thirty to fifty repetitions daily can strengthen and tone the muscles involved in maintaining bladder health. These exercises may also prevent the loosening of vaginal muscles that can contribute to prolapse of pelvic organs. One of the best things about Kegel exercises is that you can do them anywhere: such as in the check-out line, waiting for a stoplight, or on the phone. To help her remember to do them, 45-year-old Debbie puts a sticky-note on the dashboard of her car that says simply "K" for Kegels. You can too!

One of the sad commentaries on our poor attention to bladder health in the past is that a quarter to a third of all nursing home admissions for women are related to bladder incontinence. There is no longer an excuse for this, and no need for women to just "live with it." Research and treatment options over the past 15 years have advanced enough to move us out of the dark ages when addressing these problems.

If you are having bladder problems not resolved by the simple measures we've mentioned, see a urologist or a *urogynecologist* (a gynecologist specializing in bladder problems). These specialists can do some very basic office bladder testing and offer a range of treatments—from physical therapy (yes, *for the bladder*—and it works very well for some women) to medications, to surgery. You owe it to yourself to at least get some testing done and to know your options before accepting that you need to wear pads every day for incontinence. And as always—the sooner you address this, the more effective these solutions will be.

Remedies for Bladder Infection

Acute bladder infections usually respond well to either conventional treatments, or a variety of herbal medicines, which a trained practitioner can easily offer. The larger problem for postmenopausal women is the *recurrence* of bladder infections, caused, as we learned, by an altered bladder environment that sets the stage for bacteria. Either local or systemic estrogen supplementation can restore an acidic pH, rebuild the bladder lining, and prevent these infections. Any of the options offered for vaginal dryness will help.

If estrogen use isn't preventing infections effectively, or if you prefer not to use estrogen, you have additional options. Naturopathic physicians and other holistically oriented practitioners can offer ways to affect the pH of the bladder via diet, lifestyle adjustments or herbs. If you still have frequent bladder infections after exhausting all these options, consider seeing a urologist to determine if there is a mechanical problem or a medical solution.

Herbal Remedies for Sexual Desire

Over the years, herbalists have employed many herbs for pre- and post-menopausal women addressing problems with sexual function. While we have limited scientific study of these agents, they do enjoy a long history of use. This is precisely why women interested in exploring these herbal options need to see a practitioner highly experienced in prescribing herbal medicine. (See "The Art of Herbal Prescribing" below.)

The Art of Herbal Prescribing

Prescribing the appropriate herb, or in many cases, combination of herbs, is a practiced art, cultivated over years of study and practice. Herbal medicine, largely an oral tradition, draws from a vast lineage of knowledge, gathered and honed over centuries, and passed on to ardent and serious students.

While herbs undeniably work via chemical constituents, they also have more subtle qualities, tangible to the experienced herbal practitioner. For instance, Chinese and Ayurvedic healers utilize the unique "heating," "cooling," "drying," or "moistening" qualities as well as their pharmacological ones. Experts in herbal medicine recognize that herbs also have certain "personalities," which make them more or less suited for certain individuals, and also in combination with other herbs.

The kind of sensitivity that ensures advanced, professional herbal prescribing can only develop in one who has spent years of study and practice in using herbs for human health. It cannot be developed from reading an article, referencing a book, or a short course of study on herbs. Therefore, when seeking an herbal solution to libido or any other issue, it's best to work with a practitioner trained in a full range of herbal medicines for this and other problems. To find a practitioner or resource, see the Resources section at the end of the book.

Phytoestrogens, such as black cohosh, red clover, and licorice, often in combination, can help some women overcome a lack of libido. Carla, a 48-year-old computer graphic artist, found that one such combination prescribed by her naturopathic physician, brought her right back up to her usual level of sexual functioning within four weeks. Among others, it contained the herb panax (Korean) ginseng. Known for its effects in helping men with erectile difficulties[40] panax ginseng, either alone, or in a combination with other herbs, can help women too. This form of ginseng does contain phytoestrogens, and can help with other menopausal symptoms too. Because it can increase blood pressure in some individuals, it's best to work with an experienced herbal clinician when using it.

Some herbalists offer the popular herbal aphrodisiac, damiana, as a "cordial," to be taken one hour before "desired result." Although damiana's exact action remains unknown, a recent study showed a hormonal effect via its ability to act like progestin by binding to progesterone receptors in the body.[41]

Most famous for is effects on memory, ginkgo's action of increasing circulation has led many natural health clinicians to propose its use in erectile dysfunction in men and lack of libido in women. A study conducted at the Institute of Sexology in Paris (which truly exists) compared the sexual response of 202 healthy women before and after supplementation with ginkgo biloba and another herb, muira puama, together in a commercial extract. After one month of supplementation, 65% of the women reported significant increases in "sexual desires, sexual intercourse, and sexual fantasies, as well as in satisfaction with sex life, intensity of sexual desires, excitement of fantasies, ability to reach orgasm, and intensity of orgasm."[42]

Another report, from the University of California, San Francisco, found that ginkgo was 84% effective in treating the sexual dysfunction caused by SSRI antidepressants (Prozac®, Paxil®). Desire, lubrication, orgasm, and "afterglow" were all enhanced.[43] While both men and women were included in this study, women had a better response to the herb than men (91% vs. 76%).

Standard doses of ginkgo are 40–60 mg, two to three times a day. You can also experiment taking it an hour before bed. As we have mentioned before, ginkgo can thin the blood, so concomitant use with blood thinners, aspirin, and blood-thinning supplements listed in Chapter 3 should be monitored.

Testosterone

All testosterone products are available through prescription only. Compounding pharmacies offer natural testosterone in pill, cream, and sublingual drop form, among others, and can also add it to natural estrogen and progesterone—which puts all hormones in a single dose. Currently, only one oral pharmaceutical preparation (which comes with estrogen, too), Estratest®, is available at regular pharmacies. Side effects can usually be avoided by making sure that blood levels never go over the reference ranges.[44]

Before giving you a testosterone prescription, your clinician should rule out other causes of symptoms (for example, relationship problems, depression, hypothyroidism). If you and your clinician still suspect a testosterone deficiency, make sure that you have the following to ensure the safety of a testosterone prescription for you:

- Blood test showing testosterone is low.
- Adequate knowledge of potential adverse effects.
- No history of depressed (good) cholesterols.

After beginning the testosterone prescription, have your blood levels retested periodically. Have your blood lipids checked after six months and then once a year. If you experience any unwanted side effects (especially lowering of voice or enlargement of clitoris), discontinue the testosterone and check with your practitioner.

Viagra

Some clinicians suggest the use of sildenafil (Viagra®), a drug approved for erectile dysfunction in men, for women complaining of lack of sexual function. Although proven effective in men, Viagra® has yet to prove itself for women. In one study, Viagra® use did increase clitoral sensation and lubrication, but overall sexual experience, including desire, quality of sexual intercourse, overall satisfaction with sexual function and orgasm, were unchanged in postmenopausal women.[45] In another, large study done in Vancouver, British Columbia, 583 women who described themselves as having sexual dysfunction were randomized to receive either Viagra® or placebo. After 12 weeks, there was no difference between the two groups.[46] Viagra® has, however, been shown to be more effective at reversing the sexual dysfunction specifically caused by the SSRI antidepressants (Prozac®, Paxil®, Celexa®, Zoloft®).[47] If you're on one of these antidepressants and can't find your libido, 75 mg Wellbutrin® may be a better antidepressant choice, rather than adding Viagra®. Side effects of Viagra® are not common, and include mild to moderate headache, flushing, nausea, abnormal vision, stomach upset, runny nose, and bladder infection.

There you have it—the range of effective treatments for sexual function and bladder health. But before you go out in search of the "magic bullet," we recommend you first sit back and look honestly about what really needs changing, and what may not. Certainly, it's important to address the health of your tissues, to prevent infection, atrophy, and pain. When it comes to sexual desire, however, understand that some changes are normal and not pathological. If you still choose to use natural or medical supports for libido, approach them from the perspective of enhancing your pleasure rather than treating a dysfunction. It's high time we stop treating the natural cycles within women's bodies as "problems," and move into an era of honoring every phase of a woman's life.

9 Mental Health and Memory

"I don't recognize myself sometimes," says Leslie, a 48-year-old social worker. "About two months ago, I started having these 'moods.' I'll get into a state where I disagree with my partner about *everything*. It comes on without warning, and goes away just as quickly. We've always had a good relationship, and she's being very patient with me, but I feel bad about some of the things I say when I'm in that mood. I wonder if this has anything to do with my screwed-up cycles." Leslie also adds that lately, she cries easily. "Silly things—like seeing a baby on television or a song on the radio—will trigger these sentimental feelings. Sometimes I can't contain myself."

Does Leslie's story sound familiar? While many women enjoy a smooth mental and emotional transition into menopause, for others, mood changes can be the very first indication that menopause is just around the corner. Menopausal women sometimes describe having less of an emotional "buffer" between their psyche and the outside world. Sensing the pull of a changing hormonal tide at perimenopause, women sometimes describe a loss of control over their emotions.

New scientific evidence is confirming the link between hormones and mood that women have long sensed. In this chapter, you will learn how hormones, genetics, attitude, and other life stressors all contribute to our moods. *Every woman deserves a high level of mental and emotional wellness in her menopausal years.* That's why we've written this chapter both for women experiencing significant mood disorders (which menopause can trigger in certain people), but also for women who feel well and yet wish to optimize moods, memory, and mental clarity.

Attitude: Menopause Inside Our Western Culture

Before we talk about how to optimize mental health, we need to acknowledge the role of attitude. We live in a culture fraught with ambiguous feelings about women's bodies, women's roles, and women's worth. The same society that values women for their reproductive capacities, historically refers to menstruation as "the curse," and child rearing still goes without "pay." Then along comes menopause and instead of the anticipation of becoming a respected elder, as we saw in Chapter 2 that women in other cultures sometimes do, Western women often dread the change, as a sign that we're no longer useful as women. The message behind every "age-defying" beauty product advertisement is that we ought to be ashamed of our age. If we're not hypervigilant, we will naturally internalize these beliefs and make them our own, and our mental and emotional experience of menopause can suffer as a result.

Expectation can translate into experience during menopause. We saw, for example, that Japanese women, who had traditionally listed shoulder pain as the most prominent menopause symptom, began complaining of more hot flashes after their physicians informed them that hot flashes were expected. Likewise in the West, if a woman learns to expect depression and physical debility, it can profoundly affect her experience of menopause. An analysis of the Massachusetts Women's Health Study found that women who *expected* menopause to cause problems were, in fact, the ones who reported more symptoms when it arrived.[1] In fact, until very recently, Western cultural belief held the assumption that women would become depressed or anxious when they could no longer bear children. This belief was so entrenched, that nobody questioned it until a decade ago. Real research into women's moods revealed some surprises.

Actual studies tell us that while many women experience mild mood or anxiety symptoms during perimenopause, *women in menopause do not have an increased rate of psychological disorders.*[2] Indeed, the incidence of mental health disturbances appears to *decrease* after menopause, and many women enjoy a sense of renewed vigor and emotional well-being. This isn't so surprising if we admit that mature women have a better sense of who they are, what they want, and how to get it, compared to younger women. Studies measuring contentment show that it's those things we tend to get better at as we age, such as managing stress and having better relationships, which determine a woman's satisfaction—and *not* menopausal status.[3]

While we learn to accept this natural transition, it's important not to deny that menopause can be a really trying time for some women. As a response to the negative images of menopause of the past, we do see a movement toward the other extreme; encouraging women to celebrate menopause as if it was the beginning of a new life. While some women find it liberating to celebrate menopause, for others, however, these notions can miss the point. For women facing very hard physical or emotional challenges, the added expectation that they *should* be having a great time at menopause can be irritating or even disempowering, rather than serving as an antidote to negative beliefs about menopause.

Every woman's menopause is her own. Some will celebrate, some will endure, and most will do a little of both. Some women will notice hardly a thing at menopause. There's no right or wrong way to approach it. Menopause is neither the beginning nor the end of life. It occurs simply as another phase of life along a developmental continuum. The challenge is to accept changes as they occur and to integrate these changes into our identity and life experience.

The Chemistry of Emotion

It may seem unusual to consider the brain as an organ actively involved in the process of menopause (we often consider the ovaries as the predominant organs involved). But the brain acts as the master computer of the whole experience—and so missing this connection means we're considering only a portion of the story. Conventional medicine is finally acknowledging and investigating the science behind the mind–body connection. We are learning how chemistry translates into many mental symptoms. The dynamic, and sometimes dramatic, chemistry of perimenopause gives us the perfect opportunity to explore this link.

Men and women have different physiologies. It should come as no surprise that we have different psychologies too. We know that women have twice the rate of depression and anxiety disorders as do men.[4] Differing levels of sex hormones lend partial explanation. Estrogen, progesterone, and testosterone dramatically influence brain chemistry and thereby have important influences in determining mood and behavior.

Any woman who menstruates can describe physical or mental changes that occur across the menstrual cycle. This does not imply pathology. It just means that she is sensitive to what's happening in her body. Though we often focus on negative symptoms, many women can also describe positive changes occurring at specific times during their cycles, like an increase in sexual mood or sensation at ovulation, or a feeling of clarity or lightness after the menses.

In their recent book, *Women's Moods*,[5] Deborah Sichel and Jeanne Watson Driscoll offer an elegant description of brain anatomy, neurochemistry, and the impact of female hormones. After we've been exposed to medical texts and research focusing predominantly on men for centuries now, work like Sichel and Driscoll's is a breath of fresh air. Finally, we're getting a real picture of what the Western medical system's "invisible woman" looks like.

As Sichel and Driscoll explain, the brain has evolved from the inside out, and can perhaps be best described as actually a "brain within a brain within a brain." The most primitive and innermost structure, the *brain stem*, governs involuntary activities such as breathing, digestion, and the regulation of heart rate. Surrounding the brain stem are structures that constitute the *limbic system*, that regulates appetite, the sleep-wake cycle, aggressive impulses, sexual activities, and the menstrual cycle. (See Figure 9.1.) As you might guess, the limbic system plays a big role when it comes to women and our hormones. Some scientists refer to limbic system as the "emotional brain." Its functions are the ones most often disrupted in depression. Finally, there's the outermost aspect of the brain, or the *cerebral cortex*. This part controls the sophisticated functions of thought, language, and problem solving.

One way that these three parts of the brain communicate with one another is by neuronal networking—that is, using receptors. In fact, this communication method works similarly to that between sex hormones and the other tissues they affect. Nerve cells in the brain release chemicals called "neurotransmitters." (See Figure 9.2.) A neighboring nerve cell

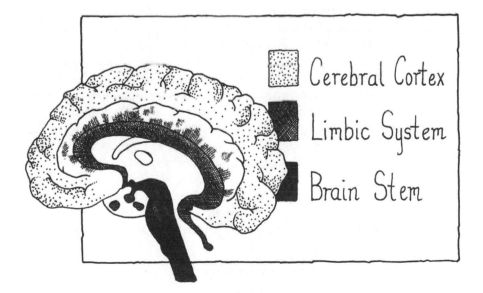

Figure 9.1. The brain stem is surrounded by the limbic system, which is surrounded by the cerebral cortex.

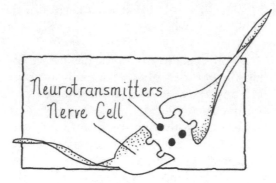

Figure 9.2.   Nerve cells transmit impulses from one another via neurotransmitters, chemicals that are released by one nerve cell and picked up by the receptors of a neighboring nerve cell.

picks up these chemicals through receptors. In this way, nerve cells transmit impulses or information from one to another.

Our brains make several kinds of neurotransmitters. We will focus on those most important for mental health: the *monoamines*. The monoamines include serotonin, norepinephrine, dopamine, and acetylcholine. These "chemical messengers" are all involved in the regulation of mood and stress, as well as movement, memory, and the menstrual cycle. All of the monoamines can affect our mental state. When they pass through the limbic structures, they affect our emotions most profoundly.

The monamine we hear most about is *serotonin*. Research has demonstrated that normal serotonin levels are associated with stable mood states and that abnormal levels are implicated in depression, anxiety, and suicidal behavior. In fact, we now understand depression as a disease of relative serotonin deficiency and dysregulation.[6] Studies have indeed shown that people at high risk of committing suicide have very low levels of serotonin.[7]

The more we learn about serotonin and brain function, the more interesting and complex the chemistry of emotion looks. Recent discoveries indicate that there may be upwards of 20 different types of serotonin receptors in the brain, each with a different effect. We likely have special serotonin receptors that specifically interact with female hormones.

Estrogen, Progesterone, and Brain Chemistry

Estrogen affects our brain's function from before birth to our final breath. Beginning from the time we are in our mother's womb, estrogen affects the organizational development of our brain.[8] Throughout our growing years, our reproductive years, and our menopausal years, estrogen (and lack of it) has a profound impact on our behavior.

Scientists have discovered estrogen and progesterone receptors throughout the brain, which implies that these hormones affect many brain functions. We find the highest concentration of these receptors in the limbic system, our so-called "emotional brain," which controls appetite, sleep-wake, aggression, and sex. This means that these female hormones have a big influence over our behavior in these areas.

The link between female hormones and moods has to do with how these hormones influence serotonin and the other monoamines. Estrogen and progesterone have the amazing ability to alter the *concentration* and *function* of these "mood chemicals." Estrogen affects mood, in part, by increasing levels of serotonin and other neurotransmitters and by altering the number and function of receptors for these chemicals. Contrarily, progesterone decreases the number of estrogen receptors, and may even dismantle some of the nerve connections that estrogen promotes. This may help to explain why some women feel depressed during the second half of the menstrual cycle or while taking progesterone supplements as part of oral contraception or HRT.[9]

In short, estrogen, through action on brain chemicals, elevates mood. Progesterone, on the other hand, tends to dampen estrogen's effects. When these two female hormones exist in optimal proportion to one another, they contribute to relatively stable moods. And when the hormone balance tips in unpredictable ways, so can our emotional state.

Change is Difficult

When hormone levels fluxuate, as they do during perimenopause, the brain constantly has to adapt. It does this by altering the number and function of receptors and making other such adjustments to our neurological hardware. Every time hormones change, our brain essentially needs to reset itself.

As you can imagine, this is easier to accomplish during small fluctuations, and more difficult to do during big ones. Also, it's harder for the brain to restabilize after a really fast change in hormone levels (such as after childbirth or oophorectomy), as compared to a more gradual one. In fact, the rate of change seems to affect stability more than the actual levels of hormones themselves do.

Although the brain is quite good at maintaining a stable state, repeated challenges to the system can take their toll. The impact of this kind of brain stress may mean that over time it takes less and less to upset the balance. In our emotional lives, this means for instance, that if a woman has had an episode of depression, her chances of having another episode increase.

Other Stresses at Menopause

The first lesson learned in any biology class is that of *homeostasis*. All living systems seek homeostasis, or "a stable state," to achieve wellness. Whatever brings *stability* to a woman's life will promote a sense of well-being. On the flip side, whatever creates flux, can lead to "dis-ease." It's little wonder that hormone fluctuations, which send serotonin and other monamine levels on a roller coaster ride, contribute to mood instability.

Hormonal fluctuations are just *one* of innumerable stresses which affect our mental health. Lack of sleep from vasomotor temperature fluctuations has been proposed as a big, although indirect, cause of depression and irritability.[10] Job, family, illness, war, and other life issues all have huge impacts. It's important to acknowledge the enormous impact of the crisis of September 11th, 2001, and all events following it, on the psyches of women today. For some, the immediate and ongoing stress of living in a changed world coincided directly with the onset of perimenopause, lowering the threshold for discomfort, and making tracking the cause of insomnia, anxiety, and other emotional challenges more difficult.

Each kind of stress may have its own neurotransmitters and pathways. Following are some potential stresses—both positive and negative—that can confound, and occasionally overwhelm, our ability to maintain mental and emotional balance:

☺	success	☹	failure
☺	performing	☹	illness/surgery
☺	travel	☹	pain
☺	job changes	☹	children leaving home
☺	getting married	☹	getting divorced
☺	pregnancy	☹	challenges with kids
☺☹	weather changes	☹	public speaking
☺☹	going back to school	☹	death of friend, family member or pet
☺☹	buying or selling a house		
☺	intense physical exercise	☺	dealing with in-laws
☺	holidays	☹	financial gain/loss
☺	emotional events	☹☺	taking care of parents
☺☹☹	retirement	☹	any major disappointment
☺	new relationship	☹	accident/injury
☺☹	learning a new skill	☹	insomnia
☺	quitting smoking, drinking	☹	war or fear for safety
☺	becoming a grandparent	☹	political strife/issues
☺☹☹	any of the above happening to a partner, child, or someone else close to you		

Menopause often coincides with changes in family dynamics, each requiring an adjustment, and therefore, each defined as "stress." Some women have children who are leaving home, an event that may trigger feelings of loss, the proverbial "empty nest syndrome." Women who have chosen to have children later in life may be raising young children during perimenopause. Yet others are becoming grandparents, which can add joy and also stress, with extra travel and time spent with new grandchildren. Finally, for many women at this time, aging parents are requiring care. This not only demands time,

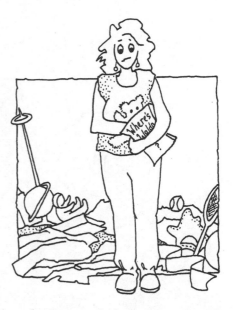

but can also add the stress of revisiting the joys and challenges of one's own child–parent relationship.

For some women, the process of encountering aging itself can be emotional and require adaptation. We come face-to-face with our own mortality at menopause as we feel new aches and pains and watch our bodies change. This can be especially hard on women who closely identify with good health and physical appearance. Also important, women desiring a pregnancy can go through much heartache over the loss of fertility. Even women who have no desire to bear children at this time can feel a sense of loss as they leave this chapter of life behind.

Change itself produces stress, and change is the hallmark of menopause. *If we don't slow down to integrate these changes, we will overload our systems.* Compared with past generations, women's lives have become so complicated, and we are generally facing so many challenges, it seems quite miraculous that we are able to withstand as much stress, and remain as stable, as we do. However, maintaining this stability may be more of a strain than we admit, or even know.

Like any organ, the brain has a remarkable ability to adapt to stress, but also like others, it has its limits. Our busy lives, and the credo to do more and more with less and less (more work, more responsibility, more striving to accomplish but also with less sleep, less relaxation, and less support from others) puts a tremendous burden on our brain, as well as the rest of our body. This strain may catch up with us in the guise of depression, unresolved grief, or severe anxiety. If you feel any of these things, ask yourself this simple question: "Am I doing too much?"

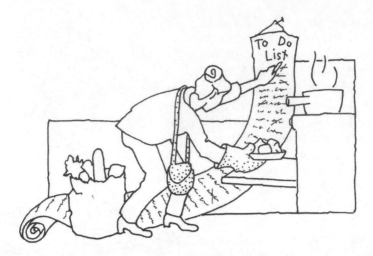

Leah

In January, Leah had just finished a big project at work and was about to embark on another one. She had just come through a rough time, with the death of her father last year, and her last child going to college. Last fall, she came down with a month-long bronchitis and it seemed that she was still catching up on regular household duties. Then, last week, one of her co-workers left, and some of his work ended up getting divvied out to her.

"I just can't seem to cope," she told her best friend. "I think there's something wrong with me. I go in to work, and know there's so much to be done, and I can't seem to get started. My sleep isn't great, and I'm eating like a fiend," she confided. "Yesterday, I went into a crying fit that lasted for twenty minutes."

In truth, there's nothing wrong with Leah. She is responding completely appropriately to the impossible demands that have befallen her. Often in life, we have the expectation that we ought to be able to "cope," when coping means not allowing ourselves the time to process and recover from significant stresses. If Leah were to decide she needed an antidepressant so she could continue working at the same pace, she would only be prolonging her state of imbalance. Leah needs to look realistically at decreasing the demands on her time, and prioritize creating the space to allow healing through integration to happen. She needs a prescription for time and self-care.

Another View of Menopausal Mood Changes

Fortunately, there is help for women feeling overwhelmed by mood changes and by other stresses in menopause. In just a moment, we will present tools for self-care for those under normal stresses, and a guide to treatment for women needing more intervention to regain mental/emotional stability. But first, we'd like to introduce an approach to perimenopausal mood changes that you won't often find at your doctor's office.

Taking an empowered approach to a hormonally influenced mood change is a radical notion. Our culture doesn't promote the benefits of having a heightened awareness of our emotions. But if you think about it, when we're in touch with our feelings, we know exactly how we feel about our job, our relationships, our roles. At perimenopause, it can be incredibly obvious to us what's working, and what's *not working* in our lives.

"Dear woman," sighs Grandmother Growth tenderly. "I see that Change has thinned the protective layers hiding your anger, your fears, your grief. Yes, I see your hidden feelings and secret desires exposed a little more with each hot flash. You may think your feelings are out of proportion, too sharp, quite insane. But, I assure you, they are only raw from neglect. Receive them without judgment, nourish them, and your 'uncontrollable' feelings during the menopausal years will lead you to the deepest heart of your own secrets."

Susun Weed[11]

Fueled by the power of our emotions, we can turn the perimenopause into a time of transformation: to change behaviors and beliefs that don't serve us, and make empowering changes in our lives. This might mean challenging negative beliefs we may hold about menopause, and consciously replacing them with positive ones. It also might mean sticking up for ourselves as we negotiate relationship, job or home issues, as Leah needs to do (see page 200). For Diane, a 50-year-old home health nurse, that meant quitting a dead-end job where she was expected to do two people's work for little compensation. "I got tired of being a doormat," she said emphatically. "Perimenopause taught me how to say 'no.' Today, I have a job I love, more time for family, and less clutter all around. There are some advantages to having a shorter fuse!"

Some women find that emotional intensity at perimenopause can inspire spiritual exploration. Indeed, some spiritual traditions refer to personal transformation as an experience of "being in the fire" of purification. Certain Hindu traditions, for example, describes the burning of impurities, or *samskaras* in the fires of purification during the process of spiritual transformation. A perimenopausal women in the midst of a mood swing or a hot flash can look surprisingly like one of Hindu's fa-

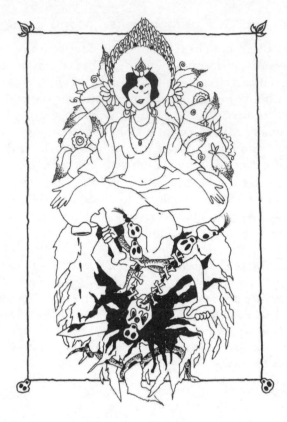

Figure 9.3.   Kali, a fierce and powerful Hindu goddess.

vorite deities, Kali—a fierce and powerful goddess who doesn't take any "guff" from anybody. (See Figure 9.3.)

Looking at her image, especially upside down, it's easy to see why the male-dominated power structures in our society would attempt to silence Kali-like energy. If our own Kali energy finds a voice, what might we cease to tolerate? What changes would we begin? The end result of using menopausal mood changes in a transformative way can be a life rearranged: simplified of emotional baggage and clutter, and redirected toward the goals that will help us fulfill our life's potential.

The Chemistry of Balance

While *perimenopause* can present the emotional changes that accompany hormonal flux, *menopause* (the cessation of menses) itself can provide a welcome respite from shifting moods. By this time, hormones have settled into their new, consistent level. We can then expect that the memory of hormonal fluctuations, and the mood disturbances which may have accompanied them, will fade into the past.

Many women say they feel more at peace now that they've gotten past the reproductive years. Cami, a 56-year-old visual artist, credits menopause with a quantum leap in her drawing skills. "I used to fuss over my drawings terribly. I'd get an idea, start drawing, then change my mind and have to erase everything. But now, I think of what I want, I pick up a pen and draw it. There's no more of this dilly-dallying around." Cami explains that she *likes* what she's drawing more since entering menopause. She believes that menopause brought more contentment and fewer conflicting emotions.

When We Need More Help

For some women, menopause or perimenopause coincides with significant mental or emotional challenges, such as depression. When this happens, it's possible to feel out of control, and necessary to get help. Fortunately, help exists, and also many treatments have improved immensely in the last ten years. We'll devote the next section to knowing what can cause actual mood disorders, how to spot them, and what natural and conventional help is available.

While menopause does not cause depression, the natural hormonal changes during perimenopause may leave some women at *higher risk* for the development of actual illness, such as depression and anxiety. The hormonal effect on neurotransmitters can then be the proverbial "straw that broke the camel's back" in terms of emotional and mental stability.

Women facing significant mental or emotional health challenges at menopause usually have other contributing factors. These include a previous history of mental health problems (especially around PMS or after childbirth), a family history of depression or other mental health problems, a prolonged and symptomatic perimenopause, and severe psychosocial stress coinciding with perimenopause, such as divorce, widowhood, other health problems, increased family responsibilities, or significant loss of role. In addition, sudden loss of the ovaries, whether through surgery, chemotherapy or radiation, may also increase the risk for depression, because the brain does not have ample time to adjust to such a rapid depletion of reproductive hormones.

It is important to note that changes in mood, anxiety or behavior also occur on a continuum. Some may be mild and amenable to refocusing on self-care techniques. Some may be more moderate and require other kinds of interventions. Some women may develop very serious forms of depression or anxiety that, left untreated, can result in severe dysfunction and even death. It's also possible for mild symptoms to progress insidiously. A woman may start out feeling mildly depressed, and if she's not alert to it and doesn't take action, depression can become her reality more of the time. Staying on the lookout for more serious problems is important in preventing a downward spiral of emotion. By using some of the self-care techniques we'll present, it's possible to catch yourself and divert a crash.

Depression and Anxiety

Everyone experiences the blues, or feelings of nervousness. Common perimenopausal mood changes (for example, irritability, anger, and mood swings) can sound a lot like symptoms of important psychiatric syndromes. Therefore, it's important to distinguish mild symptoms of anxiety or depression from syndromes that may require more intervention. Let's find out how.

The difference between relatively minor perimenopausal symptoms and more serious mental illness has a lot to do with how *functional* a woman feels. Women with major depression or anxiety disorders have difficulty functioning in their day-to-day lives. They are much more likely to require medical intervention to regain health.

Western psychiatry uses a classification system called the *DSM* (*The Diagnostic and Statistical Manual of Mental Disorders*) to help quantify problems that constitute "mental illness."[12] It is a useful device, though not without its limitations. Naming a problem, and realizing that other people experience it too, can offer assurance to anyone suffering. However, a diagnosis can't tell us if and how these feelings interfere with our daily lives. Use the following information to guide you in knowing whether or not mood disturbances you may be having may require more help.

Mood Disorders

There are several types of mood disorders. Of these we will discuss four: *major depression, dysthymia, bipolar disorder, and premenstrual mood dysphoric disorder (PMDD)*.

Major depression is a very serious illness, notable for disturbances with a number of symptoms that may include changes in sleep, appetite, and concentration. People with major depression can experience a loss of pleasure or interest in activities, pervasive feelings of hopelessness and despair, and suicidal thoughts. Symptoms must be present consistently for at least two weeks. Often debilitating, major depression can seriously disrupt a person's life.

Dysthymia is a kind of chronic but milder type of depressive disorder. The same kinds of symptoms as in major depression occur, but to a less disabling degree. People with dysthymia can generally attend to life's responsibilities. They may, however, have a higher risk of developing major depression. When these occur together we call it "double depression."

Bipolar disorder is characterized by the experience of both high and low moods, although the "highs" may not always be pronounced. Hormonal changes frequently affect this problem.

Premenstrual mood dysphoric disorder (PMDD) is a type of depression notable for its appearance late in the second half of the menstrual cycle—sort of like a "super PMS." Symptoms look quite similar to those of major depression, but resolve with the onset of menses. About 3–5% of women who menstruate meet criteria necessary for a diagnosis of PMDD. A much more common situation involves women who experience premenstrual worsening of another disorder (depression, bipolar disorder, anxiety, eating disorder, etc.).[13]

The following is a list of several important symptoms that commonly occur in depression:

- Pervasive feelings of sadness or despair
- Changes in sleep (either too much or too little)
- Disturbance of appetite or significant changes in weight
- Loss of pleasure or interest in usual activities or hobbies
- Difficulties with concentration or memory
- Feelings of helplessness, hopelessness, or significant guilt
- Changes in sex interests or drive
- Thoughts of death, including suicide, or harm coming to self or others

If two or more of these symptoms seem to apply to you, please discuss them with a clinician trained in mental health.

Another Culture's Take on 'Depression'

Tierrona Low Dog, M.D., a family practitioner and Native Lakota herbalist who practices integrative medicine in Albuquerque, New Mexico, tells of her people's approach to "depression." According to Low Dog, the Lakota people look upon what medicine calls a pathology as actually a "journeying time," a time when a person travels deep into the center of her or his being. The Lakota honor this experience for the wisdom it will bring to the tribe when the person emerges from the journey. Native peoples, Low Dog explains, pray, cook, and care for one journeying and care for his or her family as well. Their reverence for this process allows the entire community to partake of the lessons received when a person has gone into the darkness and safely returned. Low Dog cautions, however, that the rates of depression and other forms of mental illness are growing among Native Americans and that an integrated approach combining the wisdom of tribal tradition with the best of current treatment options will likely lead to the best results.

Anxiety Disorders

Women sometimes complain of anxiety in perimenopause. It's helpful to be able to distinguish between minor anxiety that can be easily treated and those requiring more intervention. We'll discuss the four most common anxiety disorders below.

Generalized anxiety disorder is characterized by a pervasive sense of worry, not helped by reassurance. Patients may describe sleep problems, feelings of being "on edge," and having difficulty concentrating or thinking of things other than their worries. *Panic disorder* often presents with the sudden onset of severe symptoms of fear, a sense of impending doom, and an urge to escape. Physical symptoms include heart palpitations, shortness of breath, nausea, and dizziness. People with panic disorder can feel anxious while anticipating a next panic attack.

People who have *obsessive-compulsive disorder* (OCD) have persistent, disturbing thoughts, ideas, or images that cause significant anxiety or distress. They may try to dispel the anxiety by engaging in repetitive acts or behaviors (compulsions). We used to think OCD was relatively rare, mainly because those with this disorder felt too ashamed of their symptoms to come forward, seeking help. We now know it to be a relatively common disorder.

Our last anxiety-related disorder, *post-traumatic stress disorder (PTSD)*, generally occurs after an exposure to a major traumatic event. Serious injury, threatened death, or witnessing a traumatic event can all trigger PTSD. People who suffer from PTSD can seem to "re-experience the trauma" through intrusive thoughts or recollections of the event, which can also recur in dreams or nightmares.

Getting Help

If you think you, or someone close to you, might be suffering from one of the mood or anxiety disorders listed above, please seek help. Reaching out for assistance can be difficult, especially for women who are accustomed to putting the needs of others before their own. Also, those who were raised to "keep a stiff upper lip," or with the fading taboos attached to mental illness may feel that asking for help is almost as difficult as weathering the difficulties. Also, it's normal to think "This shouldn't be happening to me." Don't let denial of your situation prevent you from obtaining the support you need and deserve.

We recommend finding a mental health practitioner with a holistic approach—meaning one who sees you not only as someone with a list of symptoms, but as someone with a full mental, emotional, physical and perhaps spiritual life. Don't hesitate to visit more than one practitioner before settling on someone you feel addresses you in your entirety.

Very effective treatments for all of the above have changed (and saved) the lives of many women. A family doctor, gynecologist, or other practitioner can either offer treatment or make appropriate referrals. Near the end of the following section, you will learn about medications that are offered to women suffering from severe mental health disturbances.

Nurturing Your Mental and Emotional Health

Today, most women generally accept the notion that a good diet and a physical exercise plan are important to one's well-being. But have you considered the necessity of a mental wellness plan? Think about it. Our society programs us for productivity. Women often have excessive demands on their time and energy—even if they enjoy what they're doing. Our work and home lives aren't going to steer us toward taking time out for ourselves.

To counteract the inherent stress of life, we recommend that each woman give some time to the care of her soul. Make room for joy. The menopause transition provides a perfect opportunity to do this. Whether you are feeling on top of the world, experiencing a few ups and downs, or perhaps suffering from a significant mental health challenge, taking time to reflect on nurturing your emotional well-being can pay off in the long run.

In *Women's Moods,* Sichel and Driscoll offer an excellent approach to self-care: their "NURSE" Program.[14] The word "nurse," they point out, in fact means to attend, minister, sustain, cultivate, and nourish. With this definition in mind, they have used it cleverly in an acronym to guide women in developing self-care strategies "to maintain your brain's optimal functioning in spite of its inherent vulnerability." The NURSE program highlights the following areas of self-care, inviting women to include aspects of each in an overall plan to support mind, body and spirit:

> N*ourishment and Needs*—Provide yourself with optimal nutrition, appropriate supplements, and if needed, prescription medications.
> U*nderstand*—Read! Educate yourself about the influence of hormones and moods. Know when psychotherapy can be helpful, and use it.

Rest and Relaxation—Make sure you're getting good sleep, and get serious about stress-reduction. Relaxation is a learned art. It requires constant practice.

Spirituality—Explore and nurture the essence of your true nature, whether through meditation, yoga, prayer, being in nature, or however else you feed your soul.

Exercise—Elevate your mood, immune function and increase physical as well as mental/emotional health with this universal tonic.

Sichel and Driscoll's NURSE program provides an excellent format for self-care, because it addresses all of the most essential elements in maintaining mental/emotional wellness. It offers a valuable guide for every woman, whether or not she is in menopause. We highly recommend it.

In our next section, we'll assist you in identifying ways in which you might consider supporting your mental wellness in menopause. As clinicians, we tend to think of supports for our patients falling into three basic categories: lifestyle choices, psychotherapy, and pharmaceutical options (including supplements). Depending on how balanced you feel right now, you may want to find support in one, two, or all three areas. Women with significant mental health challenges will probably need to address all three areas.

Lifestyle

Everyone can benefit from a healthy lifestyle. Choices we make daily have powerful implications in maintaining mental and emotional balance. The worksheet on page 209 will allow you to assess which areas of your lifestyle are creating balance in your mental wellness, and which could use improvement. This exercise creates the foundation for creating a mental wellness plan.

In pencil, put a checkmark beside each behavior noting whether you agree or disagree with each statement. Next to the ones you check "disagree," think about what you might do that would turn it into a true statement. For example, if you check "disagree" beside the statement "I have a stable sleep/wake cycle," you might write "talk to my doctor about sleep remedies" to the right. If possible, bring this list with you to a

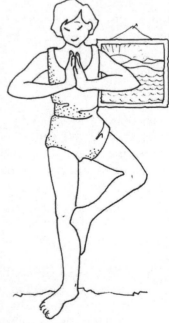

visit with one of your health care practitioners, and ask for their help in any areas where you need support.

Nurturing a Healthy Lifestyle

Read each statement and mark whether you agree or disagree with it. If you disagree with it, note to whom you could turn for help and what that help might be.

	Agree	Disagree	How might I find support in this area?
1. I have a stable sleep/ wake cycle.			
2. I have a healthy diet.			
3. I exercise regularly.			
4. I avoid the use of substances that can contribute to problems.			
5. I employ regular relaxation techniques and nourish my soul frequently.			
6. I spend time with people I enjoy.			

Congratulate yourself for your success regarding anything that you checked "agree." (Really . . . do it! It's important to celebrate our accomplishments.) Now, congratulate yourself for your courage to identify weak points in the areas where you checked "disagree." It is a strong woman who can identify where she needs support and asks for it. Take a few more minutes to flush out the boxes on the right side of this table, to brainstorm on places where you might find that support. Refer back to this list occasionally, updating your responses. In time, you may find that you could agree with all the statements.

Psychotherapy

Psychotherapy can take many forms. Basically, psychotherapy refers to the opportunity to process your thoughts and ideas with someone you don't need to take care of. Traditional psychotherapy may be offered individually, in family or couple's treatment, or in group therapy that is either professionally led or peer supported. Nontraditional forms include dance or art therapy and certain forms of body-centered therapy, among others.

You definitely don't need to be suffering from a mental illness to benefit from psychotherapy or counseling. Psychotherapy itself exists on a continuum from a relaxed approach aimed at optimizing one's self-awareness and personal growth, all the way to very intensive psychoanalysis—the proverbial "on the couch" treatment used for everything from personal growth exploration to treatment of severe psychiatric illness.

Many women utilize the less intensive *supportive psychotherapy* when they feel a need for insight and suggestions, or seek to change patterns of negative thought or behaviors. When menopause coincides with major shifts in relationships, career or health, psychotherapy can provide a much-welcomed "hour of clarity" amidst the upheaval. The insights gained can be long-lasting. Giving ourselves the space to be heard and supported by a good counselor can be a way of nourishing our souls. When important decisions face us, supportive psychotherapy can aid us in making choices that support our continued well-being.

Psychotherapy has also proven useful to patients with depression or other mental illness. Recent studies have validated the effectiveness of certain techniques for specific types of disorders. *Short-term cognitive therapy*, which helps patients identify and change distorted thought patterns that trigger or perpetuate distress, has been compared favorably with antidepressant medication in effectively treating mild to moderate depression.[15] A special type of therapy combining aspects of cognitive behavioral and feminist therapy with Zen meditation, known as *dialectical behavioral therapy*, has been shown to be effective in treating people with borderline personality disorder. *Psychodynamic therapy*, a derivative of psychoanalysis, has been shown to be successful in treating people with panic disorder.[16] Personality problems may respond to the type of intensive psychotherapy known as *psychoanalysis*.[17,18] During psychoanalysis, in which a client may meet with a therapist several times per week, a client often "transfers" patterns of behavior onto the relationship with her analyst, who then helps the client understand and consciously challenge self-defeating behaviors.

If you wonder whether or not you might benefit from some form of psychotherapy, talk with your practitioner about it. For some women, psychotherapy can be an important component to overall well-being. Then, if you decide to give it a try, it's crucial that you find a therapist who you really like. Obtain two or three names from someone you trust—such as your health practitioner or a good friend. Have a short chat on the phone first, asking the therapist about his or her experience with the issues important to you. Interview a few different practitioners to find the right "match." A good therapist will appreciate and encourage this approach. Once you've made a good connection on the phone, schedule an initial appointment with one or two practitioners. Your first visit may be an introductory session—a time to "feel out" how well you might work together. Go with an open mind and a willingness to be honest. Taking the time to find a therapist that you "click" with will pay off in the long run.

Supplements

Natural remedies can also be used to facilitate mental wellness at menopause. If you are feeling mentally and emotionally balanced and want to try some of the gentler natural products listed below for only minor mood disturbances (namely the B vitamins and essential fatty acids), you probably don't need an assessment beforehand. However, we do feel that if you are dealing with moderate to severe mood disturbances, you do need a careful assessment by a qualified professional. Self-treatment with over-the-counter products, or simply buying what the health food store clerk or pharmacist recommends, completely bypasses the essential step of an evaluation. At best, you might be wasting money on a product that's ineffective or inappropriate for you. At worst, you could unknowingly take something that is contraindicated or interacts badly with other medications or supplements you may be taking. Self-diagnosis and self-medication can sometimes result in patients not receiving the appropriate care for their condition.

In Chapter 3, we listed many important natural remedies for "Perimenopausal PMS." Refer back to this chapter for information about optimizing exercise, diet, and phytoestrogenic herbal combinations, all of which are broad remedies that address the sum total of perimenopausal symptoms. Also in Chapter 3, we discussed vitamin B_6, calcium supplements, and vitex, which treat symptoms specific to PMS. It's worth considering these remedies even before menopause if you have mood aggravations before your menses. Also, the phytoestrogenic remedies can help in any mental/emotional situation where estrogen has proven effective. Phytoestrogens are weaker than estrogen replacement. Therefore, expect their action to be milder than estrogen. They may or may not be enough to solve your particular mood disturbance. An experienced practitioner can give you an idea of whether or not they will likely work for you and a six week trial will usually determine whether or not you will need something stronger.

Additional natural remedies can offer more specific help if moods are the chief, or only concern. Also, women already in menopause or peri-menopausal women whose mood disturbances aren't necessarily tied to their cycles can find best relief with the following remedies. Note that many treatments listed below help with both anxiety and depression.

We've arranged treatments from gentlest to strongest in effect. In many cases, natural remedies may be appropriate for women with mild peri-menopausal mood disturbances, while women who suffer from mental ill-ness will likely need conventional help. However, consulting with a well-trained herbalist, a naturopathic physician or a conventional provider familiar with these remedies will help ensure that you will be directed to-ward a remedy effective for you.

B Vitamins

Natural health practitioners often recommend a complex of the B vita-mins for their patients who complain of a wide range of nervous-system or stress-related problems. The effectiveness of a B-complex for anxiety, de-pression or other emotional disturbances is mainly based on patient re-ports and from inferences about related issues.

We know that vitamin B_6 is involved in the function of serotonin and GABA, two brain chemicals that impact depression and anxiety. B_6 has also been shown in animal studies to lower blood pressure by decreasing the "fight-or-flight" activity of the nervous system, which could potentially explain its calming effect.[19] As we saw in Chapter 3, a review of vitamin B_6 in nine published trials showed its effectiveness in treating premenopausal depression.[20]

Several of the B vitamins have been shown to enhance the activity of an-tidepressant medications. Only 500 micrograms of folic acid (technically a B vitamin) greatly improved the antidepressant activity of fluoxetine (Prozac®) in 127 patients with major depression in a randomized, pla-cebo controlled trial.[21] In another study, 10 mg each of vitamins B_1, B_2 and B_6 enhanced the effect of tricyclic antidepressants in geriatric patients with depression.[22]

B vitamins are water-soluble, which means they do not tend to accumu-late in the body. Most B complex supplements contain 50–100 mg of $B_{1, 2, 3, 5}$ and $_6$, along with 400 micrograms of folic acid and about 1 mg of B_{12}. Overdosing any B vitamin can lead to nerve toxicities. However, taken at the doses recommended above, and in this balanced form, side effects or adverse interactions are uncommon. A B complex is one of the gen-tlest, safest remedies to try for taking the edge off perimenopausal or menopausal emotional disturbances.

Omega-3 Fatty Acids

Nerve cell membranes contain high amounts of *omega-3 essential fatty acids,* which are now being studied for their impact on psychiatric disorders. Some researches have suggested a relationship between omega-3 fatty acids and the all-important serotonin, as well as other mood-affecting neurotransmitters. People with postpartum depression and schizophrenia can have low levels of omega-3 fatty acids. In one experiment, treatment with very large doses of fish oil helped maintain the mood stability of men and women with bipolar disorder.[23] While we don't advocate fish oil as a proven treatment for serious mental illness, we can nonetheless acknowledge that essential fatty acids probably play a role in mental stability.

You'll find omega-3 fatty acids in cold-water fish and flax oil. Many companies make supplements from these sources, and also from extracts of borage, hemp, black currant, and evening primrose. Some people experience mild gastrointestinal side effects with these, especially with fish oil. (Hint: To avoid the relatively unpleasant sensation of fishy-smelling burps—take fish oil before a meal.) Omega-3 oils have extremely low toxicity, even at high doses. Modest doses range from 1,000–3,000 mg per day.

St. John's wort

St. John's wort (*Hypericum perforatum*) is a sun-loving, Western plant that blooms in July, near the holiday of St. John the Baptist. An abundant herb, it grows profusely in wide-open prairie and field lands. Extracts of the flowers and leaves of St. John's wort contain *hypericin* and *hyperforin,* two chemicals thought to be important in its antidepressant activity. St. John's wort has been shown to affect mood by at least two mechanisms: by inhibiting reuptake of serotonin,[24] and by inhibiting the enzyme that breaks serotonin down. This enzyme, monoamine oxidase, is often called MAO.

Many supplement manufacturers standardize their St. John's wort and other supplements in an effort to guarantee quality. Although it is a valiant attempt to ensure quality, many herbal practitioners hold that

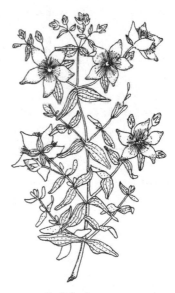

St. John's wort
(*Hypericum perforatum*)

standardization offers more hype than hope. The case of St. John's wort offers a good illustration of this issue.

For several years, herbal researchers believed that *hypericin* was the main medicinal constituent in St. John's wort. Accordingly, supplement companies standardized their extracts to contain quantifiable amounts of hypericin. Later studies refuted hypericin as the important ingredient, and declared *hyperforin* the chemical responsible for the herb's activity. Supplement companies then changed their products to be standardized for a guaranteed amount of hyperforin.

The truth about herbal medicine is that no one chemical gives a plant its medicinal action. Herbs, like foods, have dozens of constituents, which tend to act synergistically in producing a therapeutic action. In this way, they are far more complicated than drugs, which contain usually one, or rarely two, active chemicals. St. John's wort may, in fact, contain more than fifteen substances that work synergistically to combat depression.[25] We are light years away from being able to reliably standardize herbal medications.

Nonetheless, most studies on St. John's wort that make it into medical literature rely on doses of 300 milligrams, standardized to a 0.3 percent content of hypericin, three times daily. In a recent review published in the *Archives of Internal Medicine*, an analysis of all scientific studies conducted on St. John's wort between 1982 and 2000 found St. John's wort effective in treating mild and moderate depression. The herb outperformed placebo, but was not as effective as a tricyclic antidepressant.[26] Trials comparing St. John's wort to the SSRI class of drugs, such as Prozac®, are now under way. One of the first reported out has found St. John's wort comparable to Prozac® in the treatment of 240 people with mild to moderate depression.[27] As more results roll in, it is likely that, as with the tricyclics, we will find that St. John's wort serves as an effective intermediary, its strength somewhere between prescription antidepressants and supplements like the B vitamins or omega-3 fatty acids.

Because it can sensitize the skin and possibly the eyes to sunlight, always wear UV protection to these areas if you take St. John's wort. St. John's wort has also recently been found to lower the blood concentrations (by speeding elimination) of several drugs, including cyclosporin, amitriptyline, digoxin, and warfarin,[28] and to decrease the effectiveness of birth control pills.[29] If you are on any other medications, make sure you check with your practitioner before adding St. John's wort.

5-HTP

5-Hydroxytryptophan or 5-HTP is a chemical occurring naturally in the body. It is made from the amino acid L-tryptophan and is converted into serotonin.

Stress, B_6 or magnesium deficiency, or problems with insulin metabolism can result in the body not completing the first step in this process—that is, converting L-tryptophan into 5-HTP.[30] Supplementing with 5-HTP, then, can elevate levels of serotonin in the body.

5-HTP has received criticism largely because of a perceived issue with safety. During the 1980s, L-tryptophan was available as an over-the-counter supplement, and was rivaling newly available prescription antidepressants in sales. In 1983, a batch contaminated with bacteria resulted in severe illness and even death in several individuals, who contracted eosinophilia-myalgia syndrome (EMS). As a result, all L-tryptophan was pulled from the market for a decade, and reappeared later as a more expensisve, prescription-only item.

5-HTP is not produced in a way that is likely to result in bacterial contamination leading to EMS. However, it still is a supplement that needs to be used under supervision, and with caution. Overdose of 5-HTP can potentially result in mental confusion, anxiety, and high blood pressure, symptoms that constitute "serotonin syndrome." 5-HTP is a strong, over-the-counter antidepressant, which can be potentially more effective than St. John's wort for some individuals, and have less side effects than conventional antidepressants. For more information on 5-HTP, consult the book with the same name, by naturopathic physician Michael Murray, N.D.[31]

Kava Kava

Many conventional drugs for anxiety have side effects or significant risks for tolerance and dependence. Hence, there's growing interest in kava kava as a potential anti-anxiety herbal medication with fewer side effects. Kava (*piper methysticum*) is a plant native to the Pacific Islands that has been used in ceremonies for thousands of years.[32] It has quickly become a favorite antianxiety remedy in the West.

The exact mode of kava's action is still under investigation and may turn out to be a combination of several mechanisms. It appears to affect two brain chemicals involved in anxiety: GABA and norepinephrine. Additionally, kava appears to act as a central muscle relaxant and anticonvulsant.[33] Most people find that a single dose induces relaxation in as little as 15–30 minutes. It is available in tea, tincture (alcohol extract), and capsule form. Corresponding doses of these forms are one cup, ½ teaspoon, or one capsule as needed, up to three times daily.

Most studies on kava utilize capsules standardized to contain 50–70 mg kavalactones (the ingredients thought to produce its effect). An analysis of the seven double-blind, randomized, placebo-controlled trials of oral kava for the treatment of anxiety up till June 1998 was performed by researchers at the University of Exeter, United Kingdom. Kava scored better than placebo in treating anxiety in all of the studies.[34]

Kava is one of the herbs being closely watched for adverse side effects and interactions. In December 2001, German and Swiss officials reported thirty cases of liver toxicity in people taking kava and called for restrictions on its use. Toxicologists in the United States analyzing the reports have found that concurrent use of alcohol and other drugs toxic to the liver probably accounted for some of these cases, while in others, the individuals likely had an allergic reaction to the kava, which wouldn't translate to a risk for the general population.[35] Nonetheless, we caution against kava use in those with liver disease and in conjunction with liver-toxic substances like alcohol and certain drugs and recommend periodic checks of liver enzymes for people who use kava daily for more than three months.

Long-term, heavy use of kava can produce a scaly skin rash known as kava dermopathy. It also can increase the action of barbiturate drugs and benzodiazepines like Xanax®.[36] Kava may aggravate depression in some individuals. Before trying it, you should consult with a practitioner familiar with kava, and clear any potential drug interactions if you take other medications.

Hormone Replacement Therapy

Some health providers feel that "stabilizing" hormone levels may help women with mood changes experienced throughout the perimenopausal transition. As we have discussed, relatively rapid changing levels of hormones that women experience in this time can contribute to mood changes, including depression and anxiety. Most scientific studies show that estrogen can enhance mood in menopausal women with mood disturbances, but that it cannot alone treat major depressive disorders.[37] Therefore, if a woman does have major depression or anxiety, she shouldn't rely on HRT alone to bring her back into balance.

Some health providers suggest a trial of low dose estrogen for women with milder mood disturbances. Used for 21 days each month (beginning on day 1 of the menstrual period flow and used for 21 consecutive days), the small dose of estrogen serves to supplement the woman's existing cycle. For some women, this affords a "calming" effect. This approach is not recommended as a long-term solution, however, and should only be used in women still having menstrual cycles, and with the supervision of an experienced clinician. Controlled studies have not been done using this approach, but some health providers have had positive results.

Low dose oral contraceptive pills (OCPs) provide another hormonal option. OCPs can "smooth out" the hormonal changes in perimenopause that may be contributing to distressing mood changes. For women who experience erratic cycles, this approach provides the additional benefit of cycle regulation, as we discussed in Chapter 3.

In addition to these benefits, HRT (as well as herbal phytoestrogens) can sometimes restore a general sense of well-being for women. Sally, a 53-year-old administrative assistant, said while she could live with her minor menopausal symptoms, HRT made her feel more like "herself." Indeed, a study of 500 women aiming to look at a general notion of "quality of life" found that women taking HRT had improvements in mood changes, sexual life issues, family life, professional life, cognitive difficulties, menopausal symptoms, sleep, and general health.[38] While neither hormones nor phytoestrogens are cure-alls, nor the answers for everyone, in some situations they may help women regain a sense of balance.

As a reminder, before starting any hormonal treatment aimed at helping moods, it's important to obtain a very clear assessment of your emotional state. This will help steer you in the right direction regarding treatment. For example, if anxiety predominates, using an antianxiety treatment will provide more relief than hormonal treatment. And always build regular follow-up visits with a practitioner into your plan.

Medications

If your symptoms are severe or have not responded adequately to more natural treatments, you may find relief using prescription medications.

Selective Serotonin Reuptake Inhibitors

Released in 1988, Prozac®, was the first selective serotonin reuptake inhibitors (SSRIs) on the market. Prozac® dramatically affected the way we looked at the treatment of depression. Prior antidepressants were often very difficult to tolerate, potentially dangerous, and reserved for only the most ill patients. After the development of the more easily tolerated SSRIs, medicine basically lowered its threshold for treating depression. As a result, people today who have more moderate illnesses may be routinely offered antidepressant medications.

SSRIs work by increasing serotonin levels available in the synapse (spaces between nerve cells) and alter the sensitivity of the serotonin receptors. It's interesting to note that SSRIs seem more effective for women than men, and especially *before* a woman's menopause, while estrogen is plentiful. SSRIs are also the conventional treatments of choice for premenopausal women with severe PMDD.[39,40] The reason for these findings is not yet completely clear, but we know it has to do with the interactions between estrogen and the neurotransmitters that effect mood. It seems that an adequate amount of estrogen is necessary for the SSRIs to have their best effect. Women with PMDD may respond positively to these drugs within a few weeks, although it may take several months to feel their full effect.

There are about 10 SSRIs on the market now including Prozac®, Zoloft®, Luvox®, Paxil®, and Celexa®. Zoloft® has recently gained FDA approval for treating post-traumatic stress syndrome. Sarafem®, promoted as a new PMDD drug, is Prozac® renamed. All provide comparable results, and most people tolerate these drugs well. A large percentage of people do experience loss of sexual desire or function. All SSRIs possess slight variations in effectiveness and side effects for different people. This means that if you don't respond to (or cannot tolerate) one of them, you may opt to try another.

Tricyclic Antidepressants

Tricyclic antidepressants (TCAs) are older medications, which drug makers discovered serendipitously in 1958. While exploring a new medicine (*imipramine*) for the treatment of schizophrenia, they noted that patients enjoyed improvement in mood, even though the drug didn't end up working for schizophrenia. There are 10 medications available in this group, which include *amitriptyline, imipramine, nortriptyline, desipramine, and doxepin.*

After menopause, TCAs appear to be as effective as SSRIs in the treatment of depression. Also like SSRIs, tricyclics are quite effective for the treatment of anxiety disorders. Tricyclics seem to exert their antidepressant effects by increasing amounts of neurotransmitters available (norepinephrine and smaller amounts of serotonin), and by altering the sensitivity of receptors to the chemical that attaches to them.

Various side effects may limit the use of these drugs in some patients. They may include dry mouth, constipation, low blood pressure, palpitations, sedation, weight gain, and others. Still, TCAs are very effective antidepressants, and may provide important alternatives for those patients who cannot tolerate, or don't respond to SSRIs.

Monoamine Oxidase Inhibitors

Monoamine oxidase inhibitors (MAOIs) were the first antidepressants to be discovered (in the early 1950s). The same as the tricyclics, MAOIs came to market through the back door. While investigators tested one such MAOI, *iproniazid,* as an antituberculosis agent, they noted that patients experienced prolonged elevation of mood (even though they did not enjoy relief from TB). The realization that MAOIs acted as antidepressants, and the knowledge that they seemed to act by making neurotransmitters more available at the synapse, formed the basis of our early hypothesis that depression results from low neurotransmitter levels.

The use of MAOIs decreased when the tricyclics became available, and even more dramatically when the better-tolerated SSRIs hit the market. People on them must follow a somewhat restrictive diet to avoid a potentially dangerous blood pressure elevation. Other side effects may include low blood pressure, sexual dysfunction, insomnia, sedation, and weight gain among others. Still, if a patient does not respond to other modalities of treatment, MAOIs can offer an important alternative.

Buproprion

The biochemical effect of buproprion (Wellbutrin®) is not completely clear, but has been hypothesized to cause increased levels of norepinephrine and dopamine, two brain chemicals involved with mood. *Buproprion* is effective for many kinds of depression, and was also recently approved as an antismoking agent. It seems to provide important relief for depression in people with bipolar disorder, because it may be less likely than other antidepressants to stimulate manic episodes.

Wellbutrin® has also been used to treat ADD, bulimia, and various kinds of anxiety disorders. It has relatively few side effects, and causes less sexual dysfunction than other antidepressants (especially SSRIs). In fact, practitioners sometimes add Wellbutrin® to other antidepressants as an antidote to these sexual side effects. It may also augment the antidepressant response of other agents. Its most common side effects include nausea and agitation. Although infrequent, seizures can occur more commonly on this drug than on other antidepressants. Therefore, people with risk factors for seizures should avoid Wellbutrin® if possible.

Venlafaxine

Venlafaxine (Effexor®) is known as a "selective serotonin-norepinephrine reuptake inhibitor." It may provide the unique benefit of effecting an SSRI response at lower doses, and a TCA response at higher doses. Besides being an effective antidepressant, it is used for treatment of anxiety, chronic pain, and ADD. Side effects most closely resemble those of SSRIs, and include nausea, sleepiness, and insomnia. Some patients have developed high blood pressure on Effexor®, and so blood pressure should be monitored regularly, especially in the early months of treatment.

Nefazodone and Trazodone

Nefazodone (Serzone®) and trazodone (Desyrel®) act on the serotonin system, but in ways distinct from the SSRIs. Both have prominent
antianxiety effects and work effectively as antidepressants. A nonhabit-
forming sedative, Desyrel® is often used as a sleeping agent in lower
doses. Most people tolerate the side effects of these medications (dry
mouth, nausea, dizziness) pretty well. Visual effects can include "visual
trails" (especially with Serzone®), which often improve over time. Sometimes vivid and disturbing dreaming can indicate the need to discontinue
the medication.

Recent reports suggest that nefazodone can cause severe liver dysfunction.[41] Therefore, you should carefully review your need for this drug with
your clinician.

Benzodiazepines

This class of medications include clonazepam (Klonopin®), diazepam
(Valium®), lorazepam (Ativan®), and alprazolam (Xanax®). They are all
very effective antianxiety agents, and may have important roles in easing
symptoms of anxiety and facilitating the early phase of treatment with antidepressants. Side effects can include sedation, dizziness, unsteadiness of
gait, and memory problems. Potentially habit-forming, it's important to
use these agents under close supervision and in the lowest, effective doses.
The longest-acting one of these, Klonopin®, may inrease bone loss, if used
long-term (see Chapter 7).

Using Prescription Antidepressant Medications

With so many agents to choose from, you can see why working with a
psychiatrist or other clinician highly trained in antidepressant therapies
might be necessary for women suffering moderate to severe mental disturbances. A good clinician may recommend one over the other because
of a patient's particular symptoms, medical history, and anticipation of
side effects. Most commonly, the clinician will recommend starting in
lower doses and increasing gradually over time to the lowest, effective
treating dose. Though a patient may experience some improvement of
symptoms in the first few weeks of treatment, it may take 8–12 weeks to experience the full clinical benefit of these medications. (This is also true of
St. John's wort and 5-HTP.) Therefore, it's important to allow for adequate time, and adequate dosing before deciding that "this medication is
not for me."

If you take either a natural or conventional antidepressant, maintain close follow-up with your prescribing clinician. Utilize other supports too (such as self-care techniques and psychotherapy). Stay clear of alcohol and other drugs of abuse while on these medications because of drug interactions, and because these drugs may inhibit the antidepressant response. Because we don't have enough information regarding safety, we do not recommend using strong herbs and supplements that treat depression (like St. John's wort and 5-HTP) together with prescription medications that you may be taking for the same reason. The National Institutes of Health is actively exploring herb/drug interactions, and we should have much more information on this issue in the coming years.

If you have responded to medications and other treatments, it's best to remain on the effective treating dose for 6–12 months before discontinuing treatment. This phase of treatment should also be closely monitored to track reemergence of symptoms, and to determine the timing of discontinuing the drug. When going off a drug, you can usually avoid side effects if you taper slowly. For patients with recurrent mood episodes, it may make sense to consider continuing to use these medications indefinitely.

Certainly, the foundation of recovery from depression, anxiety, or other mental/emotional disturbances is supported by a balanced approach and should not rely on medications alone. Indeed lifestyle changes, and gains made in psychotherapy continue to provide support long after discontinuing a drug, as Sharon proved (see below). In addition, they may help you avoid recurring problems.

Sharon

Sharon was a successful, bright, upper middle class woman who could not tolerate the notion that she was suffering from depression. Depression, she thought angrily, happens to other people—not someone who supposedly "has it all," as she was often described. During two years of denying her problem, Sharon suffered considerably from feelings of isolation, desperation and hopelessness.

Sharon eventually recovered from her bout with mental illness, thanks to her husband who insisted she seek help. Her family doctor prescribed medication while she pursued psychotherapy to address the issues underlying her illness. Within two years, Sharon was able to go off the medication.

"I know this may sound incredible," she reflected, after her recovery, "but I'm almost grateful to my depression. I used to feel so separate from other people—like I was better than them, truthfully. I guess I used to feel that the world revolved around me, my family, how nice our house was, and how well I dressed our kids. I feel more connected to people now—from all walks of life."

In experiencing the suffering of her own depression, Sharon had actually developed a tremendous compassion for other people. Today she feels that life has more breadth and depth than before her depression, and she is able to find meaning in simple things, like connections with other people.

Menopause and Memory

Many women describe a change in the way they think as they traverse perimenopause. They may describe difficulties finding a word, memory impairment, or poor concentration. For some, these changes are reminiscent of the kind of forgetfulness they may have experienced after childbirth, during lactation, or in the days directly leading up to their period. The common denonimator in all of these situations is a drop in estrogen levels.

Since 1950, scientists have been studying estrogen's impact on mental function. One of the earliest of these studies showed that elderly women who received estrogen injections actually increased their IQ test scores after 6 months.[42] In the half century that has followed, numerous other studies have been performed, about half showing that estrogen improves some aspects of cognitive function, and the other half demonstrating no such benefit.

The different outcomes of the studies may have to do with what the researchers actually measured as "memory."[43] Psychologists now describe memory as not only a single function, but several. They have been able to determine which aspects of memory hormones, like estrogen, affect, and which aspects change simply by virtue of our normal aging processes.

One of the world's leading researchers in this field is Dr. Barbara Sherwin of McGill University in Montreal. Dr. Sherwin has conducted research showing that women deprived of estrogen lose some of the ability to recall recently learned verbal information. In extensively reviewing the research of others in this area, Sherwin has consistently found that tests measuring women's verbal and short-term memory show a decline at menopause. A recent analysis of 17 randomized, controlled studies found that HRT did help with verbal memory *in certain patients*—specifically if a woman was suffering from other menopausal symptoms.[44]

If you can't recall somebody's name, pause in search for a word, or end up saying "you know, the whatchamacallit!" you can probably attribute that to lower estrogen levels.[45] Likewise, if you walk into a room and forget why (a short-term memory phenomenon), blame it on menopause! Sherwin and others have concluded that estrogen supplementation may help to maintain aspects of short- and long-term verbal memory in women at this time.

Other aspects of our memory and mental function have more to do with normal aging than with menopause per se. Information learned visually (such as someone's face) and spatial memory (as in giving someone directions to your house) do *not* correlate with estrogen levels.[46] (In fact, some studies have found that estrogen supplementation actually impairs spatial memory.) There is conflicting information about whether or not menopause has an impact on our ability to perform logical thinking, do math problems or have fast reaction times.

Estrogen has a number of effects that might explain why low or falling levels correspond to verbal memory problems. First, estrogen increases blood flow to the brain, which is awfully important when it comes to thinking. Second, estrogen aids in the organized flow of information (neurotransmitters) between brain cells. Third, estrogen helps us make a neurotransmitter called *acetylcholine*, which carries complex information such as words.[47] Given the fact that we are just beginning to study the role of female hormones and brain function, it's highly likely that we'll find many more links between estrogen and cognition in the future.

Estrogen and Alzheimer's Disease

Alzheimer's disease is the most common form of dementia in the Western hemisphere, with an incidence of over 5% of the population after age 70, and 24–40% after age 85.[48] Although some of the earliest signs can overlap with the loss of verbal memory (word recall) that occurs normally for many perimenopausal women due to low estrogen levels, additional functions of daily living become affected in Alzheimer's patients. Unlike normal memory disturbances, the memory impairment of this dementia can interfere with spatial or visual memory, and the ability to reason. Thus, people with Alzheimer's may get lost while driving, forget a face, or have trouble with instructions.

A handful of research linking estrogen and Alzheimer's disease has garnered enormous public attention. There is a connection: estrogen is involved in controlling the production of a protein involved in Alzheimer's dementia known as apolipoprotein E (apoE). Whether or not that translates directly into ERT preventing Alzheimer's disease is yet to be determined.

Very few studies on the matter have been performed to date. Some have found that women on estrogen were less likely to get Alzheimer's disease.[49,50] Another very small study found that women with Alzheimer's dementia improved their mental function when they were given estrogen.[51] However, a recent large study found no difference in Alzheimer's incidence between postmenopausal users and non-users of HRT.[52] Another study published in *JAMA* did not support its purported ability to slow the progression of Alzheimer's disease.[53] It is safe to say that our knowledge regarding the use of estrogen for Alzheimer's prevention is yet in its infancy. Yet, if you have a strong family history of Alzheimer's (which does have a genetic component) and are considering whether or not to take hormones, it's worth talking with your clinician about this. Note that the selective estrogen-like drug raloxifene doesn't offer help in this department. A recent three-year study of over 7,000 women found no benefit in terms of cognitive function for raloxifene over placebo.[54]

Many women are concerned about a rather rapid decline in memory, and worry that they are showing signs of Alzheimer's disease. This is *not* the case. Rest assured that the loss of verbal recall and short-term memory that most women routinely experience near menopause are not early Alzheimer's signs.

Ginkgo, Memory, and Alzheimer's

At 200 million years of age, ginkgo biloba is certainly one of the oldest surviving species of plants known to possess health benefits. It works by improving circulation, both to the brain and to the periphery of the body. Capsule doses of ginkgo are usually 120 mg per day, in two or three divided doses.

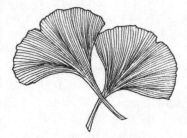

Several studies have shown the benefits of ginkgo biloba for memory. A four-week study in 1996 of patients with Alzheimer's type dementia found significant benefit of ginkgo over placebo.[55] A year long study, published in the *Journal of the American Medical Association* in 1997, confirmed ginkgo's long-term benefit in Alzheimer's patients.[56] Most studies on ginkgo are positive in this area, showing a 25% improvement in memory, concentration, and alertness within a 4–6 week period of use.[57] When compared to today's pharmaceutical drugs for Alzheimer's disease (tacrine or donepezil), ginkgo scores comparably in effectiveness, but has many fewer side effects.[58] Not all studies agree that ginkgo is effective for dementia, however.[59]

Ginkgo biloba (*Ginkgo biloba*)

Ginkgo does have blood thinning properties, which can also explain its effectiveness in patients who have problems with blood clots. However, this same action makes ginkgo contraindicated for patients on blood thinners, those with a history of hemorrhagic stroke, or for patients undergoing surgery. People with epilepsy should know that two cases have been reported that implicated ginkgo in re-triggering epileptic seizures.[60] Other adverse reactions may include mild gastrointestinal complaints and extremely rare allergic skin reactions.

Soy Isoflavones and Alzheimer's

A recent study indicated that soy may potentially be protective against Alzheimer's disease. Dr. Helen Kim of the University of Alabama divided 45 monkeys who had had their ovaries removed into three groups. Group one was placed on a diet high in soy isoflavones, group two on a diet without isoflavones, and group three on a regular diet and Premarin®. At the end of three years, the monkey's brains were analyzed for the content of special proteins essential in the development of Alzheimer's disease. Only those in the high soy isoflavone group had lower amounts of these proteins.[61] More studies are now needed in this area to uncover the effect of soy on the development of Alzheimer's disease.

Coming of Age

Thank goodness, we can now throw out the erroneous notion that menopause causes depression, and laugh at the suggestion that our lives are over after our reproductive years. More accurately, in menopause, personal creativity replaces "hormonal responsibility." When we put the ebbs and flows of our cycles behind us, we can harness more energy for self-development and spiritual growth. Author Gail Sheehy refers to this time as a "Second Adulthood."[62]

Yes, there can be challenges. It's normal to expect temporary mood fluctuations as hormones rise and fall with the tide of perimenopause. But are these always bad? The next time you have one, ask yourself "what constructive change could these emotions fuel?" They might be revealing a truth too long hidden.

It's also important to know the limits of emotional or cognitive changes we can accommodate. The wise woman knows that when she's overwhelmed, she gathers support. When we just can't maintain our balance, we gather information, guidance if needed, and use the excellent natural or conventional medicines available to us. Women with a history of depression or anxiety, or those who go through surgical menopause, especially, should stay tuned to their emotional state and seek help right away if mood disturbances set in.

Women now can expect to live one-third of their lives after menopause. This time can signal a maturing of our psyche, a coming into one's own, a time for putting those decades of life experience to work for us. We know who we are. We know what works, and what doesn't; what's important, and what isn't. We tell it like it is. At menopause we can choose to step into what Susun Weed calls our "crowning years"[63] wearing our wisdom proudly.

10 Breast Health

"**B**reasts are the most public, private parts of our bodies," writes Meena Spadola, author and producer of the documentary film *Breasts*.[1] We wear them right out front. Our culture fixates on them as defining womanhood and sends women mixed messages about whether we should flaunt—or hide them. It's little wonder that most Western women have an ambiguous relationship with their breasts.

"I believe that every woman has a breast story," Spadola continues, "and I don't mean a story *about* her breasts. I mean the story *of* her breasts." In the context of our culture, our breast story likely contains elements of pleasure, pain, nurturing, fear or judgment—and for some: loss. Losing a breast, or two breasts, to cancer can be particularly hard for Western women who inherit the culture's breast obsession. This would be a large enough trauma—but then comes the reality of facing life and death. As Harriet, one of the women interviewed by Spadola puts it, "You don't know until you die of something else that you've survived breast cancer."[2]

Breast cancer is the most common cancer in women in the United States with more than 180,000 diagnoses each year. That's the bad news. The good news is that we are diagnosing breast cancer earlier, and newer treatments include both less radical surgery and more successful medical therapies. According to the American Cancer Society, *more than nine out of ten women who discover and treat their breast cancer early are cancer-free five years later*. This means that many more women are surviving breast cancer and living well into the menopause years. Today, there are over 1.6 million women surviving breast cancer in the United States.[3]

Many women have concerns about the links between hormone replacement and breast cancer risk. Also, many women can't take hormones because of a personal or family history of breast cancer or other problems. In this chapter we'll explain what is known to date about this risk, and discuss alternatives to hormones for women wishing to stay off them. But before we delve into treatments, let's briefly review some important information about breast cancer risk, diagnosis, and treatment.

Preventing Breast Cancer

Most of the risk factors for developing breast cancer are out of our control. By far the most important risk factors for developing breast cancer are being a woman and growing older. Other known *unmodifiable* risk factors for breast cancer include prior breast cancer, a mother, sister or daughter with breast cancer, onset of menopause after age 55, and specific changes in genes.[4]

We do have the power to change other risk factors for breast cancer. Obesity, alcohol consumption, hormone use, radiation exposure to the breast, delayed childbearing and not having carried a pregnancy to full term are some areas believed to affect one's lifetime risk for breast cancer. Let's look more closely at each.

Childbearing

There's good news for natural mothers: childbearing decreases risk of breast cancer, possibly for three reasons. First, women who carry a pregnancy end up having fewer menstrual cycles than women who don't. This means the breasts are "exposed" to fewer cyclic estrogen changes over a lifetime, which decreases the risk of breast cancer. Next, going through a full term pregnancy causes the breast cells to fully "mature," through a process known as *differentiation*. These mature, fully differentiated breast cells are less vulnerable to the effects of future estrogen stimulation with menstrual cycles. Finally, high levels of *progesterone* produced in pregnancy may change the breasts cells' sensitivity to estrogen that provides some protection from breast cancer over time.

Radiation

Repeated exposure to radiation in the area of the breasts may increase the risk of breast cancer in the future. Here, we're talking about radiation treatments to treat cancers, like Hodgkin's lymphoma (which can be located in the chest)—*not* the radiation from mammography. We'll talk more about mammography later. During radiation treatments, the same high doses of radiation that are used to kill cancer cells can cause damage to the DNA of breast cells, setting up a scenario for breast cancer to develop.

Alcohol

Many things can go wrong in a body that could eventually activate abnormal breast cell growth. Alcohol has a unique ability to negatively affect *several* mechanisms for the initiation of breast cancer. Alcohol may increase breast cancer risk by:

* increasing the levels of estrogen in the blood
* stimulating liver metabolism of cancer causing substances
* easing the transportation of cancer-causing substances into breast cells
* activating *prolactin* release (a breast-stimulating hormone)
* impairing the immune system's ability to remove precancerous cells
* reducing our body's uptake and use of protective nutrients[5]

Diet

Author and naturopathic physician specializing in the treatment of breast cancer, Steve Austin, N.D., writes "Tell me what a culture eats, and I'll tell you its breast cancer risk."[6]

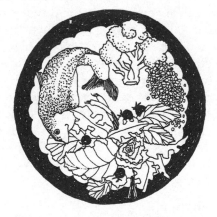

Dr. Austin is referring to the observation that cultures in which people consume unprocessed foods, lots of fresh fruits and vegetables, and very little fat and animal products experience less breast cancer than those on less healthy diets.

In general, traditional Asian diets are associated with very low risk of breast cancer, Mediterranean diets with moderate risk, and Western diets with a high risk. Sadly, we are now witnessing the increase in incidence in breast cancer in countries like Japan, as they adopt our Western lifestyle and dietary patterns.[7,8] A variety of studies have implicated red meat, saturated fat, alcohol, pesticides, and a high total calorie intake with higher breast cancer rates, while fiber, vegetables, soy foods, and those containing omega-3 fatty acids may be protective. We'll look at each of these separately.

Fiber

According to some studies, women who eat high fiber diets cut their risk of breast cancer roughly in half.[9,10] Fiber from vegetables and fruits show the greatest correlation with breast health.

One explanation for fiber's benefit has to do with the way a portion of our estrogen leaves the body via the digestive tract. On its way out, fiber traps estrogen and carries it out of the body with the stool. (See Figure 10.1.) In the absence of fiber, the more "free-floating" estrogen can be re-absorbed by the blood vessels that line the gut, and re-enter circulation. This "recycling" of estrogen means that our bodies (including, of course, our breasts) get exposed to this estrogen all over again.

Vegetables

A report in the *Journal of the National Cancer Institute* identified that women who ate their vegetables had lower rates of breast cancer.[11] In particular, vegetables high in the carotenes lutein, beta-carotene, and zaxanthin were beneficial. 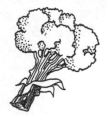 This study did not find added benefit from taking vitamins C or E, or folic acid in supplements. It seems that for breast cancer, the whole orange, not just vitamin C, helps keep us healthy.

Among vegetables for breast cancer protection, one family reigns supreme. Broccoli, cabbage, brussel sprouts, kale, and kohlrabi all belong to the broccoli family, and all assist in estrogen

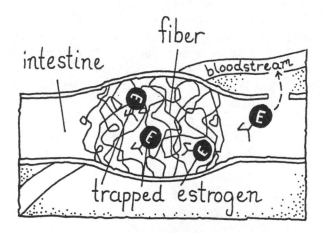

Figure 10.1. Fiber traps estrogen and carries it out of the body with the stool.

metabolism. A chemical found in this family of vegetables, known as *diindolylmethane,* speeds up the pathway that breaks down estrogen, rendering it inactive on breast tissue. The overall effect for someone who consumes a lot of these vegetables may be to decrease one's exposure to estrogen, and thereby decrease breast cancer risk.

There is controversy over the potential role of pesticides sprayed on vegetables and fruits regarding breast cancer risk. The most newsworthy of these chemicals are the organochlorine pesticides, like DDT, which can bind to estrogen receptors, including those in the breast. Although banned in the United States 25 years ago, DDT is still produced here and exported to countries from which we import produce. DDT and its by-products stow away in our fat tissue, and so concentrate in fatty places like the breast. Higher concentrations of DDE, a breakdown product of DDT, were recently found in the blood among Egyptian women with breast cancer when compared to women with normal breasts.[12] Breast feeding, which can deplete women of some of the fat in their breasts, may lower levels of DDT and DDE, and also lower breast cancer rates.[13]

The largest study to date assessing these types of pesticides and breast cancer, the Nurses' Health Study, doesn't support a correlation.[14] Upon a closer look however, it seems that factors, such as diet, ethnicity, body fat, menopausal status, breast-feeding history, and estrogen receptor status in women tested can all affect whether or not DDT and other estrogen-mimicking chemicals will impact breast cancer risk.[15] Timing of exposure affects risk too, as illustrated by a study of women farmers from North Carolina who had higher breast cancer rates if they had been exposed to DDT between ages 9–16.[16]

Organochlorines comprise but a few of the hundreds of pesticides and industrial chemicals that live in our environment and enter our bodies every day. While relatively few (compared to the numbers which are produced) chemicals have been proven to cause cancers, neither have they been proven safe. Chemical manufactures are not required to do exhaustive testing to prove the safety of a chemical before releasing it to the market. Rather, the "burden of proof" falls upon those concerned about its safety. If you are inclined to play it safe, you can consider peeled fruits and vegetables (like oranges and avocados) as better than unpeeled ones. Better yet, consider purchasing certified organic produce, now guaranteed pesticide-free due to strict, new organic standards in the United States.

Soy

This humble legume is the hottest food in research nowadays. Large population studies linking soy consumption to decreased rates of many kinds of cancers have fueled much of the interest. Scientists have set out to uncover what the active components of soy are, how they work, and how they can alter our risks of cancer.

In Chapter 4, we learned that soy helps with hot flashes and other vasomotor symptoms in menopause. The compounds responsible for this benefit are soy's phytoestrogens, *genestein* and *diadzein*, which bind to estrogen receptors in the body. When our own estrogen wanes, consuming these weaker plant estrogens can, in part, make up for the loss, allowing our bodies to feel like there's more estrogen around.

Researchers now believe these phytoestrogens explain, in part, why soy-eating populations have lower breast cancer rates. However, some recent reports have also indicated that these same phyto-estrogens can actually *increase* the growth of estrogen-sensitive breast cancer cells in animals.[17] This has led to a lot of confusion for patients. Are soy foods helpful or harmful for breast cancer?

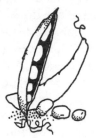

The answer depends on when you eat it, and whether or not you have active breast cancer. Soy has consistently been found to be beneficial in *preventing* breast cancer. For women who already have had breast cancer, or who have a strong genetic predisposition, the safety of soy is unknown. Let's take a close look how soy may prevent breast cancer.

As we advance our understanding about soy's phytoestrogens, we are seeing that how soy affects breast cancer risk has a lot to do with *timing*. Preliminary animal studies show that dietary exposure to genistein during gestation or before puberty protects against the chemical induction of breast cancer.[18,19] One explanation offered for this is that genestein causes some of the same types of changes in the breast that occur during pregnancy—which, as we discussed above, decreases a woman's breast cancer risk. Animal studies tell us that eating soy at puberty causes breast cells to more rapidly differentiate into mature, normal breast tissue.[20] This is an important point, because *poorly* differentiated cells are much more aggressive than mature, or differentiated cells if they become cancerous.

A second important thing to know about the timing of phytoestrogen consumption is this: consumed *over a lifetime*—especially all throughout the reproductive years, when our own estrogen levels are high, soy's phytoestrogens act to block our own estrogen from landing on estrogen receptors. This means the body has less exposure to the stronger estrogens, which lowers breast cancer risk.

While these explanations for the observed protective effects of soy are still under investigation, they do make physiologic sense. If further studies find soy's protective effects to hold true, then the recommendation for all females would be to start eating soy in childhood, replacing much of our meat based diets with the protein in soy (which is probably a healthy thing to do anyway).

It is important to note the lower breast cancer rates found in women who consume soy products occur in cultures where soy is eaten during a *whole lifetime.* We can't say that women who begin eating lots of soy products for the first time at menopause are going to receive the same benefits as lifetime soy eaters. One recent report did indicate that postmenopausal breast cancer patients had lower urine levels of soy's phytoestrogens diadzein and genestein than controls.[21] However, it's likely that the women without breast cancer had been consuming soy long before menopause, which could have accounted for their reduced risk.

The issue, again, is timing. First of all, by menopause, obviously our breasts are done "maturing," so genestein's effect on the creation of normal, mature breast tissue won't carry over into menopause. Second, the estrogen-blocking effect of soy's phytoestrogens may not benefit menopausal women, because we don't have much of our own estrogen around anymore. The possible exception to this might be in the case of obese women, who make considerable quantities of estrogen in fat tissue. There is speculation that for obese women, phytoestrogens could still decrease the "exposure" that the breasts have to the stronger estrogen, and be protective.

Soy's phytoestrogens are just a part of the story regarding its anti-cancer effects. Phytoestrogens aren't the only active components of soy. Another chemical in soy, *lignans,* have the ability to speed up the breakdown of estrogen in the liver, rendering it inactive on breast tissue. There are hundreds of studies being done currently on the exciting anticancer effects of the chemicals in soy foods. No doubt you will continue to see these benefits touted in magazines, on television, and even in your supermarket.

In summary, *soy foods consumed over a lifetime decrease one's likelihood of developing breast cancer.* We are unsure about whether or not this benefit extends to menopausal women. There is no plausible evidence that menopausal women who do not have breast cancer should avoid soy, and its many health benefits extend far beyond that of the breast. (Later in the chapter, we'll discuss soy use in women with diagnosed breast cancer.) We do recommend putting soy in context, however. When attempting to mimic the traditional diets of cultures where breast cancer is low, such as that of Asian women, keep a balanced approach. Fish, fresh vegetables, and few processed foods may have as much to do with the health benefits of these diets as does soy.

Fats

There has been much written about the potential role of dietary fat and breast cancer risk. So far, studies conflict and there is no definite conclusion about whether or not fat in general increases risk. One potential problem with these studies is that most lump all fats into one category. But as our knowledge of nutrition becomes more sophisticated, we now recognize that all fats are not created equal. The "bad fats," found in most animal products except fish (including red meat, eggs, and dairy products) have very different qualities when compared to the "good fats," from cold water fish and vegetable sources.

Salmon, mackerel, cod, halibut, and sardines are high in the healthy omega-3 fats. These "good fats" have been shown to inhibit the formation of blood vessels to newly growing tumors,[22] thus preventing their growth. Besides this "tumor-starving" action, dietary omega-3 fatty acids have been shown in laboratory tests to prevent normal cells from turning into cancer cells, block the growth of cancer cells, and help the body destroy cancer cells through a process known as *apoptosis*.[23] One study found that omega-3 fats, in combination with a purified extract of genestein from soy, suppressed the growth of breast cancer cells.[24] Omega-3 fats can also benefit the immune system by increasing the number of T-helper cells, a type of white blood cell that helps the body recognize foreign cells. As you can see, eating fish might well contribute to the low rates of cancer among those that eat a traditional Asian diet.

We also know that body fat itself makes estrogen, and that obesity increases breast cancer risk. Certainly, a high-fat diet can contribute to obesity. Americans typically consume between 30–45% of their calories as fat—most of it saturated animal fat. For a better approach to diet, limiting fat to 15–25% of calories, and selecting omega-3 "healthy fats" from fish may decrease risk of cancer as well as other chronic diseases.

Caffeine

Some authors claim that caffeine increases your risk of breast cancer. There is no evidence that this is true. Caffeine can contribute to fibrocystic changes in the breast, an extremely common thickening of normal breast tissue. Since these lumps are often tender, especially around the period, eliminating caffeine, from all sources (coffee, tea, including green tea, chocolate, and colas) can make a woman with tender breasts more comfortable.

Not surprisingly, when breasts are less tender and lumpy, women are more apt to do breast self-examination, and feel more confident about what they're feeling. Therefore, although caffeine does not have any direct impact on the development of breast cancer, remaining caffeine-free, if you are prone to fibrocystic breast lumps, can potentially make it easier for you to detect a real problem early.

Hormone Use

One of the most important issues for menopausal women, and in medicine today, is the evolving understanding of just how much (and which kinds of) estrogen affects breast cancer risk. Here's the current state of our knowledge.

Birth Control Pills

There has long been controversy about the possible link between birth control pills and breast cancer. After all, birth control pills do contain both estrogen and progestin. After many large studies over 40 years, there is no consensus on whether birth control pills increase a woman's risk of breast cancer. One thing is for sure: if birth control pills do have an effect, it is of small magnitude because it is so hard to prove.

As with every medication (and birth control pills are a medication), each woman has to weigh the potential risks and benefits of its use. On the positive side, birth control pills do provide excellent contraception and several other important noncontraceptive benefits including decreasing the risk of ovarian cancer, pelvic infections, and anemia, as well as cycle regulation. On the negative side, some women experience side effects such as breast tenderness, weight gain or headaches. Women can often eliminate these problems by switching to a different brand. The *potential* increase in breast cancer risk is probably too small to be factored into the equation.

Hormone Replacement Therapy

As studies continue to be published, more data points to the fact that longer-term use of hormone replacement in women after menopause increases the risk of breast cancer. One of the studies recently addressing the question of hormone replacement and breast cancer risk was published in the *Journal of the American Medical Association* (*JAMA*) in 2000.[25] This study included over 46,000 postmenopausal women and showed a slight but not statistically significant increase in risk of breast cancer over time in HRT users. Statistics say that breast cancer happens to one in ten—or 10 out of 100 women who live to age 80. (Remember though—because you are an individual and not a statistic, your personal risk factors will obviously adjust this number.) HRT increases this risk to 14 out of 100 women who would get breast cancer if they remained on HRT for more than five years. This translates to a 40% increase risk. In summary, five years of HRT does cause a small but noticeable increase in breast cancer. Less than 5 years' use of HRT (used primarily to control bothersome symptoms of menopause) conveys little or no increased risk.

Exercise

The largest study on exercise and breast health (using data from the Nurses' Health Study) has added to the growing evidence that routine exercise has a modest, but measurable benefit in terms of breast cancer risk reduction.[26] Exercise may lower breast cancer risk by reducing our number of ovulatory menstrual cycles and, thus, reducing the cumulative exposure to progesterone and estrogen.[27] Exercise's ability to enhance the immune system may also explain its effect.[28] And, women who exercise tend to

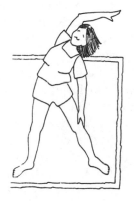

have lower body fat. As we saw above, fat tissue produces estrogen, which increases our overall exposure to this hormone, and may contribute to breast cancer risk.

Emotions

We hear a lot about how emotions influence our health in general. It shouldn't be surprising to hear then, that emotions might also affect our breast health. Interesting research has found that the psychological profiles of women with normal breasts, fibrocystic breasts, and breast cancer differ. Even more, there is evidence to suggest that one's state of mind can help determine how aggressive a breast cancer is, if it develops, and also our chances of survival.

In one study, women with all levels of breast health were asked to describe their own personality traits. Women with normal breasts fell into the category of "calm, relaxed, outgoing, and able to express anger."[29] Those with fibrocystic breasts had self-descriptions that indicated they were more tense and restless, and also more expressive, both of friendly emotions and anger, when compared to women without fibrocystic breasts. Women with breast cancer indicated they were less assertive, and more prone to hold emotions inside, such as anger. In the same study, the women with healthy breasts had less of a need for neatness and order than women with breast cancer or fibrocystic breasts.

There is also some evidence that one's personality could influence how aggressive a cancer is, if one were to develop. A group of Swedish researchers who had previously noted that personality traits correlated to the aggressiveness of certain types of brain tumors brought their research into the realm of breast cancer, where they obtained similar findings. Women with breast cancer who had an "outstanding psychological profile marked by extreme emotional reactivity as well as by genuine creativity" had more poorly differentiated ductal carcinomas.[30] As mentioned earlier, the more poorly differentiated the cancer cells are, the more aggressive the cancer is.

The emotional make-up of a woman at the time of a diagnosis of breast cancer can have an impact on her long-term health. Israeli researchers conducted an 8-year follow-up study of 40 women with a diagnosis of breast cancer and found the degree of psychological distress, anxiety, hostility, and paranoia experienced by patients at time of diagnosis correlated to how well they remained. The more anxious women were when diagnosed, the shorter they survived.[31] Also, emotions experienced during the months and years following a diagnosis of breast cancer have a strong correlation with survival. Researchers from George Washington University Medical Center found that women with metastatic breast cancer who did not suppress their emotions lived longer.[32] A study in the United Kingdom found that depression, and also the degree of helplessness or hopelessness a woman with metastatic breast cancer felt had a negative impact on her long-term survival.[33] Other studies have supported these findings, showing that women who are able to express their emotions have better survival rates.[34] Although there's much more study that needs to be done before we can come to any conclusions, the research so far supports the notion of healthy, balanced expression of emotions for breast health.

When we hear information like this, it's important to avoid the pitfall of blaming a woman with breast cancer for emotionally generating her problem. First of all, there are so many causes of breast cancer, almost no one can be sure what caused any one particular case. Secondly, blaming the victim is one way we attempt to push away our fears about death and disease. It's also a way to shirk responsibility from contributing to the culture's lifestyle, environment, and dietary patterns that increase breast cancer risk. Where information linking breast health and emotions *can* be helpful, is in motivating us to reflect individually on our emotional state, and take action to maintain our mental health. You might ask yourself "How could my state of mind be affecting my health?" Often, women have an instinctive knowledge of this link—and what we need to do about it.

Calculating Breast Cancer Risk

The National Cancer Institute (NCI) has developed a breast cancer risk assessment tool called the Gail Model. This tool involves a questionnaire addressing many of the above risk factors that provides an estimate of a woman's risk of developing breast cancer over the next five years and for her lifetime. This tool may be helpful to all women but is particularly helpful for women with multiple risk factors who may choose to participate in some medical prevention studies available for women at high risk of breast cancer.

The Gail model only lists factors which have been absolutely proven to increase risk, and for which researchers are able to fairly accurately calculate the risk of developing breast cancer using mathematics. They include age, race, age of first menstrual period, number of first degree relatives (mother, sister, daughter) with diagnosed breast cancer, age of first full term birth, and history of breast biopsies or abnormal tissue.[35] (The factors still under investigation, such as the role of diet and exercise, are not included.) Using responses to these questions, the NCI can calculate one's risk of encountering breast cancer within five years, and also by age 90. Log onto their handy website at http://www.nci.nih.gov for your own calculation, or phone them at 1-800-4CANCER for more information. Also, many OB-GYN offices have a special calculator with which to complete this assessment tool for you.

It is important to recognize that the risk of developing breast cancer (which is reported to be a risk of 1 in 10) is a *lifetime* risk. This means that you need to live to age 80 to be in the 1 in 10 risk group. The National Cancer Institute has also broken down a woman's risk of breast cancer by age. A woman's risk of getting breast cancer is:

- 1 in 2,525 by age thirty
- 1 in 217 by age forty
- 1 in 24 by age sixty
- 1 in 14 by age seventy
- 1 in 10 by age eighty

Again, keep in mind that these are statistical averages and your individual risk will vary.

Breast Cancer Screening

In the United States there are three basic components to screening for breast cancer: breast self-examination, clinical breast examination, and mammography. The American Cancer Society has recommended that women (over the age of 20) do a monthly breast self-examination, have a yearly breast examination by their medical provider, and have yearly mammography screening beginning at age 40.

Breast Self-Examination

Some recent discouraging reports state that breast self-examination doesn't decrease deaths from breast cancer. However, we recommend you not give up this screening method. For one thing, finding a cancer at an early stage can allow for more breast-conserving surgery.

Many women readily admit they don't know what a "normal" breast looks and feels like. Interviews with women who do not perform breast self-examination say that they are afraid of what they'll find, and also that they're not sure what they're looking for.[36] Other women fear breast self-examination as "looking for a problem" (see page 241). Let's discuss these points, and hopefully clear up some of these doubts.

Breasts are primarily comprised of fat and gland tissue. (See Figure 10.2.) The glands are made up of lobules or small clusters of tissue designed for milk production. For lactating women, milk is made in lobules deeper in the breast, then delivered to the nipple via milk ducts.

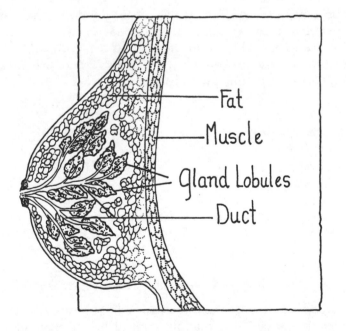

Figure 10.2.   The anatomy of the breast.

Just as women have many different sizes and shapes of breasts, they have different feeling to the breast tissue. Graphically speaking, breasts usually feel like lumpy mashed potatoes. Some women have breasts that are very soft and have minimal "lumpiness." Others have breasts that literally feel like bags of marbles (and are understandably more challenging to examine). You will likely find areas in your breasts that feel thicker or lumpier than others.

The best time to do your breast exam is at the end of your menstrual period, to avoid the lumpiness and tenderness that can increase before the menses. If you are not having regular periods, you might just choose the first of each month as your breast exam day.

To visually examine your breasts, stand in front of a well-lit mirror, such as one in the bathroom. Note that your breasts are probably (at least) slightly different from one another. This is normal—for, like fingerprints, no two breasts are exactly alike. Look for any changes in how your breasts look: lumps, dimpling, puckering or skin that resembles that of an orange peel. Place your hands on your hips and tighten the chest muscles, then relax and stretch the elbows behind you—looking for the same changes. (See Figure 10.3.) Raise your arms slowly overhead and see if both of the

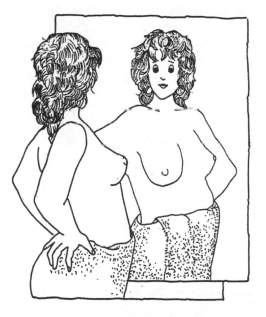

Figure 10.3.   Place your hands on your hips and tighten your chest muscles, then relax and stretch your elbows behind you to look for changes in the appearance of your breasts.

breasts rise on the chest, or whether one stays fixed in position. Normally, both breasts rise when the arms are lifted.

Some women find it helpful to do the feeling portion of the breast exam in the shower. Other women prefer to check the breasts while lying down. The important thing is to get familiar with your own breasts and be complete in feeling all the breast tissue.

One reliable way to examine the breasts is by using a back and forth pattern, moving horizontally across the breast, as shown in Figure 10.4. This method allows a woman to keep track of what she has already felt, and not leave any portions of the breast unexamined. Begin in the upper-outer portion of the breast, which extends all the way into the armpit. Place the flat portion of the middle three fingers on the skin, at an angle that's very close to the skin. (This makes the exam much more comfortable than using the tips of the fingers and "poking" into the breast.) Press downward, tractioning the skin and moving the fingers in small circles to feel the tissue underneath. Make a few circles with minimal pressure, a few with moderate and some with more pressure, feeling at superficial, moderate, and deep levels of the breast. As you get good at doing this, the process of feeling the breast in one area takes about two seconds.

Drag your fingers horizontally an inch toward the breast bone, and feel on all levels here. Repeat this action, using the pattern in Figure 10.4 to feel the breast tissue all the way to the breast bone, then beginning on the row below it, until you have completed feeling the whole breast.

Normal, fibrocystic changes tend to be mobile, tender, smooth lumps that get bigger or more tender before the period, and less so during menstruation. A distinct lump or a thickening that feels different than the sur-

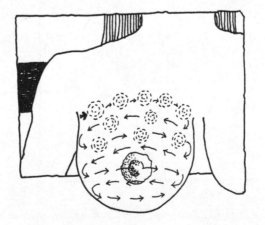

Figure 10.4.   Recommended pattern for breast self-examination.

rounding tissue warrants further investigation. This includes any distinct 3-dimensional change in the breast—meaning an area which seems to protrude outward rather than remaining relatively flat and smooth. New lumps which are firm or rough, rather than soft and smooth should be noted. If you find an area like this, it does not mean that you have cancer. It does mean that you need to have it evaluated by a health provider. *The vast majority of these findings do not indicate cancer.* In the minority of cases that do, early detection can be lifesaving.

The most important part of doing a breast self-exam is recognizing a persistent *change* in your breast (not including the monthly fluctuations that correspond to cycles). If you regularly examine your breasts, you will know them better that any health practitioner—and detect changes well in advance of any scheduled check-up.

Reframing the Breast Self-Examination

For some women, breast self-examination feels like "looking for a problem," and causes fear and consternation rather than reassurance. If you're among them, or if you think you won't realistically be faithful about breast self-examination, we have an alternative: the "Monthly Self-Appreciation and Massage." Taking aside five or ten minutes a month to give our breasts positive attention can benefit us on many levels.

The breast self-massage, according to author Susun Weed, "allows us to recognize normal breast changes without fear, and gives us time to respond thoughtfully to abnormal changes."[37] Like breast exam techniques, there are many ways to do breast massage. Weed includes a good one in her book *Breast Cancer? Breast Health!*[38] Basically, any pattern you use can encourage the normal function of lymph tissue and bring relaxation to the tissues. Stroking the tissue in the direction of the armpit will encourage drainage of lymph tissue. When we keep lymph channels open, we promote free movement of the white blood cells that scout for, and destroy abnormal cells.

Treat yourself to some nice massage oil, maybe even a candle, and always perform a breast massage in a relaxed environment. Although it may seem foreign at first, developing this kind of nurturing self-care can sometimes be an antidote to fears that may surround our breasts.

As you massage your breasts, note their unique geography. Your breasts are different from anyone else's. Here comes the most important part: take a moment to appreciate your breasts. As an active affirmation, tell them one thing you appreciate about them. Maybe it's how they make you look in your favorite dress. Perhaps they provided nourishment and transferred a healthy immune system to your child, or brought pleasure to you or your partner.

Approached in a positive light, some women will feel more inclined to really commit to the health of their breasts, and establish this routine check-in. When we know our breasts because we touch them regularly, we are more apt to notice changes. More as a by-product than as a goal, early detection of problems from an attentive, caring breast massage can help us maintain breast health.

Clinical Breast Examination

The clinical breast examination by your health provider is an important part of breast screening. Because the incidence of breast cancer increases with age, screening should continue life-long. The American Cancer Society recommends that from age 20–30 you have a clinical breast exam by your health care provider at least every 3 years and after age 40 each year. If you are still cycling, scheduling your visit for breast examination for the days right after your period can allow this exam to be more comfortable for you.

Mammography

Next in the screening category is the issue of mammography. Many women feel that they are at low risk for breast cancer and choose not to have mammogram screening because they have no family history of breast cancer. Unfortunately, a lack of family history of cancer by itself does not guarantee low risk. In fact, more than 80 percent of women who develop breast cancer have no family history of the disease. It is true that women who *do* have a positive family history for breast cancer have a higher risk of developing it, and the more close family members with the diagnosis (mother, sister, daughter), the higher the risk for the individual woman. You should discuss with your health provider your personal history and risks for breast cancer and decide on a screening interval that is appropriate for you. And again, since breast cancer increases with age, mammogram screening should continue life-long.

Many women are alarmed at the number of their friends and acquaintances that have been diagnosed with breast cancer. Some women believe that we are seeing an increased rate of breast cancer overall. Most authorities attribute part of the rise in breast cancer diagnoses to the increased number of mammograms being done; therefore, we are finding more breast cancers than we would have otherwise known about. Many new federal and state programs have been funded in the past 10 years that provide breast cancer screening for underinsured or uninsured women. As a result, women who would have foregone mammography in the past, are getting them—and breast cancers that would have gone unnoticed until they got much bigger are being found. So even though it *seems* like more breast cancer is occurring, it's really that breast cancer is getting *diagnosed* more frequently right now. The best part about the programs that fund mammograms for those who couldn't afford them, is that they allow us to find breast cancers at an earlier stage than they might have otherwise been found, meaning more women survive their disease. Recent studies of the effectiveness of mammography show that breast cancers are being found at an earlier stage, allowing for more breast-sparing surgery and likely better overall survival from breast cancer.

One issue for women in regard to mammography is the worry about exposure to radiation with yearly tests. Indeed, one should be wary of unnecessary exposure to radiation. Over the past 40 years, the amount of actual radiation exposure from mammography has decreased significantly. According to Susan Love, author of *Dr. Susan Love's Breast Book,* the amount of radiation exposure from one mammogram is less than the amount of radiation you would get by walking nude on a beach for 10 minutes.

Since the damage from radiation can cause free radicals, it may not be a bad idea to have some antioxidants in your system before you go, if you are concerned about the exposure. Several studies have documented the protective effects of antioxidants like vitamins C and E and beta-carotene against radiation damage. Although none of these studies have specifically been done on protection during a mammogram, it certainly can't hurt, and just might help, to take a dose of 2,000 mg of vitamin C two hours before your appointment.

About 15–20% of women who have mammography, actually will need to return for extra tests. This includes ultrasound, or additional views on mammography. *About 80% of abnormal findings on mammogram are not cancer* but are areas in the breast that require further testing to make a diagnosis.

One final point about mammography: like every test that you may have done, it is not 100% accurate in detecting breast cancer. If you or your health practitioner identify a breast lump yet the mammogram is "normal," the lump should have further evaluation with either ultrasound testing or biopsy.

Other Screening Techniques

For a number of years, researchers have been looking for an alternative to the radiation of mammography for breast screening. Thus far, things that have been tried include computed tomography (CT), thermography, magnetic resonance imaging (MRI), and position emission tomography (PET) scanning.

None of these techniques have yet proven superior to mammography in finding breast cancers. Each one of these options has a downside that precludes its use in breast cancer screening. For example, CT scanning uses far more radiation than mammography. Thermography (based on cancers giving off more heat than normal tissues) misses some cancers that do not give off heat. MRI is good at finding cancer, but unfortunately also highlights lots of other benign or normal tissue thickness. Thus, using MRI would cause women to undergo many more invasive tests than need be. It is also much more expensive than mammography. Finally, PET scans are not very good for showing exact abnormal areas clearly so that a biopsy could be done. As you can see, we have a way to go to find a more optimal breast screening tool.

Two up-and-coming techniques are on the horizon: digital mammography and ductal lavage. *Digital mammography* may soon offer much clearer pictures than conventional mammograms, without any increase in radiation exposure. In digital mammography, the film normally used for recording the breast image is replaced by an electronic X-ray detector. The electrical signal from the detector is digitized and stored in computer memory to form a digital image. This image can then be displayed and adjusted interactively by the radiologist to facilitate detection of small breast cancers. The National Cancer Institute (NCI) and the American College of Radiology Imaging Network (ACRIN) are launching the first large, multicenter study to compare digital mammography to standard mammography for the detection of breast cancer. The Digital Mammographic Imaging Screening Trial (DMIST), involving 49,500 women in the United States and Canada, will compare digital mammography to standard film mammography to determine how this new technique compares to the traditional method of screening for breast cancer.

For women who have a genetic marker for breast cancer, a new procedure known as *ductal lavage* may soon offer more thorough screening when mammogram and examination are normal.[39] Because more than 95 percent of all breast cancers begin in the cells lining the milk ducts, it makes sense to look for them there. With ductal lavage, a hair-thin catheter is inserted into a milk duct opening on the nipple (after application of anesthesia!) and a small amount of ductal cell fluid is withdrawn. A pathologist examines this sample for normal, precancerous, or cancerous cells.

In a recent clinical study, ductal lavage was performed on more than 500 high-risk women at nineteen prestigious breast cancer centers. Even though all of the women had had normal mammograms and physical exams within the twelve months prior to the study, atypical or precancerous cells were found in 15 percent of the breasts studied and cancerous cells in 5 percent.[40] (While most atypical cells do not actually progress to cancer, women with atypical cells are at a higher risk of developing cancer.) As noted breast cancer authority and author Dr. Susan Love says on her website, "With ductal lavage, we can find cells that are just *thinking* about becoming cancer." For more information on ductal lavage, visit www.susanlovemd.com.

Vasomotor Symptom Relief and Breast Cancer

If you have had, or know you're at high risk for breast cancer, you have likely been told that you should not take estrogen. In general this is the wisest course of action. However, there are currently several studies under way to address the safety of estrogen use in breast cancer survivors. Some health care practitioners believe it safe for these women to use a short course of estrogen, and factor in quality of life issues if symptoms like intense hot flashes, night sweats, and sleep disturbance are too uncomfortable, or prevent normal functioning,[41] and don't respond to alternatives.

Also generating concern among breast cancer survivors and their health care practitioners are black cohosh, red clover, and soy, all popular remedies among menopausal and perimenopausal women (see Chapter 4). We've undertaken to answer these concerns by analyzing all the data available to date regarding the safety of these products in women with a history of breast cancer.

Black Cohosh

While *Cimicifuga racemosa,* or black cohosh, works well for most women with vasomotor symptoms, its *effectiveness* for women with a breast cancer history probably depends on what other therapies they may be on at the same time. Columbia University recently undertook the first randomized, controlled study of black cohosh in breast cancer survivors. Symptoms like hot flashes did decrease, but not any more than in women taking placebo.[42]

In the above study, two-thirds of the women were on the powerful antiestrogen tamoxifen, which significantly contributes to hot flashes. One could certainly argue that tamoxifen confounded the results of this study, and call for a study of breast cancer patients who are not on tamoxifen, which hasn't yet been done. It makes sense to infer that women on tamoxifen will likely find little benefit from taking black cohosh, while women not on tamoxifen may see more benefit.

The good news is that black cohosh *appears* safe for women with a history of breast cancer. (Please note that the data here still relies on laboratory and animal studies—and we'll have definitive answers regarding human studies in the future.) Although black cohosh does possess a phytoestrogen named actein, the herb has demonstrated a lack of estrogenic effects in animal and other laboratory experiments.[43,44] Extracts of black cohosh have been applied to breast cancer cells in a laboratory, and shown to inhibit their growth.[45,46]

Scientists hoping to answer the question of the safety of black cohosh for women with breast cancer presented their findings at the 23rd International Symposium on Phyto-Estrogens at the University of Ghent, Belgium, in January 1999. One group had tested the German extract called Remifemin® with estrogen receptor-positive breast cancer cells in a laboratory, and found the herb did not stimulate growth of the cancer cells. Then, this same black cohosh extract was applied, along with estradiol to the cancer cells, and was found to inhibit the estrogenic growth effect of the estradiol. Finally, black cohosh extract was applied along with tamoxifen and estradiol to breast cancer cells, and was found to enhance the antiproliferative effects of tamoxifen.[47,48]

Recently, scientists have discovered that the body has at least *two types* of estrogen receptors. The pharmaceutical industry has used this finding to create a new class of estrogen-like drugs: *selective estrogen receptor modulators*, also called SERMS (see Chapter 11). SERMS have different actions, depending on their effects on these two types of receptors. Some herbal researchers speculate that black cohosh's anticancer effect is like that of the SERMS, a so-called phyto-SERM; that it behaves like an estrogen to relieve symptoms, but like an anti-estrogen to block cancer.

Red Clover

Red clover (*Trifolium pratense*), on the other hand, may not be as safe in breast cancer. In a recent laboratory study, breast cancer cells responded similarly to red clover as to estradiol.[49] The most prominent phytoestrogen in red clover, *formononetin,* promoted growth of breast cancer in mice. It should be noted that the concentration of red clover required to achieve this was several thousand times that of the estradiol, however.[50]

Soy

There's all kinds of conflicting information regarding the use of soy in breast cancer. Some articles tell women about soy's miraculous anticancer properties, and promote its use in cancer. Other sources warn against the danger of making an active breast cancer grow. When a woman has a diagnosis of breast cancer, the last thing she needs is a bunch of conflicting information about whether or not she should be eating soy! Let's see if we can straighten this issue out.

The confusion has arisen not only out of conflicting studies, but more often, out of misinterpretation of the data. It is pretty easy for anyone with a strong belief to interpret studies in a way that supports their belief. This is nothing new—it happens all the time in both natural and conventional medicine. Looking more deeply at the research, patterns begin to emerge. A little earlier we discussed how consuming soy over a lifetime has a protective effect against breast cancer. We also stated that the added benefit to breast tissue of healthy women who just start consuming soy at menopause is probably less, although it is likely a very healthy food for most women. However, *the safety of eating or supplementing with large amounts of soy products for women with known breast cancer is uncertain.*

Here's the story: Yes, the chemicals found in soy, when studied in a laboratory, have many, many anticancer properties. These include its antioxidant properties,[51] its ability to inhibit the formation of newly growing blood vessels to tumors[52,53,54] (a mechanism that cancer researchers are excited about these days), and its ability to induce cancer cell destruction.[55] But here's the caveat. *Different doses of genestein are proving to have different effects.*[56] Most of the positive studies are done on individual constituents in soy, such as genestein, given as a purified, high-dose single chemical. While the lower doses of genestein that we are able to get through diet do seem to prevent normal breast cells from transforming into cancerous ones, dietary levels do not show the ability to inhibit mature, breast cancer cells.[57]

Also, while very high concentrations of purified genestein do seem to slow down breast cancer cell growth, lower doses might actually cause breast cancer cells to grow.[58] The upshot of this is, women with breast cancer could potentially be encouraging its growth unless they ingested high amounts of purified genestein—and no one knows exactly how much that needs to be yet.

There's another issue here, too. According to animal studies, whether soy acts to inhibit or encourage growth of breast cancers depends on the concentration of estrogen in the system. Genestein increased the growth of human breast cancer tumors in mice that had their ovaries removed (you could think of them as "menopausal mice"), but not in mice with ovaries.[59] Other studies have found supporting data—that genestein can block the ability of estrogen to make breast cancer cells grow *if* there's estrogen around, but not if there's not.

You can think of phytoestrogens like this: if there's lots of estrogen around, they tend to weaken estrogen's effect. If there's not a lot of estrogen around, phytoestrogens may increase the estrogenic effects in the body. This may not be good for women with breast cancer—especially those in menopause. There are many beneficial effects of soy foods for other health issues, and in weighing these, some women may choose moderate consumption.

What we know about soy in active cases of breast cancer comes from laboratory and animal studies. It may not turn out to be the same for women. There are currently studies under way to evaluate this issue. Until they are published, and soy's safety in breast cancer seems more likely, we recommend that women with breast cancer be cautious about their soy consumption. Certainly, women should not consume supplemental soy powders or extracts until such time as we know what concentrations are likely to be beneficial, rather than detrimental.

Even if soy turned out to be safe for women with breast cancer, there is a question of whether or not it would even be effective for menopausal symptoms if a woman is on tamoxifen, which most breast cancer survivors take after initial surgery and chemotherapy and/or radiation. We know tamoxifen is an estrogen-blocker, meaning it stops estrogen from getting onto receptors. This is what causes many of the side effects of this drug, such as hot flashes. Tamoxifen can block soy phytoestrogens as well.

A study done at the Mayo Clinic found that 150 mg of soy isoflavones per day given to 155 women with breast cancer did not result in a lessening of their hot flashes.[60] The majority of the women studied (68 vs. 32) were taking tamoxifen. The same group published a study of vitamin E for hot flash reduction in breast cancer survivors. They found that vitamin E did *slightly* lower hot flashes. Here, 60% of the women were on tamoxifen.[61] In the face of tamoxifen's induction of hot flashes, these remedies provide little to no relief.

Nonhormonal Remedies for Vasomotor Symptoms

Simple options for temperature control include layered clothing, using a wet washcloth around the neck and purchasing a small fan and placing it on your desk or next to the bed. As we discussed in Chapter 4, you can sometimes control vasomotor symptoms by avoiding triggers such as hot rooms, alcohol, caffeine, and spicy foods, getting aerobic exercise, and using regular relaxation techniques including yoga, breathing exercises, and visualization.

If these measures do not provide enough control of hot flashes or night sweats, a few nonhormonal remedies may help.

Kava Kava

As discussed in Chapter 9, kava kava is very effective at relieving anxiety. Kava has also been used for hot flashes and night sweats. A German study found it to be helpful for both physical and emotional symptoms at menopause.[62] One advantage of this herb is that it contains no phyto-estrogens and, therefore, has no potential ability to fuel the growth of breast cancer. Note that kava should not be used with any other antianxiety medications or alcoholic beverages, or by persons with established liver disease.

Clonidine

Clonidine is a medication generally used to control high blood pressure. It seems to work by changing the brain chemistry that allows hot flashing to occur, resulting in decreased flashing by up to 50%. The major side effect of this medication can be dizziness from a drop in your blood pressure if you have normal blood pressure.

Selective Serotonin Reuptake Inhibitors

SSRI antidepressants such a Prozac®, Zoloft®, Paxil®, Serzone®, and Celexa® have been found to decrease flashing, some by up to 60%.[63] They can be a good choice, especially if a woman dealing with breast cancer is battling depression and hot flashes simultaneously. Side effects on low doses of the medications are generally minimal but may include insomnia and decreased sex drive.

Safe Treatments for Vaginal Symptoms

For women with a history or high risk of breast cancer, there are several excellent remedies for vaginal dryness, which can lead to discomfort during intercourse. These include:

- *Vaginal lubricants* as needed during sexual activity.
- *Vitamin E capsules,* which can be opened with several pin-pricks and inserted into the vagina, or the oil rubbed into the vulvar area. Insert one opened gel-cap nightly for two weeks, then use once per week as maintenance. Wear a pad, and underwear you won't mind staining on the nights you use vitamin E.
- *Regular sexual stimulation,* which promotes your own moisture.

If these are not adequate for comfort, you may consider several of the low-dose, topical estrogen treatments discussed in Chapter 8. Low dose estrogen which is applied to the vaginal area, has very little absorption into the rest of the body. Particularly the option of using estriol, the weakest of the estrogens, is a good one. Vaginal tissues respond readily to this weak estrogen, and low doses can relieve vaginal symptoms in as little as two weeks.

The Essence of Healing

Breast cancer is never easy. No woman who's gone through it would tell you that she'd ever want to do it again. And yet, many women with breast cancer are able to use this extreme challenge to create positive change in their lives. A diagnosis of breast cancer can prompt a woman to reassess what's important and to live her life more deliberately. Nancy, diagnosed with breast cancer at age 60, used the opportunity to heal an emotional rift between her and her daughter. "You suddenly get in touch with what's important," she explains. "I became less interested in 'being right' and more interested in sharing myself." Bea experienced a new depth to her relationship with her husband after her diagnosis of breast cancer. "I was really worried about how he would feel about me losing a breast. His tenderness showed me that it was *me* he was in love with, not my body. I'd say our relationship is more deliberate and deeper than ever."

Often, a breast cancer diagnosis motivates someone to pursue a very healthy diet, supplements, counseling, exercise, and other healthy activities. Women without breast cancer could learn much from watching and listening to their sisters, mothers, daughters, and friends who have gone through this challenge. The consistent message spoken and shown by those who encounter this challenge and pursue healing is this: *life is precious.* Why wait for a diagnosis of breast cancer before reassessing our life's priorities, and responding accordingly? If you were suddenly diagnosed with breast cancer, how would your diet and exercise routines change? What would you spend your time doing? Who would you spend time with, and how would the quality of that time change? For Nancy, it took breast cancer to spur her to reach out to her daughter, and to make important dietary changes, both of which enriched her life. If you're a woman without breast cancer, what would it take for you?

11 Hormone Replacement Therapy

Hormones are molecules that convey messages from one part of the body to another. We sometimes call them "chemical messengers" for this reason. Because hormones travel via the bloodstream, their messages can travel anywhere the blood flows. For example, one hormone abundant in childhood, known appropriately as "growth hormone" routinely makes the voyage from the brain to all growing body parts (including the most distant bones of the toes). Likewise, the hormone insulin leaves the pancreas every time we eat, and pays a visit to every metabolically active cell in the body. We owe much of the smooth functioning of our bodies to these miraculous and mobile little packages of information.

Reproductive, or sex hormones (mainly estrogen, progesterone, and testosterone) belong to a special family known as *steroid* hormones. All steroid hormones, by definition have similar chemical structures, using cholesterol as a starting-block. We actually need some cholesterol in our bodies to manufacture steroid hormones.

Figure 11.1 shows the structure of our three all-important sex hormones, along with cholesterol. Notice that it only takes minor variations to change a hormone from progesterone into testosterone and estrogen. (It's pretty amazing to see that the molecular differences between men and women boil down to only a couple of atoms!)

Sex hormones usually get carried around in the bloodstream by carrier proteins. These carrier proteins are known as sex hormone binding globulins, or SHBGs. You could actually think of SHBGs like little busses that cart hormones around.

Just as people passing through on a bus are basically watching the scenery, hormones that stay on their carrier proteins are merely watching

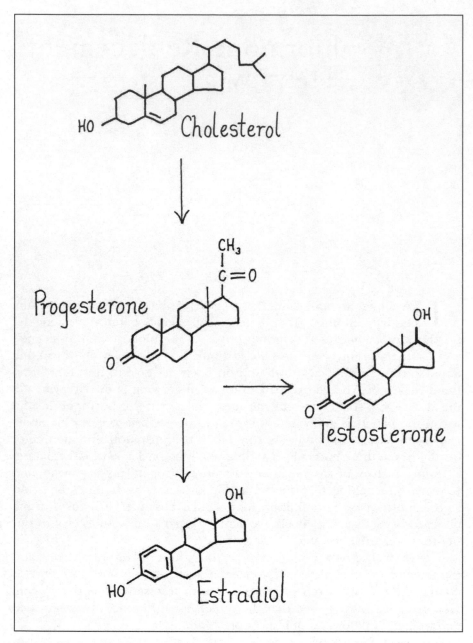

Figure 11.1.   The molecular structures of cholesterol, progesterone, testosterone, and estradiol.

the tissues pass by, and not affecting them. Only when a hormone "gets off the bus" can it deliver its message to the tissues. For example, estrogen riding on SHBG can pass right by the breast or uterus and not affect it. But if estrogen detaches from its carrier protein, it can deliver a message to these tissues. As we've mentioned earlier, hormones communi-

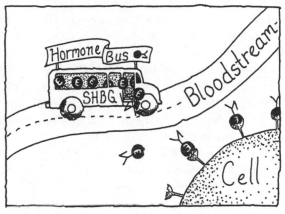

cate their messages by docking onto a receptor on the tissue's surface, into which they fit like a key into a lock.

Hormones and Lookalikes

We've talked about the fact that hormone receptors are shaped so that only "their" hormone can fit just perfectly onto their surface. For instance, progesterone and testosterone each have their own receptors, and can't bind to those of estrogen.

But, wait! We've also learned that the estrogen receptor, in particular, can accommodate some other molecules, like phytoestrogens. As it turns out, we now know of dozens of chemicals from hundreds of sources that can, and do, bind to estrogen receptors in the body.

This fact is keeping the natural and conventional remedy-makers busy, as they scramble to either discover or invent ever more intriguing "estrogenic" compounds for the booming menopausal market. But before any of us goes rushing headlong into taking *any* of these estrogenic compounds, especially over the long term, it would be wise for us to look at the bigger picture. Let's step back and see what we know so far about taking in estrogenic compounds as medicine or food, keeping in mind that taking ERT has been possible for less than a century. Perhaps even more important, let's find out what we still *don't* know about the effect of taking external estrogenic compounds into our own bodies.

The first synthetic compound discovered to act like estrogen in the body was diethylstilbestrol (DES), which was synthesized by British scientist and physician Edward Charles Dodds and his colleagues in 1938. Over the next three decades, doctors prescribed DES to 5 million women, mainly to prevent miscarriages, but also to suppress milk production after childbirth and alleviate hot flashes and other menopausal symptoms. It was touted by the pharmaceutical industry as a wonder drug, and at one time was promoted to obstetricians as an agent to ensure bigger, healthier babies for all pregnant women.[1] A generation later, we discovered the real impact of DES, as an abnormally high number of the *daughters* of women on DES came down with a relatively rare form of vaginal cancer. Some of the women developed added reproductive problems, such as an abnormally shaped uterus, which increases the risk of miscarriage. DES also contributed to abnormalities in sperm production in sons of women who took the drug.

As discussed in Chapter 4, the first estrogen-like compounds found in *plant* form were discovered during the 1940s, as sheep farmers in Western Australia planted red clover for feed. The sheep enjoyed this new delicacy, and red clover became their central food. Soon, however, infertility among the flocks appeared, and within 5 years, farmers were no longer able to breed their sheep. Following several years of research, scientists traced the problem back to the sheep's diet of red clover. As it turned out, one of red clover's ingredients, *formononetin*, could bind to estrogen receptors, which in this case interfered with the sheep's ovulation. Consumed in enormous quantity, this first known phytoestrogen acted like a contraceptive. Some scientists hypothesized that clover contained phytoestrogens as a survival strategy—to decrease the population of its predator!

Over the years, we've come to find that some pesticides, like DDT, endosulfan, and kepone (linked in some studies to increased rates of breast cancer),[2,3,4] bind to human estrogen receptors. So does dioxin and polychloro biphenols (PCBs), industrial waste products now ubiquitous in our environment and under investigation for their role in birth defects for certain animal populations.[5]

The potential ability of several industrial or agricultural chemicals to act on the estrogen receptors and affect fertility, sexual development, and behavior- and hormonally related cancers, has led to initial investigations by the National Academy of Sciences to assess the real threat of these "endocrine disrupters." However, it will be many more years, perhaps more than a generation, before we know the real impact of estrogen-like compounds in our environment, and not all the evidence is unanimous in assigning blame at this point. Also, information about any of their potential health hazards may encounter resistance. As then vice president Al Gore pointed out about these *xeno-* (or foreign) *estrogens* in 1997, "Because industrial chemicals have become a major sector of the global economy, any evidence linking them to serious ecological and human health problems is bound to generate controversy."[6]

Plant-based hormone-like compounds, like phytoestrogens (including formononetin from red clover, genestein from soy, and sitosterol from alfalfa) are under investigation for their various health benefits—but also as to whether or not they could contribute adversely to human health. So far, most of the phytoestrogens look pretty safe, and in fact have many healthy antioxidant and anticancer effects. However, as we saw in Chapter 9, *formononetin* from red clover, and soy's isoflavones may not, in fact, be safe for women with breast cancer. In addition, some practitioners question the use of soy for women with uterine fibroids, or endometriosis, because of the potential of phytoestrogen stimulation of these problems.[7,8] So far, these cautions are mainly theoretical.

There's a lot we don't know yet about consuming estrogen-like molecules. We are at the beginning—not at the end—of a push for more information about estrogenic compounds in our environment, our foods, and in the remedies we take. While consumers drive the current rush to find estrogen-related treatments for menopause—from both natural and pharmaceutical sources, it's also important to realize the newness of this whole arena.

Pharmaceutical drugs, whether conventional or natural, obviously fall into a different category from foods. The estrogens in HRT are, on average, 1,000 times stronger than even the strongest of phytoestrogens. It makes sense then that estrogen itself has a stronger impact on our long-term health when compared to that of phytoestrogens. For example, actual HRT has a much greater potential to increase bone density than any phytoestrogen. Correspondingly, its risks are greater.

We have yet to witness the long-range results of so many women using hormone replacement. Never before in the history of our world has this occurred. Will HRT turn out to be one of the greatest contributions to public health since immunizations? Many people think so. Or will we one day regret involving so many millions of women in this grand hormonal experiment?

In an effort to answer these questions, researchers have enrolled 25,000 menopausal women in a 10-year study of ERT. This trial, the Women's Health Initiative (WHI), will test the effects of ERT in many long-term, as well as short-term health conditions. If the results turn out to be positive, it is expected that HRT will be promoted as a "major preventive public health strategy for all postmenopausal women."[9] Results of this study won't be available until after 2005. Until then, it's important to remember that many questions about long-term hormonal therapy remain unanswered.

Making Your Choice

The discovery of estrogen receptors in almost every tissue in the body has led some scientists and doctors to propose that postmenopausal ERT can delay the effects of aging for every woman who can take it.[10] Many women are already experiencing considerable pressure from their doctors to use HRT. Sue is one such person. Having just experienced the loss of one of her best friends to breast cancer, Sue was wary about her gynecologist's recommendation. "I told him that I was uncomfortable with taking hormones," she relates. "He didn't ask me why, or give me any alternatives. He just bristled and was very short with me. I felt judged and disrespected."

We maintain that a woman's choice whether or not to take hormones—especially long-term—is a very personal and individual one. This choice deserves careful joint contemplation by a woman and her practitioner, *after* a thorough assessment of the risks and benefits hormones will likely give to her. *No* practitioner can promise you that any estrogenic or other type of medication, taken long-term, will absolutely be safe and without risks. We simply don't have all the answers to these questions, and we may not, during your menopausal lifetime. Precisely for this reason, *your intuition ought to be included, along with any advice from your practitioner, when deciding whether or not to take hormones.*

By now in this book, you have had the opportunity to assess your risk factors for osteoporosis and heart disease. In our final chapter you'll learn how HRT may affect other long-range health concerns which may or may not affect you. After you've done all the reading you can to inform yourself about your options, then schedule some time with your practitioner and request a conversation about these benefits versus risks. If you need to, don't hesitate to ask for some time to process the information you've learned and talked about, so that the choice you arrive at is indeed one you feel good about. Also important, while you listen to the advice, read up on the options, and weigh all the factors—don't forget to ask yourself—"Does this *feel* right to me?"

Short-Term Use of HRT

Distinguishing between short and long-term use of HRT can help a woman simplify her decision-making process. For women who just want to treat symptoms and either do not wish to use natural approaches (such as diet, herbs, supplements, and exercise) or are not helped by them, HRT is an option. From our review of the current literature, *using HRT for under five years, does not increase breast cancer risk.*

Following, we've summarized the benefits and risks of short-term HRT.

Short-term HRT is useful for:

• Menopausal symptoms not helped by natural therapies

The potential risks of short-term HRT include:

• Blood clots
• Gallbladder problems
• Increase in asthma symptoms (currently under investigation)

The nuisance side effects of short-term HRT include:

• Vaginal bleeding, possibly requiring further investigation
• Headaches
• Bloating
• Breast tenderness

A 1995 study found that asthma risk increased in women using post-menopausal HRT and that the risk increased further in users of longer duration.[11] However, other studies have shown just the opposite—that estrogen acts like an anti-inflammatory. In one study, women with asthma were able to wean themselves off high-dose steroids when they went on estrogen.[12] While the jury is out, it's wise to watch closely for any worsening of symptoms if you have asthma and begin HRT.

Long-Term Use of HRT

HRT use over five years does slightly increase breast cancer risk. The studies that show this have used Premarin® or conjugated equine estrogens as the standard. Below, we will discuss different forms of natural estrogens and what we know about them in terms of breast cancer.

New data suggests that long-term use of estrogen alone may increase the risk of dying from ovarian cancer. A study looking at 211,581 women over 10 years found that deaths from ovarian cancer increased the longer a woman remained on estrogen, and those using it over 10 years more than that doubled their risk.[13] Since most women on estrogen also take progesterone, the results of this particular study may not apply to most women who take HRT. (Progestin may be one reason why birth control pill use decreases ovarian cancer risk.) A prior article, which analyzed the pooled data from 17 studies on this subject *did*, however, conclude that estrogen with progestin use beyond 10 years was associated with an increased risk of developing ovarian cancer.[14] When the results of the large Women's Health Initiative trial come in, we'll be able to make more definitive statements about the impact of HRT on ovarian cancer risk. For now, it looks like (as in the case of breast cancer) there may be a small but noticeable increase in risk of ovarian cancer if a woman uses HRT for more than 10 years.

As for the benefits of long-term HRT, osteoporosis prevention rises to the top of many women's lists. Although HRT provides more benefit to the bone if it is begun at the onset of menopause, HRT use beginning between the ages of 65 and 74 still protects against hip fractures.[15] As to cardiac protection, we no longer recommend HRT as a front-line therapy for heart disease prevention. Estrogen's impact on Alzheimer's disease, which we discussed in Chapter 9, is still under investigation. Following is our summary of the benefits and risks of long-term HRT:

Long-term HRT is useful for:

- Osteoporosis prevention
- Prevention of colon cancer, macular degeneration, Alzheimer's (potentially)
- Heart disease protection in women without established disease

The potential risks of long-term HRT include:

- Slightly increased risk of breast cancer
- Slightly increased risk of ovarian cancer
- Increase in asthma symptoms (currently under investigation)
- All risks listed for short-term HRT

The nuisance side effects of long-term HRT include:

- All risks listed for short-term HRT but reduced

There is no consensus about how long women should take HRT. That's a good thing—because a lack of standard in this situation illustrates the fact that each woman is unique.

The Many Forms of Hormones

If you have chosen either short-term or long-term hormone replacement, the next step is to choose the form in which you want to take it. In the past, most menopausal women in the United States were routinely offered oral Premarin® (conjugated estrogen from horse urine) along with synthetic progestin, such as Provera®. Today, women are demanding more choices. They often cite personal philosophy, convenience, effectiveness, and lack of side effects as motivating their choices. The next section will give you the knowledge you need if you decide you want to be involved in choosing a hormone product.

Estrogens

Most conventional estrogen preparations are based on the structure of estradiol. In fact, many forms of estrogen today are biologically identical to the estradiol that your body produces. In other words, it's easy to find a "natural estrogen" that any practitioner licensed to do so can prescribe. Table 11.1 lists several of the more common oral forms of estrogen that conventional providers prescribe. Later, we will discuss forms of estrogen commonly prescribed by natural medicine providers.

Table 11.1. Selected Plant-Derived Oral Estrogen Compounds

Brand Names	Form	Dosage
Estrace®	estradiol	0.5–2.0 mg
Ortho-est®	estrone sulfate	0.625–1.25 mg
Estratab®	esterified estrogen	0.3–1.25 mg
Ogen®	piperazine estrogen sulfate	0.625–1.25 mg
Menest®	esterified estrogen	0.3–2.5 mg
Cenestin®	conjugated estrogens	0.625–1.25 mg
Estinyl®	ethinyl estradiol	0.02–0.05 mg

The doses in Table 11.1 are equivalent to 0.3–1.25 mg of Premarin®, the standard upon which the majority of large studies have been performed. As women are becoming more active in choosing the forms of estrogen they want to take, pharmaceutical companies have responded by putting out many forms of more natural, plant-derived hormone products which have the same effectiveness as Premarin®.

Many women find taking conventional estrogen in a patch form more convenient than oral prescriptions. Several of the more common patch forms of estrogen prescribed by conventional providers are listed in Table 11.2. Patches are placed on the abdomen or buttock and changed on an average of once or twice per week. Local skin irritation is an occasional side effect.

Table 11.2. Selected Estrogen Patches

Brand Name	Form	Dosage
FemPatch	estradiol	0.05–0.1 mg
Alora	estradiol	0.05–0.1 mg
Esclim	estradiol	0.025–0.1 mg

Estroderm	estradiol	0.05–0.1 mg
Vivelle	estradiol	0.025–0.1 mg
Vivelle dot (smaller patch)	estradiol	0.037–0.1 mg
Climara	estradiol	0.025–0.1 mg
Estradiol (generic)	estradiol	0.5–0.1 mg

People with either a family history or existing condition of high triglycerides should know that estrogens can increase this problem. Also, a history of abnormal breast tissue (see Chapter 10), gallbladder disease, or blood clots may make estrogen therapy contraindicated for you. Migraine sufferers also may find their headaches exacerbated by estrogen use. If any of these problems pertain to you, discuss them with your practitioner before deciding whether or not the benefits of ERT outweigh its risks.

Some providers who use both natural and conventional forms of estrogen report that women have fewer side effects with natural forms of estrogen. If one form of estrogen produces unwanted side effects, your health practitioner can help you find another that may indeed work better for you. Table 11.3 provides a reference for dose equivalents should you choose to switch from one form of estrogen to another.

Table 11.3. Relative Potencies of Various Oral Estrogen Preparations

Estrogen Preparation	Dose Equivalent
Micronized estradiol	1.0 mg 1x/day
Conjugated estrogens (Premarin®)	0.625 mg 1x/day
Ethinyl estradiol	5.0 mcg (micrograms) 1x/day
Tri-est	1.25 mg 2x/day

As women become increasingly conscious of the risks of hormones, they are demanding safer forms of therapy. One way the research community has tried to address this is by testing the effectiveness of lower doses of estrogen. An important study, done in 1997 by a group at the University of California Medical School at San Francisco, found that *half* the amount of estrogen given to 406 postmenopausal women for two years produced positive effects in bone and lipid changes.[16] The women did not experience overgrowth of the uterine lining, even without the addition of a progestin or progesterone to their regimen.

The hormone used in this study was a plant-based esterified estrogen. Similar studies using half doses of conjugated equine estrogens have been inconclusive with regards to preventing osteoporosis. Another contribution from this study addresses the issue that women often forego the benefits of HRT if they can't tolerate taking hormones. "Many women drop out of therapy after a short time because they don't like the side effects," commented the study's chief investigator, Harry K. Genant, M.D. However, Genant and his colleagues found the plant-based hormone used in this study caused less problems with headache, nausea or breast tenderness than typically found with conjugated estrogens. They proposed that women might stay on their HRT if it caused less problems.

If you are concerned about the negative effects of hormones, but still want their benefits, talk to your practitioner about low-dose HRT. Your practitioner will need to follow you closely in this, somewhat unproven, area. Appropriate monitoring for results on bone, via DEXA and possibly, urine NTx testing, as discussed in Chapter 7, can help guide you and your practitioner to make sure that this approach is working for your bones. We do advise adding a progesterone agent to your regimen until the safety of low-dose estrogen alone on the uterine lining has been more completely documented.

Estriol

So far, we've been discussing the most potent form of estrogen that the body makes: estradiol, along with its synthetic equivalents. However, estradiol is just one of *three* known estrogens that are found naturally in the body. Women have significant quantities of two other estrogens, *estrone* and *estriol*, circulating in their bloodstreams.

Over the last three decades, interest in the weakest estrogen in the body, estriol, has mounted. Estriol is mostly a breakdown product of the two stronger estrogens, estradiol and estrone, which the body keeps in equilibrium. (See Figure 11.2.) There is also evidence that estriol may be synthesized directly from the same building blocks that make the other two estrogens.[17]

Varied sources estimate that estriol is somewhere between one-quarter and one-twentieth the strength of the other two estrogens. It's relative weakness, and a few provocative studies, which we'll mention in a moment, have led some clinicians to wonder if estriol could be a safer form of estrogen than estradiol or its analogues.

Oral estriol is effective in relieving hot flashes, insomnia, vaginal dryness, and many other symptoms of menopause.[18,19] Doses are usually 2 mg/day, but have been increased to as much as 8 mg/day with side effects limited to transient vaginal bleeding. Topical preparations of estriol have

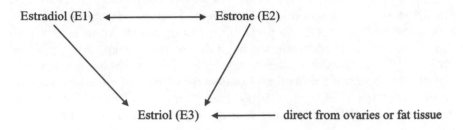

Figure 11.2.   Estriol is primarily a breakdown product of estradiol and estrone.

also effectively treated vaginal dryness, as well as improved overall skin elasticity and premenstrual acne.[20]

In Chapter 7, we discussed the scientific evidence for estriol's effect on bone. To summarize here, estriol has shown promise in some, but not all, of the small studies that have tested its effect for treating or preventing osteoporosis. It is still considered an unproven therapy in this area. Women choosing to use it for bone protection should be monitored very closely via DEXA testing and possibly urine NTx testing (see Chapter 7) to verify whether or not estriol is working for them.

Regarding heart health, we again have just a handful of studies from which to glean estriol's effect, although these preliminary results look positive. A Chilean study found that estriol has an important antioxidant ability with LDL—although less so than estradiol.[21] Small studies have found estriol at 2 mg/day to decrease total cholesterol, increase HDLs, and actually *decrease* triglycerides (in contrast to conjugated estrogens, which raise them)[22,23] for women between 70–84 years old. Other preliminary studies suggest that estriol may not have the same blood clot problem as estradiol.[24]

Regarding the safety of estriol, it has been shown not to affect blood pressure, weight, Pap smears, and mammograms in postmenopausal women taking between 2 and 8 mg/day of estriol for 6 months.[25] The safety of "unopposed" estriol in uterine cancer risk has yielded conflicting results, so we do recommend using some progesterone agent along with any systemic estriol supplementation.

In January of 1978, a provocative commentary appeared in the *Journal of the American Medical Association*. Entitled "Estriol, the Forgotten Estrogen?" its author, Dr. Alvin Follingstad of Albuquerque, New Mexico, made a case for using estriol, even when HRT was contraindicated, such as with breast cancer.

Follingstad pointed out studies in which populations with low breast cancer rates showed higher urinary output of estriol.[26] He also cited the work of Henry M. Lemon, M.D., who showed that estriol reversed breast cancer in animal studies.[27] When Lemon and colleagues tested estriol for safety in women with existing breast cancer, they unexpectedly observed that 37% of those women actually went into remission while on estriol. (It is curious to wonder why this particular study of Lemon's was never published.) Follingstad asked his AMA colleagues more than two decades ago, "Do we indeed have a safer and possibly a noncarcinogenic estrogen that has been neglected, one that can be administered orally, maintains its unique identity, and is as effective as estrone or estradiol?"[28] Natural medicine clinicians and only a handful of researchers have been trying to answer that question ever since.

Studies of estriol have been limited to small numbers of women, and absolute safety is, therefore, unknown. Supporters of estriol frequently point to studies that have shown populations with a high urinary output of estriol to correlate to lower breast cancer rates. But estriol (a breakdown product of estradiol and estrone), leaving the body via the urine, doesn't tell us how much was actually in circulation in the bloodstream. Unfortunately, no studies exist which correlate blood levels of estriol with breast cancer rates. Also, in contrast to the findings of regression of breast cancers in women on estriol by Lemon, another group found that estriol, like estradiol and estrone, indeed activated breast cancer cells in a laboratory. When the estrogen-blocking drug, tamoxifen, was added to this experiment, it was not able to keep estriol from activating cancer cells.[29] Clearly, much more investigation needs to be done before we can say whether or not estriol is safe for women with breast cancer.

Tri-est/Bi-est

"Tri-est," or triple estrogen, is a compounded prescription HRT, comprised of all three of the estrogens the body makes. It became popularized by pioneer nutritional medicine physician Jonathan Wright, M.D. Tri-est formulations typically contain 10% estradiol, 10% estrone, and 80% estriol. Dr. Wright supports this particular formulation with the argument that it reflects the ratios of the estrogens in normal, cycling women. Urinary levels, and his recent study involving blood level testing of estradiol, estrone, and estriol support this ratio.[30] The logic behind Tri-est is that women are receiving mostly estriol—the potentially safer estrogen which we just discussed, with a little of the stronger estrogens thrown in to presumably give it more kick—to help with symptom control and also bone protection.

To date, there are no significant studies that have been done on Tri-est. (For a discussion of why there are so few studies done on natural alternatives, see page 264.) This fact limits our ability to make strong statements regarding its effects and safety. However, it certainly is possible to determine many of their effects in individual women, by watching what happens to symptoms and following the various parameters that assess the desired result. For example, if a woman is taking Tri-est for bone health, bone density, and urine cross-fiber, testing can give you an indication whether or not it's working.

Why are there so few studies on natural alternatives?

Industry estimates put the research costs of bringing a new drug to market between $350 and $500 million dollars.[31] Drug companies can afford to invest in these studies because they are guaranteed to recover their investment by maintaining exclusive rights to sell a new drug (patent rights) for several years before the drug becomes generic.

In the United States, any compound found in nature, such as estriol and phytoestrogens, cannot be patented. Very few drug or supplement companies can afford to "bring to market" a natural compound by fronting the research dollars required before the FDA will approve the use of a certain remedy.

By contrast, natural products are eligible for patent in Germany. Many German drug and supplement companies can fund these studies, for they will then have exclusive rights to sell a particular formulation of a natural substance. Much of our knowledge about herbal and other natural remedies comes from these German studies.

Funding for studies continues to be a controversial area of discussion. Many consumers wonder about the link between using pharmaceutical industry dollars to validate pharmaceutical approaches to health, and call for more independent funding sources for research. It may, in fact, require a major change in the way medical research is funded in the United States before natural (unpatentable) approaches ever earn the research attention they deserve, and that consumers and practitioners are now demanding.

Tri-est is available through compounding pharmacies, which can literally make any dose your practitioner orders for you. Many women find it helpful to be on a form of HRT that is amenable to small increases or decreases in dosage. While the usual starting dose of Tri-est is 1.25 mg two times per day, an experienced practitioner can easily adjust this dose, using your symptoms and hormone levels as guides. See page 291 for the contact information of a compounding pharmacy in your area.

Tri-est is most commonly given orally, and can be compounded in the same capsule with progesterone or other hormones that we'll discuss below. Tri-est and all compounded hormonal preparations can be delivered orally, via capsules, under the tongue as drops or dissolvable pellets, or topically as creams or vaginal suppositories. The abundant and creative delivery methods of Tri-est increases the chances of finding an appropriate and individualized form of HRT.

All naturopathic physicians are trained in the use of Tri-est. However, only those naturopathic physicians in states licensing naturopathic medicine can write this prescription. If you can't find a practitioner who is familiar with Tri-est and can prescribe it, you may need to do a little legwork if you think this form of HRT is for you. For some women, teaming up with a naturopathic physician and a conventional provider who are willing to exchange information and work together on your behalf is the ticket. For others, find a conventional practitioner who is willing to learn about how Tri-est works. Compounding pharmacists are usually more than happy to provide practitioners with information.

Although we usually hear of Tri-est in terms of natural HRT from compounding pharmacies, many practitioners have begun favoring a slightly different preparation, dubbed *Bi-est*. Bi-est contains estriol and estradiol only, usually in a ratio of 80/20. Some natural medicine practitioners prefer to leave estrone out of the prescriptions because of estrone's reported stronger effect on breast cancer cells. While an intriguing idea, we really don't know if this makes much of a difference, simply because the body readily converts estradiol into estrone and vice versa. Therefore, there may be very little difference between Tri-est and Bi-est after all.

For selected forms of natural HRT used by natural medicine practitioners, see Table 11.4.

Table 11.4. Selected Forms of Natural Estrogens Used by Natural Medicine Practitioners

Brand Name	Form	Dosage
Ostaderm® cream	1:1:8 ratio of estradiol, estrone, and estriol	2 mg total estrogens + 65 mg progesterone per ½ teaspoon
Tri-est oral capsules	1:1:8 ratio of estradiol, estrone, and estriol	1.25 mg 2x daily
Bi-est oral capsules	2:8 ratio of estrone and estriol	1.25 mg 2x daily
Estriol oral capsules	Estriol	1–2 mg 1–2x daily

Progesterone/Progestins

In Chapter 1, we learned that our ovaries make progesterone after ovulation for women who are still cycling. Progesterone performs a crucial function there; to stabilize the endometrium that has grown in response to estrogen stimulation.

In menopausal estrogen supplementation, progesterone is usually added to the formula, mainly for the purpose of protecting the uterine lining. Without progesterone, "unopposed estrogen," supplementation can lead to overgrowth of the endometrium and possibly uterine cancer. When both estrogen and progesterone are given, we trade in the common term "ERT" (estrogen replacement therapy) for the broader term "HRT," or hormone replacement therapy. HRT refers to the fact that the prescription contains more of the complete balance of the female hormones. Table 11.5 presents a sampling of estrogen/progesterone combination products and what they contain.

Your practitioner may choose to add progesterone to your HRT either continuously, or conversely, in a cyclical fashion, which mimics the body's own timing, depending upon whether or not you're still having periods. Cyclical progesterone is more likely to promote regular bleeding, whereas continuous progesterone works better for women who have long stopped having periods. These indications are not carved in stone, however, and there are many good reasons why your practitioner may recommend one style over another. The most important thing to address is that you are getting enough progesterone to safeguard against overgrowth of the uterine lining.

Progestins

In contrast to natural estrogen, which is readily absorbed by mouth, natural progesterone is relatively difficult to absorb orally. To address this, pharmaceutical companies have developed a class of synthetic compounds that behave like progesterone, but are much easier to get into the bloodstream if taken in a pill form. These compounds, *progestins,* have been the only form of progesterone available in regular pharmacies until very recently. They include drugs like Megace®, Cycrin®, Amen®, and Provera®.

Many women tolerate progestins well. Others may have problems with bloating, breast tenderness, drowsiness, depression, or bleeding irregularities. Two progestins, medroxyprogesterone acetate and norethindrone acetate, have been specifically designed to resist breakdown into metabolites that can cause dizziness and drowsiness.[32] Progestins have also been shown to blunt the positive effect on blood cholesterol that estrogens can achieve. Asthma, epilepsy, migraine headache, and heart failure have been known to worsen in rare cases of women on progestins.[33]

For women who cannot tolerate side effects of oral or transdermal progestin or progesterone, there now exists another option—the progestin intrauterine device (IUD). Mirena®, an IUD which contains levonorgestrel (a synthetic progestin) is used for contraception, but may turn out to be a good choice for HRT in some women. Its protective effect on the endometrial lining is not yet established, however. Studies coming soon will most likely confirm this effect.

Because of potential side effects, most clinicians do not prescribe a progesterone agent along with estrogen for their patients who have undergone hysterectomy. After all, without a uterine lining to protect, isn't progesterone just an unnecessary addition?

In most cases, the answer to the above question is "yes." However, some women can potentially benefit from the addition of a progestin or progesterone even if they don't have a uterus. This includes primarily women with a history of endometriosis or women at high risk for osteoporosis. In the case of endometriosis, which is an abnormal growth of the same type of tissue which lines the uterus in areas outside of this location, adding a progestin for 6–12 months can potentially keep this tissue from causing symptoms. For osteoporosis protection, despite a lack of absolute proof, there is nonetheless some evidence that progestin or progesterone may positively increase bone density.[34]

Table 11.5. Selected Estrogen/Progesterone Combination Products

Brand Name	Form
Oral	
Ortho-Prefest®	1 mg bio-identical estradiol + 0.9 mg norgestimate
Activella®	1 mg bio-identical estradiol + 0.5 mg norethindrone acetate
Femhrt®	5 mcg ethinyl estradiol + 1 mg norethindrone acetate
Prempro®	0.625 mg conjugated equine estrogen + 2.5 mg medroxyprogesterone acetate
Premphase®	0.235 mg conjugated equine estrogen + 5 mg medroxyprogesterone acetate
Transdermal	
CombiPatch®	0.5 mg bio-identical estradiol + 0.14 mg synthetic progestagen
CombiPatch®	0.05 with 0.25 mg norethindrone acetate

Natural Progesterone

Micronized progesterone is the preferred progestin until new information points
to another choice.

                    Ken Gray, M.D., World Congress on Osteoporosis 2000

As women have become increasingly interested in natural medicine, the desire for a form of natural progesterone has grown. Since 1980 in Europe, *natural micronized progesterone* has been available. In this form, progesterone is delivered in small enough molecules to at least partially evade destruction in the gastrointestinal tract. Taken in doses of 200 mg 12–14 days per month or 100 mg every day (for cycling vs. menopausal women, respectively), natural micronized progesterone does enter the bloodstream at levels sufficient to protect the lining of the uterus.

Until recently in the United States, oral natural progesterone was only available in specialized compounding pharmacies. Today, it is also available at regular drugstores, with the brand name Prometrium®, and any clinician who works with women's health should be familiar with it. Because Prometrium® contains a base of peanut oil, women with a peanut allergy should avoid it.

Women often report a preference for natural progesterone over its synthetic counterpart. In a study at the Mayo Clinic, 176 women on micronized natural progesterone who had previously taken synthetic progesterone as part of their HRT were surveyed. After one to six months, the women reported an overall 34% increase in satisfaction on natural progesterone when compared to their previous prescription of progestin.[35] The natural progesterone also controlled breakthrough bleeding better than progestin. Lead researcher, Dr. Lorraine A. Fitzpatrick, believes the metabolites of synthetic progestins account for many of their side effects. By contrast, she explains that "With natural progesterone, the substances are believed to be the same as if you were making the hormone yourself."

Other reports have echoed the findings at Mayo. Natural micronized progesterone has been shown to be void of side effects common to synthetic derivatives, such as fluid retention, breast tenderness, weight gain and depression.[36] Recent reviews of the topic point out that "all comparative studies to date conclude that the side effects of synthetic progestins can be minimized or eliminated through the use of natural progesterone."[37] These findings on natural progesterone have led many physicians to conclude that natural micronized progesterone is, in fact, a better choice than progestin for menopausal HRT.

Natural progesterone may rank superior to progestins when it comes to the heart, too. All hormones delivered by mouth go through extensive breakdown in the intestines and liver. Paradoxically, this metabolism issue is the reason why orally administered estrogens improve lipid profiles, and why oral progestins blunt the effect. Several metabolites of progestins are close cousins of testosterone, which may partly explain why progestins can increase the (bad) LDL cholesterol, and reduce (good) HDLs. In one study, women who took a low dose of natural micronized oral progesterone 23 days of the month along with 0.625 conjugated equine estrogens showed a better lipid effect than progestins normally produce.[38] In another study, women on natural progesterone with conjugated estrogens had decreased cholesterol levels after one year, while the group on synthetic progestin did not. Both those on progestin and those on natural progesterone saw a rise in (good) HDLs.[39] It is conceivable that more study of *natural* progesterone may again flip our (currently unfavorable) view of HRT on heart health.

Women on natural progesterone may notice side effects of either gastrointestinal disturbance (because larger doses are needed for absorption) and/or the same drowsiness or even depressed mood that appear sometimes with progestin. Many women report either minor side effects that disappear within a few weeks, or none at all. Taking the hormone at night, before bed, can eliminate the occasional problems with drowsiness.

Natural Progesterone Creams

In Chapter 2, we addressed the potential use of progesterone creams for "perimenopausal PMS" and bleeding problems. For women in menopause, the benefit of progesterone creams alone (without estrogen) is unclear. As we mentioned in Chapter 7, progesterone creams do not provide reliable protection against osteoporosis. Anecdotal patient reports about their effect on hot flashes, libido, vaginal dryness, and other symptoms are not yet verified by studies.

In the past ten years, very aggressive marketing campaigns have convinced many menopausal women that natural progesterone cream is a risk-free, natural alternative to conventional hormone replacement for menopause. *Natural progesterone creams are not risk-free.* Their over-the-counter availability has led to an attitude that they do not require supervision. Natural progesterone is a steroid hormone. You should always talk to your clinician about this, as well as any other hormone, before you begin taking it. If you choose to use it, there are a few things that you should know. This section will provide you with guidelines for the safe use of progesterone cream, as well as information about how well it actually works.

Progesterone applied to places such as the forearms, chest, belly, and thighs via a cream does make it to distant places—such as the saliva and blood. We are less certain about *how much* progesterone is absorbed in cream form, *how long* that process takes, and how much of it gets to various tissues. A small Australian study found that a *single* dose of 64 mg of natural, micronized progesterone did show up in the saliva, but not in the blood or urine.[40]

Whereas a single dose of progesterone cream may not make it into the bloodstream, repeated use apparently does. A study of 19 women supplemented with 40 mg/day for 42 days showed a small rise in serum progesterone levels.[41] This study also showed that there was no difference in blood levels whether women applied the cream all at once, or in two divided doses.

In another study, six postmenopausal women on estrogen patches applied 30mg/day of progesterone cream for two weeks, and doubled their dose for the next two weeks. Blood levels of estrogen and progesterone both rose accordingly. This trial, done at Oregon Health Sciences University, noted that blood progesterone levels differed from one woman to the next in the same way that estrogen levels did. However, like estrogen, blood progesterone levels were consistent within each woman. The researchers concluded that natural progesterone cream did effectively deliver progesterone into the body.[42]

Blood levels of any supplemented hormone are affected both by how fast we absorb them, and how fast we break them down. Progesterone takes a long time to cross the skin and make it into the bloodstream, and not so long to be then carried to the liver to be broken down. Skin permeability does not allow the 25 mg/day that the body would normally produce during peak luteal phase to be absorbed.[43] In other words, because the skin absorbs progesterone so slowly, levels of this hormone never get as high as they would in a normally cycling woman.

If you're a perimenopausal woman, still cycling (making your own progesterone) and not taking estrogen, the questions about progesterone absorption aren't usually that important. However, if you are in menopause (and therefore not making your own progesterone) and on some form of actual estrogen (even in cream form), this question becomes critical in terms of protection from uterine cancer. To ensure safety, we have to guarantee that enough progesterone actually gets to the uterus.

No standard for blood levels of progesterone have been set for guaranteeing endometrial protection. Even if progesterone cream administration resulted in pretty decent blood levels of progesterone (which it doesn't seem to), we wouldn't know what blood levels to look for. Therefore, *we caution any postmenopausal woman on estrogen that progesterone creams are not guaranteed to protect you from endometrial overgrowth or cancer.* If you are taking estrogen, and are completely intent on taking progesterone in cream form, it is prudent to have an endometrial biopsy taken at least once per year, and more often if abnormal bleeding occurs. If you take estrogen, we think you're better off avoiding the problem, though, and using a delivery method of natural progesterone proven to protect the uterus.

Also, you may have noticed that the studies that have been done on natural progesterone cream involve tiny numbers of subjects: 6 women here, 19 women there. Until interest in progesterone cream attracts big research dollars, we'll only have what amounts to preliminary data. Much larger studies need to be conducted before we can say with any assurance what effects natural progesterone cream has in menopausal women.

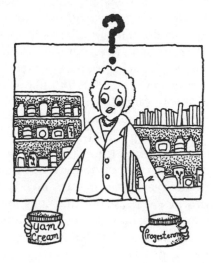

One final point about natural progesterone creams: all products are not created alike. In fact, the progesterone content of over-the-counter creams varies widely—from less than 2 mg to over 400 mg per ounce. If it isn't labeled, you may need to call the manufacturer to find out the amount of progesterone contained in any certain brand.

The best advice on the use of over-the-counter progesterone products is simply this: don't do it without adequate supervision. If you cannot be guaranteed that a wild yam cream (see below) is progesterone-free, don't take that either. Remember that progesterone is a steroid sex hormone— in the same category as estrogen and testosterone. It has risks and contra-indications. For example, some breast cancers are progesterone-sensitive, and therefore may possibly grow faster by using these creams. A woman should take a steroid hormone only if she knows about its risks and has good supervision. Prudently prescribed and followed, natural progesterone can be a very valuable remedy. Improperly used, it may be unsafe.

Wild Yam Cream

"Wild yam creams," popular over-the-counter remedies marketed to women for hormonal symptoms, have created confusion for many women. Some distributors have actually advertised that wild yam extract converts itself into progesterone in the body. Some authors have also made this statement.

Wild yam contains a chemical known as diosgenin, a compound used as a laboratory starting point in the synthesis of progesterone. Laboratory manipulation turns diosgenin into progesterone, but your body can't. *The conversion of wild yam extract into progesterone in the body is physically impossible.*

Misinformation has led some practitioners to refer to the whole product line as "the yam scam."

Wild yam, in its natural plant form, has been used medicinally by native North and South Americans for hundreds of years. It acts as an antispasmodic and relaxant, and as such is great for uterine and abdominal cramps. It may have other actions upon women's hormonal environment that we do not yet understand, but it doesn't increase a woman's levels of progesterone. A recent double-blind, placebo-controlled, crossover study (in which each group of women had three-month trials of both wild yam cream and placebo) found no improvement in menopausal symptoms with wild yam cream.[44]

Here comes another twist: many so-called "wild yam creams" on the market are just that—creams containing wild yam only. However, *some* of these creams are actually spiked with progesterone. Because levels below a certain concentration are deemed in the "cosmetic" rather than "therapeutic" category, the FDA does not require these progesterone-enhanced products to disclose that they contain actual hormone. In other words, you won't always know by reading the label whether or not a cream has progesterone in it. Many women, such as Felicia (see below), are, in fact, taking progesterone, a steroid hormone, without knowing it!

Felicia

At 48, Felicia suffered from severe PMS. After reading some consumer information about wild yam cream for PMS, she decided to give it a try.

During her first month on the cream, Felicia felt a marked improvement in her previous symptoms. By the second month, however, she noticed that while she wasn't as irritable anymore, she found herself feeling a little more depressed than usual. She decided to get some guidance.

Felicia went to her holistic chiropractor and relayed her story. "Let's see what's actually in this cream," he said. He telephoned the manufacturer and learned that this "wild yam cream" actually contained 400 mg of natural progesterone per ounce of cream, and that Felicia was actually taking about 60 mg of progesterone daily, in cream form. Because one possible side effect of progesterone is depressed mood, Felicia's chiropractor recommended she find another approach to her PMS. She was grateful to find the cause of her blues, and a little angry that the label of her "wild yam cream" did not mention any contents of progesterone.

Progesterone Gel

Gynecologists currently use a prescription gel form of progesterone, administered vaginally, called Crinone® for fertility and cycle regulation in premenopausal women. In the future, Crinone® may become FDA approved for HRT. This form of delivering natural progesterone is showing much more promise than progesterone cream applied to the skin for predictability and absorption. Blood levels of progesterone go up higher when women use it vaginally as compared with even intramuscular injections, which are highly absorbed. Even better yet, there's direct transport from vagina to uterus.[45] This may mean that women will need to take relatively little for progesterone to do its all-important job of protecting the endometrium from too much estrogen stimulation.

If inserting a vaginal gel seems less convenient than popping a pill—consider this: Swiss researchers found that women only needed to insert vaginal progesterone gel either days 1–10 of the month *or* just twice per week during the whole month to protect their uterine linings from continuous estrogen.[46]

Androgens

Androgens are the steroid sex hormones that we typically link to men. However, researchers, clinicians, and women themselves are getting increasingly interested in the role they may play in women's health. Let's explore what we now know about these hormones, and in particular, testosterone and dehydroepiandrosterone (DHEA).

Testosterone

Testosterone is the most famous androgen. Until recently, testosterone was indeed thought of as important only to men. Recently, however, researchers have found that testosterone is important in women's sex drives, sense of well-being,[47] and perhaps also bone density.[48] Some researchers suggest that even PMS may relate to lack of testosterone in women.[49]

As we learned in Chapter 8, menopause has not been shown to universally cause testosterone levels to drop.[50] Nonetheless, some individuals can develop signs of testosterone deficiency, and even demonstrate low blood levels of this hormone. For women who have a true deficiency, testosterone supplementation can sometimes be helpful. Natural testosterone can frequently be compounded into a natural HRT prescription or prescribed separately. It is also available in pharmaceutical combination with estrogen. In Chapter 8, we detailed the use, dosing, and effects of testosterone replacement for women with a loss of sexual desire, which is by far the most popular reason it is prescribed for menopausal women.

Dehydroepiandrosterone

Dehydroepiandrosterone (DHEA) is another so-called "male" hormone that is receiving new attention. It is actually a precursor of both estrogen and testosterone, into which very tiny amounts get converted. In addition, DHEA is involved in numerous functions, ranging from insulin regulation, to immune system enhancement, to metabolism. DHEA seems to play a supporting role—kind of a "behind the scenes" hormone, in these functions. Of course, it is always possible that DHEA only *appears* to be a minor player because of our lack of knowledge about it. We are only beginning to understand this hormone, and to ask the question of whether or not it has a place as a treatment option in menopause.

DHEA levels in women, as well as men, decline gradually with age. Unlike estrogen, DHEA does not drop dramatically right at menopause. An Australian study found that women's DHEA levels were more closely related to their body mass than to their menopausal status: the larger women were, the more DHEA they made.[51]

Despite the fact that menopause itself does not cause a drop in DHEA, some clinicians find that this is a convenient time to measure it, and consider supplementing women with DHEA, as part of a "total hormone picture." Some reasons one might consider testing DHEA levels include signs of androgen deficiency, such as extreme fatigue or loss of sexual desire. Of course, it is important to consider thyroid, depression, diabetes, and other important clinical entities before assuming that low DHEA is at fault.

DHEA has been studied for its effects on menopausal symptoms. A dose of 50 milligrams per day of DHEA given to women for six months resulted in significant improvement in all menopausal symptoms, especially vasomotor symptoms such as hot flashes. Despite the fact that estrogen levels had risen in these women, they did not show any increase in endometrial tissue growth.[52]

DHEA has also been studied for its effect on bone. Specifically, we have preliminary evidence that elderly people with low blood DHEA levels can enhance their bone density by supplementing with DHEA. In a study of 20 women and 16 men, with an average age of 74, 50 mg/day of DHEA given over six months, increased bone mineral density by 1.6% of the total body and 2.5% in the lumbar spine.[53] The researchers hypothesized that DHEA's effect here may have to do with its conversion to testosterone.

One word of caution here: DHEA has been shown to have negative effects on blood lipids in some women, and to date, there is a lack of study regarding how much DHEA is actually safe for women. Therefore, if you are considering its use, it's a good idea to have your blood lipids checked before and after beginning the medication. In most cases, only women who have already demonstrated a deficiency in blood levels of this hormone should consider using it, and levels should be monitored to prevent overdosing. Currently, we lack data regarding the safety of long-term dosing of DHEA.

Designer Estrogens

Every woman who considers hormones in menopause is faced with the dilemma of weighing their pros and cons. "If only there were a way to receive the benefits without the risks . . ." The pharmaceutical industry has been investigating (albeit not altruistically) a way out of this bind. The discovery that estrogen receptors in different parts of the body are not exactly alike prompted much research. What if we could design a molecule that acted like estrogen some places, and didn't act like estrogen other places? That offered benefit to bones, heart, and for symptoms, with none of the risks?

Look out—here come the designer estrogens!

Selective Estrogen Receptor Modulators

Beginning with tamoxifen, which was approved by the FDA in 1977, scientists created a class of drugs known as the Selective Estrogen Receptor Modulators, or SERMS. These drugs bind to estrogen receptors, but have different effects, depending upon which tissue they act.

Tamoxifen, which is used most popularly as an anti-breast cancer drug, binds to estrogen receptors in breast tissue but does not activate it. This is extremely helpful for women who have a history of an estrogen-sensitive breast cancer. Any estrogen that happens to be floating around in her bloodstream (such as that from fat tissue production), is blocked from binding to breast tissue if tamoxifen is occupying that receptor site.

However, while effective at treating and preventing breast cancer, tamoxifen has an opposite effect on the uterus. Women taking it experience an increase in endometrial cancers (12 more cases per 1,000 women) than women not on tamoxifen.[54] Statistically, this number is outweighed by tamoxifen's effect of decreasing breast cancer recurrence, and this fact underscores its near universal recommendation in breast cancer.

Tamoxifen has an effect similar to estrogen's in reducing (bad) LDL cholesterol by about 20%. But unlike estrogen, it does not increase HDLs. A very small amount of evidence indicates that tamoxifen may help bone, but we'll have to stay tuned to find out more on this issue. Also, serious blood clotting problems have cropped up in 10 more cases per 1,000 women when tamoxifen use is compared with placebo.[55] As you can see, while it indeed works as an effective drug in the treatment of breast cancers, tamoxifen is not our answer in the search for "the perfect estrogen" for menopausal women.

Like tamoxifen, raloxifene (Evista®) was first developed as a potential treatment for breast cancer. However, its initial approval by the FDA in 1997 was actually for the prevention of osteoporosis. Raloxifene is a step closer to our "perfect designer estrogen." It has a positive effect on bone growth and lipids (though less so than HRT), while decreasing risk of breast cancer and not affecting uterine cancer rates. Clinical studies over a two year period, which involved 12,000 women in 25 countries, showed that raloxifene increased bone mass by 2–3%.[56] That's about one-half as effective as estrogen. As we saw in Chapter 7, alendronate (Fosamax®) is also more effective than raloxifene in this department. Still, raloxifene can be considered a good choice if your goal is to prevent bone loss, rather than necessarily add density.

Small studies have reported that raloxifene lowers LDL cholesterol, although less so than HRT. To further investigate its impact on heart health, the drug's producer, Eli Lilly & Company, is conducting a study of raloxifene in 10,000 women over age 55 who have high risks of heart disease. At the end of this 7½ year trial, we should have more definitive answers about raloxifene's effect on lowering cardiovascular risk.

So far, it's sounding like raloxifene is a less potent, safer analogue to estrogen. There are a few glitches, however. Raloxifene may actually increase hot flashes. It also does increase risk of blood clots. Finally, raloxifene, as all the SERMS, doesn't have a long track record. Many researchers are cautioning against adopting them as viable alternatives to HRT because of the limitations of our knowledge. For now, we can say that raloxifene is a good choice for women at high risk for breast cancer who want a proven, conventional treatment for osteoporosis.

"PhytoSERMS"

While the search for the "perfect estrogen" continues, research into the various effects of different phytoestrogens speeds along too. As it turns out, neither are all *phytoestrogens* created equal. Rather, like estrogens, phytoestrogens also act differently in different tissues.[57] This means, for example, that one may have effects in the breast and not in the uterus, and vice versa.

Much of the research on plant estrogens in health centers not only on locating the tissues where various plant estrogens work, but on what *concentrations* have positive or negative effects in terms of activating receptors. It's becoming quite clear that dietary concentrations affect tissues very differently than do those found in high-dose extracts (as we learned in Chapter 10).[58] For example, an isoflavone found in licorice was found to have different effects on breast tissue, depending on the concentration.[59] The same was true for the effect of genestein (from soy) on uterine tissue.[60] In addition to breast and uterine tissue, ongoing research is gradually enlightening us as to the effects of various concentrations of different phytoestrogens on heart, bone, brain, blood vessel, vaginal, skin and other tissues. Today, the race to find an ideal, safe, selective "estrogen" from the plant world rivals that of the pharmaceutical world. What we are witnessing is none other than the quest for the perfect "PhytoSERM."

Tailoring an HRT Regime for You

It's little wonder why the majority of women "placed" on hormone replacement therapy at menopause discontinue within two years. Women have largely not been invited to become active participants in the decision-making process around whether or not to take them. Neither have the majority of practitioners encouraged their patients to learn about all of their choices, whether conventional or natural.

Whatever choice you make around HRT, it's important that you feel you are making an informed decision. This means being presented with options and clear information—both about what we know, and *don't* know about hormones. Most important, you both *deserve* and *need* to be included in this critical decision-making process. Finding a practitioner who has the ability and interest to spend time with you and welcomes your participation can go a long way toward helping you make choices that feel right.

Sue, who we met earlier in this chapter, had been turned off by her doctor's abrupt proclamation that she needed to be on hormones, and his lack of interest in discussing the matter further. She made an appointment with a different practitioner and explained her hesitation about hormones to her new doctor. "This one took the time to hear about my fear of breast cancer," she said. "She talked to me about the real risks, and we also decided to get a bone density test to see if I really needed hormones or not. When it came back, I saw that I wasn't as immune to osteoporosis as I had thought. She also took the time to help me find a dose and a form of hormones that I felt were the safest possible ones. I feel a lot better about taking hormones now."

Because Sue's second doctor had spent some time with her, hearing her concerns and doing a more thorough job of assessing her actual situation, Sue could get on board with her eventual decision to take hormones. As an active participant in the process, she is now much more likely to follow through with her plan. Even if she and her new doctor had decided that she would be fine on herbs, calcium supplements, and exercise, she would have been much more likely to stick to them and reap their benefits than if she had only been left with the less-positive experience with her former doctor.

Because so many different forms of hormones are now available, there

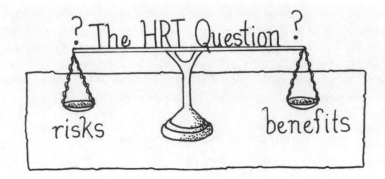

is even more reason to take time to evaluate your options, even if you have already decided to take hormones. Depending on your personal philosophy or your experience with previous hormone prescriptions, you may want to discuss whether natural or conventional hormone preparations would work best for you.

Lastly, you do have options regarding how to take the hormones. The most common methods of taking hormones are pills and patches, and just about every provider is familiar with these delivery methods. If you are interested in alternative delivery methods, work closely with your practitioner to make sure your prescription is working. Remember also that hormone prescriptions are changeable. You may start out with one form, and decide to try another if it causes unwanted side effects for you.

The decision whether or not to be on hormones is an important one. Even women who decide to take hormones for a short period of time are subjected to increased medical visits and are at increased risk of medical procedures, such as endometrial biopsy, if bleeding or other adverse reactions become a problem. Some women resist this kind of increased dependence on the medical system. There's a definite trade-off in regard to using hormones. HRT can be an important part of a wellness plan, and even a lifesaver for some—and it does come with some potential risks. Each woman will need to decide, in the balance, which way the scale tips for her.

For women making a decision about long-term therapy, it is especially important to take time, gather information, get a thorough assessment, and feel good about the support and the advice you are getting. The more thoughtful your decision-making process is, the better your chances are of actually following through on a plan that will work for you.

12 New Frontiers

Hormone replacement is a hot topic in research nowadays. With women living longer and continuing active lifestyles (and also with money to be made in the pharmaceutical industry), research dollars abound for those studying other ways to put HRT to use in menopausal women. Most of the new discoveries—but not all—show HRT's health benefits. We are learning that HRT affects areas of the body such as the colon, eyes, ovaries, lungs, and even teeth and gums. These findings will soon expand the discussion of HRT use in postmenopausal health beyond just that of osteoporosis and heart disease. For a glimpse at what lies ahead, let's take a look at emerging research to get a peek into what the future holds for long-term HRT use in menopause, and what natural alternatives might contribute in these same areas.

Colon Cancer

Colon cancer is the third most commonly diagnosed cancer *and* the third leading cause of cancer deaths in women (after breast and lung cancer) in the United States. Statistically, the "average" (whoever that is!) woman has about a 6% chance of developing colon cancer in her lifetime, which means about 1 in 16.[1]

Having a positive family history of colon cancer, and especially having a known inherited genetic problem linked to colon cancer, puts someone at much higher risk for the disease. According to data published by the Memorial Sloan Kettering Cancer Center in New York City, genetic make-up accounts for approximately 50% of colon cancers. The other 50% are attributed to lifestyle patterns, including diet, weight, and exercise; and therefore highly preventable.[2] Some researchers put the impact of life-style even higher than genetics.[3]

Initial screening for colon cancer involves a simple home-collection kit which tests for blood in the stool. Two much more invasive techniques, known as *sigmoidoscopy* and *colonoscopy* employ the use of a thin tube containing a camera which a doctor inserts into the rectum, allowing her or him to visualize the actual bowel wall. Alternatively, some doctors may choose to recommend a special kind of X-ray instead of sigmoidoscopy or colonoscopy.

Admittedly, none of these tests sound appealing. However, they are the best means of detecting colon cancers early—when they are *highly curable.* We are moving into an era in which colon cancer screening may become just as important as screening for breast or cervical cancer. We expect that within 10 years, we'll see screening colonoscopy recommended routinely beginning at age 50 for everybody. Fortunately, if you have a "clean" colonoscopy or barium enema and you do not have a known genetic pre-dispositon to colon cancer, these tests will probably only need to be done every 10 years. Your primary health care provider can recommend the exact interval of screening for you, based on your medical history.

Hormone Replacement Therapy and Colon Cancer

While colon cancer isn't typically what one would consider a "meno-pausal" issue, growing evidence of the impact of HRT on its risks may soon influence women's decisions about whether or not to take hormones long-term. Studies in the last ten years indicate that hormone replacement therapy may help protect women against colon and rectal cancer. In the Minnesota Cancer Prevention Research Unit Case-Controlled study published in 1996, women on hormone therapy had a 66% lower risk of having precancerous *polyps,* or growths in the colon when compared to nonusers. Women who stayed on HRT longer than 5 years had the lowest risk—and this lowered risk persisted for up to 5 years after stopping HRT.[4] A similar trend was seen in follow-up in the "Leisure World Study" where more than 7,700 women were followed for 14 years and the rate of colon and rectal cancer was decreased by 35% in those women who were currently using HRT or had recently used hormone therapy.[5] In addition to these two individual studies, there are two large meta-analysis studies (compilations of other studies that show trends) that report a 35–55% reduction in colorectal cancer in women who are currently using HRT or have recently used HRT (having stopped within the past 5 years).[6]

You might ask "How can hormones decrease colon cancer risk?" The real answer is—we don't know. Scientists have posited a few theories, however. The first involves the way hormones affect the *bile acids.* Bile is a strong, green digestive fluid made by the liver, and stored in the gallbladder, which literally gets squirted into the bowel when we eat. As a necessary digestive "juice," bile helps us digests fats. Unfortunately though, even the normal process of digestion involves its transformation into acids that can produce cancers. It seems that hormones like estrogen and progesterone can decrease the concentration of the bile acids and therefore provide some protection to the cells lining the inside of our colon.[7] Questions about what other effects this action may have on digestion remain unanswered.

A second theory by which HRT may protect against colon cancer is via estrogen's direct action on the cells that line the inside of the colon. Estrogen has been shown to act as a "tumor suppressor," actually blocking the growth of colon cancer cells.[8] Whether these or other mechanisms end up explaining HRT's effect on colon cancer overall, the evidence seems to point toward prevention.

Exercise and Colon Cancer

While HRT may decrease risk of colon cancer by 35–55%, exercise may have at least as much effect. Researchers at Brigham and Women's Hospital and Harvard Medical School analyzed the research published up till 1997 regarding physical activity and colon cancer. After excluding all other variables (such as diet) from the studies, they found that *people who had a high level of physical activity consistently had a 50% lower risk of colon cancer as compared to those more sedentary.*[9]

Diet and Colon Cancer

Our affluence in the West may come with a price on our colons. Relative to "developing" nations, which have lower rates of colon cancer, *Westerners eat from a menu that basically defines every food pattern proposed to increase colon cancer risk.* The Standard American Diet (nicknamed the "S.A.D." by nutritionists) contains a virtual parade of potentially risky foods: high intake of meat, fat, chemicals and alcohol, along with low intake of vegetables and whole grains. While the evidence links some of these factors more strongly than others, some patterns have emerged which can guide us in being safe, rather than sorry, with our diets.

First on the list of suspicious foods is *fried meats*. Every kind of fried meat (even fish) provides a primary dietary source of chemicals known as *heterocyclic amines*.[10] Studies have shown consistent generation of colon cancer when animals are exposed to these chemicals in their diet.[11] The obvious moral difficulties with testing this out in humans may make data in people slow in coming. Therefore, many researchers and nutritionists say "Why wait?" Broiling and baking meat, poultry, and fish saves the worry and may augment your health. (Hint: When grilling, wrap meat in tinfoil first to prevent charring, which causes heterocyclic amines to form.)

While initial reports found *fruits and vegetables* to be protective against colon cancer, more recent data has toned down these claims. An analysis of the Nurses' Health Study found no correlation between intake of fruits and vegetables and risk of colon cancer.[12] Other studies, while still showing a protective benefit of these foods on colon cancer risk, state that it may be less than once thought.[13] However, because of the known health benefits on breast, heart, and many other parts of our bodies, we still recommend a healthy amount of vegetables as a regular part of a diet.

Essential fatty acids from fish and vegetable sources rank as healthier than saturated animal fats in regard to colon cancer.[14] *Alcohol* in general has been correlated with increased rates of colon cancer, although red wine may be less damaging.[15] *Grains* may be protective in colon cancer. The Japanese have seen their incidence of colon cancer increase dramatically between 1950 and 1995. Researches have found a dietary correlation. They identified a "drastic" reduction in cereals during this time as the primary dietary change.[16] Other investigations have found rye bread[17] and wheat bran[18] to lower colon cancer incidence.

The effect of *chemicals* in our diet, such as pesticides, preservatives, and coloring are currently under study.[19] Preliminary data in small studies have linked colon and rectal cancer to higher blood levels of pesticides DDE (DDT),[20] beta-hexachlorocyclohexane (beta-HCH), and hexachlorobenzene (HCB).[21] The data on chemicals and colon cancer risk is small, and the risk so far unproven by conventional standards. Increasing our awareness of the potential effects of chemicals will certainly hasten further study.

Combined Benefits of a Healthy Lifestyle on Colon Health

In medicine we tend to separate out factors (such as dietary components, exercise, and weight) to understand their individual contribution to health and disease. However, it's important to keep a global perspective on how our lifestyle choices affect health.

Most women have had the experience of making one healthy change, and watching others come along with it. Data accumulated by the Memorial Sloan Kettering Cancer Center support a *combined* protective effect of several lifestyle factors in colon cancer risk. In other words, together, high fat intake, inadequate consumption of fruits and vegetables, and lack of physical activity may combine with being overweight to contribute to the generation of colon cancer.[22] Therefore, healthy choices that we make overall can augment one another.

Also, it's more important to establish healthy lifestyle *trends* than it is to focus obsessively on "getting everything right." Kicking back with some Ben and Jerry's once in awhile isn't going to do you in. (But the attitude that you can't relax dietary rigor once in awhile might!) Rather, it's what you do *most* of the time, not every minute, which can help determine your health in the long run.

Osteoarthritis

Many women experience minor aches and pains that seem to come on right about the same time as perimenopausal symptoms. We believe that *osteoarthritis* may account for at least some of these aches. Osteoarthritis results from the normal wear-and-tear of our joints over time. Because we live in a world with gravity—just the mere act of living on Planet Earth will induce some degree of this wear and tear for everyone. In fact, the only species thought to not see the effects of osteoarthritis are those which typically hang from trees upside-down—such as certain species of bats!

Osteoarthritis is more prevalent in women than men, and *increases* corresponding with the onset of menopause.[23] Studies of populations show that women on estrogen experience less osteoarthritic change, via X-ray, than nonusers. In actual clinical trials (where one group receives estrogen and the other doesn't) however, results are inconsistent, and do not always show a protective effect.[24]

Estrogen may benefit some joints more than others. In one study, women who took long-term estrogen replacement had significantly more cartilage in the knee.[25] In another study, estrogen therapy did not cause any significant improvement in osteoarthritis in the hand, however.[26]

Significant advances in the conventional treatment of pain from osteoarthris occurred in 2001, with the release of COX-2 inhibitors (Vioxx®) for osteoarthritis pain-management.[27] Both the gastrointestinal system and people's pocketbooks fare better on these medications, when compared to the previously recommended pain medications for osteoarthritis (ibuprofen, aspirin derivatives, and Tylenol®.)

Glucosamine Sulfate and Osteoarthritis

Natural health care providers have long recommended a supplement called *glucosamine sulfate* for joint health and for osteoarthritis in particular. A recent study of 212 people with osteoarthritis, reported in the prestigious medical journal, the *Lancet*, found that people taking 1,500 mg of glucosamine sulfate over three years significantly benefited from the supplement.[28] Similar to the effects of estrogen, not only did their symptoms improve in a short time, but unlike those in the placebo group, X-rays confirmed that they did not lose any cartilage during the three years. Some practitioners claim that they even see a regrowth of some cartilage on X-rays in their patients on long-term glucosamine sulfate, but these results have yet to be confirmed by study. These and other findings has led the American College of Rheumatology to take a serious look at this once-shunned natural remedy as a potential first-line treatment for osteoarthritis.[29]

Glucosamine sulfate may work by providing the building blocks for the body to make or maintain cartilage. Other reports show that it may also improve the synovial fluid in the joints, which keeps our creaky moving parts lubricated.[30]

Lifestyle and Osteoarthritis

Maintaining healthy body weight is very important for minimizing the effects of osteoarthritis, particularly in the knee and hip joints. Gentle stretching and yoga done correctly can keep joints mobile and healthy. Improper use of joints, either through misalignment, inadequate footwear during certain exercises, or repeated impact, can cause problems for some individuals. Finally, injuries can greatly hasten joint destruction. Prompt attention to injuries can help prevent some long-term damage.

If you have issues with osteoporosis *and* osteoarthritis—you'll need to find a balance between impact activities that build bone and healthy joint maintenance. A consultation with an osteopathic physician can help set you on the right track. These physicians can often provide treatments not only for symptomatic improvement but also recommend physical therapy and exercises aimed at keeping your joints healthy for a long time.

Periodontal Health

Speaking of bones—there are some very important issues that can affect areas of bone that we don't usually hear about in relationship to menopause. In the past 10 years, new information has surfaced about the effect of aging on the mouth, especially in women.

There are several factors to consider in looking at the mouth as we age. First is how loss of bone, or osteoporosis, effects tooth retention. We usually think about the spine or hip as prime areas of concern for osteoporosis—and indeed, they are. However, osteoporosis can also affect the jaw bone during that same bone loss process after menopause.

Hormone Replacement Therapy and Periodontal Health

Research has shown that women taking HRT improve their tooth retention.[31] The Nurses' Health Study found that women on estrogen experienced one-fourth less tooth loss than women not on estrogen.[32] For them, stronger bone was more able to hold onto teeth.

In addition to the issue of bone loss, there are changes in the gingiva or gum tissue surrounding the tooth with aging. Just as there are estrogen receptors and effects on the skin, there are estrogen receptors and effects on the gums. As estrogen levels decline, the oral tissues become thinner. This process increases a woman's risk of gum recession and infections. Women may notice both more bleeding and gum tenderness after menopause.[33] This thinning of the mucous membrane in the mouth is analogous to the thinning of the vaginal skin that occurs after menopause.

One final mouth symptom to mention that occurs with onset of menopause is a condition called "burning mouth syndrome." In this situation, women experience an intense sensation of dry mouth. This is caused by a significant lack of saliva, which is related to the decrease in hormonal stimulation of the mucous membranes. HRT generally does reverse this symptom problem.

Diet, Lifestyle, and Periodontal Health

Lifestyle factors can affect health of teeth and gums more than estrogen, however. Proper tooth brushing, regular visits to the dentist, and adequate nutrition can help ensure oral health. The fact that smoking is the single biggest risk factor for periodontal disease adds to the innumerable reasons to steer clear of cigarettes. Fiber, calcium intake, and dietary vitamin B_2 have been correlated with healthy gums.[34] And at least one study has found a significant correlation between stress levels and inadequate coping skills and progression of periodontal disease.[35]

Eye Health

For most women, aging brings visual changes. Although technically normal, a decrease in eyesight ability can be frustrating. Most of our eye changes are not related to hormones. However, one may be: age-related macular degeneration (AMD). Important to note, AMD is the single greatest cause of blindness in the United States today.

The inside of the eyeball is filled with a viscous fluid. A trained clinician can actually look into your pupil through this fluid to see the back of your eyeball. In the very back, on the inside, sits a very important region of darker-pigmented tissue—the *macula*. The macula allows us to clearly see objects which lie right in front of us. The macula depends on many tiny blood vessels, which come into this area. If the blood vessels become weakened or damaged, the macula degenerates. Thus, macular degeneration results from damage to these blood vessels. Heredity, high blood pressure,

and atherosclerosis are risk factors for the disease. In susceptible individuals, damage from metabolic waste products and free radicals can impair
function of the macula.

Natural Prevention of Macular Degeneration

Natural medicine has much to offer in the prevention of macular degeneration. Dietary antioxidants, found in fruits and vegetables, have
been shown to protect the pigmented tissue in the retina, and have been
proposed to slow down free-radical damage to arteries.[36, 37] Specifically, dietary vitamin E has correlated to decreased incidence.[38] Dietary nutrients
known as *bioflavonoids*, which are found in the intensely pigmented fruits
and vegetables such as squash, sweet potatoes, blueberries, and cherries
may also be protective of this tissue.

It is important to realize that with AMD, as with any kind of slow, degenerative process, *prevention*, via long-term use of fruits and vegetables
which contain many antioxidants and bioflavonoids, is likely to be much
more effective than supplementation after the fact. However, for people
who already have AMD, there is some evidence that a broad-based antioxidant supplement can slow down visual changes.[39] Ginkgo also holds
promise in this regard,[40] and another herb, bilberry (Vaccinium) is reported by some practitioners to also help, although its effectiveness in
AMD needs to be verified in studies.

Hormone Replacement Therapy and Macular Degeneration

Several studies have shown that women who use HRT have less of this
problem of age-related macular degeneration. This translates into better
vision in their later years. One study found that current users of HRT had
a 70% decreased risk of AMD and that former users had a 40% decreased
risk of the problem.[41] Another large case-controlled study showed that
current HRT users had half the risk of developing AMD compared to former HRT users and nearly a three-quarter lower risk compared to women
who had never used HRT.[42] The reason HRT may keep the macula healthy
is unclear.

Other Eye Changes

Other tissue-related changes in the eye, leading to decreased eyesight,
have shown a correlation to estrogen levels. These include cataracts, glau-
coma, and diseases of the retina.[43] The data shows that cataracts have the
greatest link to estrogen. Smoking and alcohol have been implicated in
cataract development. Researchers from the University of Wisconsin fol-

lowed cataract development in 3,684 residents of a small town over five years. They found that persons who took vitamin supplements containing vitamins E and C for 10 years had a 60% lower incidence of cataracts.[44]

It's worth noting that tamoxifen, the "anti-estrogen," seems to have the opposite effect on eye health, when compared to estrogen. Decreased visual acuity, edema accumulation in the macula, and cataract-like changes have been noted by women on tamoxifen. Most of these changes, other than the damage to the lens that can lead to cataracts, reverse once a woman stops tamoxifen. Women on this drug should have routine eye check-ups.

Some women at menopause complain of "dry eyes." In fact—estrogen might be related here too. Right after deterioration of visual acuity, a sensation of dryness in the eyes ranked second on the list of eye changes that some menopausal women noticed in one study.[45] Some compounding pharmacies have begun experimenting with creating eye drops containing tiny amounts of estrogen for treatment. Saline eyedrops are always appropriate—and always make sure that you are well-hydrated.

The Fountain of Youth?

When one hears all about the possible roles of estrogen in the body—from bones and brain to teeth, eyes, memory, and colon—it's easy to think we should all be on it forever! (Also, please remember not to talk yourself into having any of these symptoms—for most women don't have them.) To keep things in perspective, there's still a lot we don't know about long-term use of hormones, which is what most of the reported benefits for various tissues requires. As mentioned in Chapter 11, we now find ourselves in the midst of a grand hormone experiment. We won't know the final results of offering this elixir to a whole generation of women until our daughters, and perhaps their daughters, reach menopause. Therefore, it's important for us to take "pause" here, and proceed with some caution before we all jump on the hormone bandwagon.

In Western culture, influenced by the way we approach science, we have a tendency to separate out factors, and seek a magic bullet for our ailments. We have a tendency to forget the interconnectedness of all things, and the way that these relationships work together to form health. Lifestyle, diet, attitude, self-care—all these things probably have more to do with our overall health than any little pill, cream, or potion. While we gather the best information that Western science has to offer us from *its* perspective, let's remember to keep our gaze on the Whole Picture.

No one is better equipped for global vision than a menopausal woman today. You've seen a lot in your lifetime. You've seen enormous changes—in lifestyle, trends, beliefs, and behaviors. If you think back on your life, it's probable that you can see at least two or three distinct lifetimes in there. Perhaps you'll embark on a new chapter in the years ahead. Using your life experience and the wisdom gained from it will serve you in making your health care choices.

Now that you've reached the end of this book and accumulated perhaps more information than you need, it's time to let go of the data, and spend time with your soul. Close the book, go for a walk, take a vacation from thinking, and come back to yourself. The information pertinent to you will resurface, and you will know where to find it. That's the beauty of feminine intuition. In our heart, mind, and belly—we *know* what's right for us. Honor that. We, and many practitioners like us, are here for your support when you need us. Remember that we are your employees—your support team, not your dictators! There are things that you know about your health that even the most astute clinician will never know. On your health care team, you make the plays. With the help of the best of all health care options at your fingertips, may the game be the richest and healthiest of your life!

RESOURCES

Practitioner Information and Referrals

Champlain Center for Natural Medicine
33 Harbor Road
Shelburne, VT 05482
(802) 985-8250
www.vtnaturalmed.com
www.DrLorilee.com

Women's Choice
23 Mansfield Avenue
Burlington, VT 05401
(802) 863-9001

American Association of Naturopathic Physicians
8201 Greensboro Drive, Suite 300
McLean, VA 22102
(703) 610-9037
www.naturopathic.org

American Holistic Medical Association
6728 Old McLean Village Road
McLean, VA 22101
(703) 556-9728

American Holistic Nurses Association
P.O. Box 2130
Flagstaff, AZ 86003-2130
(800) 278-2462
www.ahna.org

Canadian Holistic Nurses Association
50 Driveway
Ottawa, Ontario
K2P 1E2, Canada
Telephone: (613) 237-2133
Fax: (613) 237-3520
Toll-free phone: 1-888-910-9998
http://mypage.direct.ca/h/hutchings/chna.html

Naturopathic Colleges and Universities

Bastyr University
14500 Juanita Drive NE
Bothell, WA 98011
(425) 823-1300
www.bastyr.edu

Canadian College of Naturopathic Medicine
1255 Sheppard Ave. East
Toronto, Ontario
M2K, E2, Canada
(416) 498-1255
www.ccnm.edu

National College of Naturopathic Medicine
049 SW Porter
Portland, OR 97201
(503) 499-4343
www.ncnm.edu

Southwest College of Naturopathic Medicine and Health Sciences
2140 East Broadway Road
Tempe, AZ 85282
(480) 858-9100
www.scnm.edu

Compounding Pharmacies

International Academy of Compounding Pharmacists (IACP)
P.O. Box 1365
Sugar Land, TX 77487
(281) 933-8400
(800) 927-4227
iacpinfo@iacprx.org

Herbal Information and Practitioners

American Herbalists Guild
1931 Gaddis Road
Canton, GA 30115
(770) 751-6021
ahgoffice@earthlink.net

Conventional Menopause Associations

International Menopause Society
c/o Monique Boulet, Executive Director
Chez Maitre M. Steyaert
Av. des Cattleyas, 3, Box 1
1150 Brussels, Belgium
++32.2.772.2183
imsociety@Filink.net

North American Menopause Society
P.O. Box 94527
Cleveland, OH 44101
(440) 442-7550
info@menopause.org

Workshops

Natural Medicine and Yoga for Menopause, Lorilee Schoenbeck, N.D.
Kripalu Center for Yoga and Health
Box 793
Lenox, MA
(800) 741-SELF
www.kripalu.org

For other workshops and appearances around the world, check
www.DrLorilee.com or www.VTNaturalMed.com.

Books

Brown, Susan. *Better Bones, Better Body: Beyond Estrogen and Calcium*. Chicago: Keats Publishing, 2000.

Cabot, Sandra. *Smart Medicine for Menopause*. Garden City Park, NY: Avery Publishing Group, 1995.

Hudson, Tori. *Women's Encyclopedia of Natural Medicine*. Chicago: Keats Publishing, 1999.

Laux, Marcus, and Christine Conrad. *Natural Woman, Natural Menopause*. New York: Harper, 1998.

Northrup, Christiane. *The Wisdom of Menopause: Creating Physical and Emotional Health During the Change*. New York: Bantam Books, 2001.

Sichel, Deborah, and Jeanne W. Driscoll. *Women's Moods: What Every Woman Must Know About Hormones, the Brain, and Emotional Health*. New York: William Morrow & Company, 2000.

Weed, Susan. *The Menopausal Years: The Wise Woman Way*. Woodstock, NY: Ash Tree Publishing, 2001.

NOTES

Introduction

1. North American Menopause Society (NAMS) estimated data. NAMS, 5900 Landerbrook Dr., Suite 195, Mayfield Heights, OH 44124.
2. NAMS estimated data.

Chapter 1

1. Baker TG. *American Journal of Obstetrics and Gynecology* 1971:110(5):746–761.
2. Chiazze Jr L. "The length and variability of the human menstrual cycle." *Journal of the American Medical Association* 1968: 203, 377.
3. Speroff L, Glass RH, Kase NG. *Clinical Gynecologic Endocrinology and Infertility* (Baltimore MD: Lippincott, Williams and Wilkins) 1999, p. 651.
4. Treolar, AE. "Menstrual cyclicity and the pre-menopause." *Maturitas* 1981;3 (3–4): 249–264.
5. Speroff L. *Clinical Gynecologic*, p. 653.
6. Treolar AE. "Variations of the human menstrual cycle through reproductive life." *International Journal of Fertility* 1967: 12, 77.
7. Bolaji II. "Sero-salivary progesterone correlation." *International Journal of Gynaecology and Obstetrics:* 1994;45(2): 125–131.
8. Yeo J. "Lab Talk." *Newsletter of the Dartmouth-Hitchcock Medical Center Clinical Laboratory* 1999: 3(2).
9. Shirtcliff EA, Granger DA, Schwartz E, Curran MJ. "Use of salivary biomarkers in biobehavioral research: cotton-based sample collection methods can interfere with salivary immuno-assay results." *Psychoneuroendocrinology* 2001; 2: 165–173.
10. Willett W, Stampfer MJ, Bain C, Lipnick R, Speizer FE, Rosner B, Cramer D, Hennekens CH. "Cigarette smoking, relative weight, and menopause." *American Journal of Epidemiology* 1983 Jun;117(6): 651–658.
11. Midgette AS, Baron JA. "Cigarette smoking and the risk of natural menopause." *Epidemiology* 1990 Nov;1(6): 474–480.
12. Torgerson DJ, Avenell A, Russell IT, Reid DM. "Factors associated with onset of menopause in women aged 45–49." *Maturitas* 1994;19(2): 83–92.

13. Torgerson DJ, Thomas RE, Campbell MK, Reid DM. "Alcohol consumption and age of maternal menopause are associated with menopause onset." *Maturitas* 1997; 26(1): 21–25.

14. Cramer DW, Xu H, Harlow BL. "Family history as a predictor of early menopause." *Fertility and Sterility* 1995;64(4): 740–745.

15. Speroff L. *Clinical Gynecologic*, p. 655.

16. Torgerson DJ et al. *Maturitas* 1997; 26(1): 21.

17. Utian WH, Boggs PP. "The North American Menopause Society's 1998 Menopause Survey. Pt I: Postmenopausal Women's Perceptions About Menopause and Midlife." *Menopause: Journal of the North American Menopause Society* 1999;6(2): 122–128.

18. Speroff L. *Clinical Gynecologic*, pp. 651–55.

19. NIA Information Center, P.O. Box 8057, Gaithersburg, MD 20898–8057.

20. Polo Kantola P, Erkkola R, Helenius H, Iriala K, Polo O. "When does estrogen replacement therapy improve sleep quality?" *American Journal of Obstetrics and Gynecology* 1998;178(5): 1002–1009.

21. Manber R, Armitage R. "Sex, steroids, and sleep: A review." *Sleep* 1999;22(5): 540–555.

22. Shaver JL, Zenk SN. "Sleep disturbance in menopause." *Journal of Women's Health and Gender-Based Medicine* 2000;9(2): 109–118.

23. Davis SR, Burger HG. "Use of androgens in postmenopausal women." *Current Opinions in Obstetrics and Gynecology* 1997;9(3): 177–180.

Chapter 2

1. Lock M. "Menopause: Lessons from anthropology." *Psychosomatic Medicine* 1998;60:410–419.

2. Lock M. "Menopause: Lessons from Anthropology." p. 412.

3. Furuta S, Nishimoto K, Deguchi K, Ohyama M. " Relationship between abnormal sensation in the throat and menopause." *Auris, Nasus, Larynx* 1996;23: 69–74.

4. Lock M. "Menopause," p. 413.

5. Somekawa Y, Chiguchi M, Ishibashi T, Aso T. "Soy intake related to menopausal symptoms, serum lipids, and bone mineral density in postmenopausal Japanese women." *Obstetrics and Gynecology* 2001;97(1): 109–115.

6. Nakamura K, Nashimoto M, Hori Y, Yamamoto M. "Serum 25-hydroxyvitamin D concentrations and related dietary factors in peri- and postmenopausal Japanese women." *American Journal of Clinical Nutrition* 2000;71(5): 1161–1165.

7. Sheehy, G. *The Silent Passage*. 1998. New York: Pocket Books, p. 250.

8. Lock M. "Menopause," p. 416.

9. Albery N. "The menopause in Japan—Konenki Jigoku." *Climacteric* 1999;2: 160–161.

10. Berger GE. *Menopause and Culture* (London: Pluto Press) 1999, pp. 38, 42, 71.

11. Berger GE. Ibid. p. 38.

12. Lock M. "Menopause" p. 412.

13. Berger GE. *Menopause and Culture*, p. 42, from Martin MC, Block JE, Sanches SD, Arnaud CD, Beyene Y. "Menopause without symptoms: The endocrinology of menopause among rural Mayan Indians." *American Journal of Obstetrics and Gynecology* 1993;168(6 Pt 1): 1839–1843.

14. Beyene Y. *From Menarche to Menopause: Reproductive Lives of Peasant Women in Two Cultures*, (Albany: State University of New York Press) 1989, p. 131.

15. Beyene Y. "Cultural significance and physiological manifestations of menopause. A biocultural analysis." *Culture, Medicine and Psychiatry* 1986;10(1): 47–71.

16. Martin MC, Block JE, Sanches SD, Arnaud CD, Beyene Y. "Menopause without symptoms: The endocrinology of menopause among rural Mayan Indians." *American Journal of Obstetrics and Gynecology* 1993;168(6 Pt 1):1839–1843.

17. Berger GE. *Menopause and Culture,* p. 40 from Ramoso-Jalbuena, J. "The climacteric Filipina: a preliminary survey of 1015 cases." *Philippine Journal of Obstetrics and Gynecology* 1991;15(2):75–88.

18. Berg JA, Taylor DL. "Symptom experience of Filipino American midlife women." *Menopause* 1999;6(2): 90–91.

19. Sommer B, Avis N, Meyer P, Ory M, Madden T, Kagawa-Singer M, Mouton C, Rasor NO, Adler S. "Attitudes toward menopause and aging across ethnic/racial groups." *Psychosomatic Medicine* 2000;62(1):96.

20. Gold EB, Sternfeld B, Kelsey JL, Brown C, Mouton C, Reame N, Salamone L, Stellato R. "Relation of demographic and lifestyle factors to symptoms in a multiracial/ethnic population of women 40–55 years of age." *American Journal of Epidemiology* 2000;152(5):463–473.

21. Berger GE. *Menopause and Culture,* p. 38 reporting on: Chirawatkul S., Manderson L. "Perceptions of menopause in Northeast Thailand: contested meaning and practice." *Social Science and Medicine* 1994;39(11): 1545–1554.

22. Kaufert PA, Lock M. "Medicalization of women's third age." *Journal of Psychosomatic Obstetrics and Gynaecology* 1997;18(2):81–86.

23. Greer G. *The Change* (New York: Alfred A. Knopf) 1992.

24. Silberman I. "A Contribution to the Psychology of Menstruation." *International Journal of Psycho-Analysis* 1950;31:266 from Freud S. *Complete Psychological Works,* (transl. Strachey J.) London: Hogarth 1961; 3(23): 226.

25. Deutsch H. from Delaney J, Lipton MJ, Toth E. *The Curse.* New York: E.P. Dutton & Co., 1976, pp. 57–58.

26. Erikson E. *Identity, Youth and Crisis* (New York: Norton) 1968, p. 278.

27. Delaney J, Lupton MJ, Toth E. *The Curse.* New York: E.P. Dutton & Co. 1976, from "Hamlet" Act 3, Scene 4.

28. Wilson RA. *Feminine Forever.* New York: Evans. 1966, p. 44.

29. Greenblatt RB in Wilson RA. Ibid, pp.13–14.

30. Wilson R. "Norethynodrel-mestranol (Enovid) for prevention and treatment of the climacteric." *Journal of the American Geriatric Society* 1966;14(10):967, 979.

31. Wilson RA, Wilson TA. "The Basic Philosophy of Estrogen Maintenance." *Journal of the American Geriatric Society* 1972;20(11):521–523.

32. Greer G. *The Change* (New York: Alfred A. Knopf) 1992, p. 119, from Wilson RA. *Feminine Forever.* p. 196.

33. Wilson RA. "Norethynodrel-mestranol . . ." p. 967.

34. Reubin D. *Everything You Always Wanted to Know About Sex But Were Afraid to Ask* (New York: David McKay Company) 1969, pp. 283, 289, 292–293.

35. Utian WH. "The fate of the untreated menopause." *Obstetrics and Gynecology Clinics of North America* 1987;14(1): 1–11.

36. Kaufert PA, Lock M "Medicalization of women's third age." *Journal of Psychosomatic Obstetrics and Gynaecology*1997;18(2):81–86.

37. Speroff L, Glass RH, Kase NG. *Clinical Gynecologic Endocrinology and Infertility* (Baltimore, MD: Lippincott, Williams and Wilkins) 1999, p. 644.

38. Utian WH, Boggs PP. "The North American Menopause Society 1998 Menopause Survey. Part I: Postmenopausal Women's Perceptions About Menopause and Midlife." *Menopause: The Journal of The North American Menopause Society* 1998;6(2): 122–128.

39. Avis, NE. "A longitudinal analysis of women's attitudes toward the menopause: results from the Massachusetts Women's Health Study." *Maturitas* 1991;13: 65.

40. Berger G. *Menopause and Culture,* p.182.

41. Kaufert PA, Lock M. "Medicalization of women's third age." *Journal of Psychosomatic Obstetrics and Gynaecology* 1997;18(2): 81–86.

42. Sheehy G. *The Silent Passage* (New York: Pocket Books) 1998, pp. 67–69.

43. Utian WH, Boggs PP. "Menopause Survey," pp. 122–128.

44. Kaufert PA, Lock M. "Medicalization . . .," pp. 81–86.

45. Healy B. *A New Prescription for Women's Health* (New York: Viking Press) 1995, p. 174.

46. Sheehy G. *Silent Passage,* p. 67.

47. Greer G. *The Change,* p. 387.

Chapter 3

1. Hudson T *Women's Encyclopedia of Natural Medicine* (Los Angeles: Keats) 1999.

2. Brown D. "Herbal Research Review: Vitex agnus castus Clinical Monograph." *Townsend Letter for Doctors and Patients* 1995;Oct(147): 138–42.

3. Weiss RF. *Herbal* A.B. Arcanum (Gothenburg, Sweden: Beaconsfield Publishers Limited) 1988, p. 317.

4. Brown D. "Herbal Research Review: Vitex agnus castus Clinical Monograph." *Townsend Letter for Doctors and Patients* 1995;Oct(147): 138–42.

5. Grieve M. *A Modern Herbal* (New York: Dover Press) 1981, p. 865.

6. Lad V, Frawley D. *The Yoga of Herbs, An Ayurvedic Guide to Herbal Medicine* (Santa Fe, NM: Lotus Press) 1986, p. 152.

7. Murray M. *Encyclopedia of Nutritional Supplements* (Rocklin, CA: Prima Publishing) 1996, p. 209.

8. Murray M. Ibid., p. 211.

9. Pederson M. *Nutritional Herbology : A Reference Guide to Herbs* (Warsaw, IN: Wendell Whitman Co.) 1998, p. 40.

10. *Drugs, Facts and Comparisons* (St. Louis Mo: A. Wolters Kluwer Co.) 2000, p. 31.

11. Pederson M. *Nutritional Herbology,* p. 40.

12. Freeman EW, Rickels K. "Characteristics of placebo responses in medical treatment of premenstrual syndrome." *American Journal of Psychiatry* 1999;156(9):1403–1408.

13. Morse CA, Cudley E, Guthrie J, Dennerstein L. "Relationships between premenstrual complaints and perimenopausal experiences." *Journal of Psychosomatic Obstetrics and Gynecology* 1998;19 (4): 182–91.

14. Larsson C, Hallman J. "Is severity of premenstrual symptoms related to illness in the climacteric?" *Journal of Psychosomatic Obstetrics and Gynecology* 1997;(3): 234–43.

15. Monteleone P et al. "Allopregnanolone concentrations and premenstrual syndrome." *European Journal of Endocrinology* 2000;142(3): 269–73.

16. Rapkin AJ et al. "Progesterone metabolite allopregnanolone in women with premenstrual syndrome." *Obstetrics and Gynecology* 1997;90(5): 709–14.

17. Michener W. "The role of low progesterone and tension as triggers of perimenstrual chocolate and sweets craving: Some negative experimental evidence." *Physiology and Behavior* 1999;67(3): 417–20.

18. Schmidt PJ et al. "Circulating levels of anxiolytic steroids in the luteal phase in women with premenstrual syndrome and in control subjects." *Journal of Clinical Endocrinology and Metabolism* 1994;79(5): 1256–60.

19. Hammarback S et al. "Relationship between symptom severity and hormone changes in women with premenstrual syndrome." *Journal of Clinical Endocrinology and Metabolism* 1989;68(1): 125–30.

20. Magill PJ "Investigation of the efficacy of progesterone pessaries in the relief of symptoms of premenstrual syndrome. Progesterone Study Group." *British Journal of General Practice* 1995;45(400): 589–93.

21. Vanselow W, Dennerstein L, Greenwood KM, De Lignieres B. "Effect of progesterone and its 5-alpha and 5-beta metabolites in symptoms of premenstual syndrome according to route of administration" *Journal of Psychosomatic Obstetrics and Gynecology* 1996;17(1): 29–38.

22. MacNaughton J, Banah M, McCloud P, Hee J, Burger H. "Age related changes

in follicle stimulating hormone, luteinizing hormone, oestradiol and immunoreactive inhibin in women of reproductive age." *Clinical Endocrinology(Oxf)* 1992;36(4): 339–45.

23. Buckler HM, Evans CA, Mamtora H, Burger HG, Anderson DC. "Gonadotropin, steroid, and inhibin levels in women with incipient ovarian failure during anovulatory and ovulatory rebound cycles." *Clinical Endocrinology and Metabolism* 1991; 72: 116–24.

24. Aganoff JA, Boyle GJ "Aerobic exercise, mood states and menstrual cycle symptoms." *Journal of Psychosomatic Research* 1994;38(3): 183–92.

25. Choi PY, Salmon P. "Symptom changes across the menstrual cycle in competitive sportswomen, exercisers and sedentary women." *British Journal of Clinical Psychology* 1995;34(pt 3): 447–60.

26. Barnard ND et al. "Diet and sex-hormone binding globulin, dysmenorrhea, and premenstrual symptoms." *Obstetrics and Gynecology* 2000;95(2): 245–50.

27. Kleijnen J et al. "Vitamin B6 in the treatment of the premenstrual syndrome— a review." *British Journal of Obstetrics and Gynaecology* 1990;97: 847–59.

28. De Souza et al. "A synergistic effect of a daily supplement for 1 month of 200 mg magnesium plus 50 mg vitamin B6 for relief of anxiety-related premenstrual symptoms: A randomized, double-blind, crossover study." *Journal of Women's Health and Gender Based Medicine* 2000; 9(2): 131–9.

29. Hudson T *Women's Encyclopedia of Natural Medicine* (Los Angeles: Keats) 1999, p. 249.

30. Hudson T. Ibid.

31. Ward MW, Holimon TD. "Calcium treatment for premenstrual syndrome. *Annals of Phamacotherapy* 1999;33(12):1356–58.

32. Thys-Jacobs S "Micronutrients and the premenstrual syndrome: The case for calcium." *Journal of the American College of Nutrition* 2000;19(2): 220–27.

33. Lock G et al. "Treatment of premenstrual syndrome with a phytopharmaceutical formulation containing vitex agnus castus." *Journal of Women's Health and Gender Based Medicine* 2000;9(3): 315–20.

34. Schellenberg R. "Treatment for the premenstrual syndrome with agnus castus fruit extract: Prospective, randomised, placebo controlled study." *British Medical Journal* 2001;322(7279): 134–37.

35. Hoffman D. *The Wholistic Herbal* (Rockport, MA: Element Books) 1983, p. 101.

36. Northrup C. *The Wisdom of Menopause* (Des Plaines, IL: Bantam Books) 2001.

37. Wyatt K, Dimmock P, Jones P, Obhrai M, O'Brien S. "Efficacy of progesterone and progestogens in management of premenstrual syndrome: Systematic review." *British Medical Journal.* 2001;323(7316): 776–80.

Chapter 4

1. Speroff L, Glass RH, Kase NG. *Clinical Gynecologic Endocrinology and Infertility* (Baltimore, MD: Lippincott, Williams and Wilkins) 1999, p. 594.

2. Raskins B. *Hot Flashes* (New York, NY: St. Martin's Press) 1987. Reprinted with permission.

3. Yen SCC. *Reproductive Endocrinology, Physiology, Pathophysiology and Clinical Management* (Philadelphia, PA: WB Saunders) 1991, p. 898.

4. Rosano GM, Rillo M, Leonardo F, Pappone C, Chierchia SL. "Palpitations: what is the mechanism, and when should we treat them?" *International Journal of Fertility and Women's Medicine* 1997;42(2): 94–100.

5. Schwingl PJ, Hulka BS, Harlow SD. "Risk factors for menopausal hot flashes." *Obstetrics and Gynecology* 1994; 84(1): 29–34.

6. Han KK, Soares JM, Haidar MA, Rodriquez de Lima G, Baracut EC. "Benefits of

soy isoflavones therapeutic regimen on menopausal symptoms." *Obstetrics and Gynecology* 2002; 99: 389–394.

7. Albertazzi P, Pansini F, Bonaccorsi G, Zanotti L, Forini E, De Aloysio D. "The effect of dietary soy supplementation on hot flushes." *Obstetrics and Gynecology.* 1998: 91(1): 6–10.

8. Schwingl PJ et al. "Risk factors."

9. Desai A. Lecture given at Kripalu Center for Yoga and Health, Lenox, MA, 1990.

10. Gannon L, Hansel S, Goodwin J.. "Correlates of menopausal hot flashes." *Journal of Behavioral Medicine* 1987;10(3): 277–85.

11. Freedman R. (Wayne State University School of Medicine, Detroit, MI) *Washington Post* (Article) Tuesday Aug. 18, 1998, p. Z16.

12. Ivarsson T, Spetz AC, Hammar M. "Physical exercise and vasomotor symptoms in postmenopausal women." *Maturitas* 1998;29(2): 139–46.

13. Hammar M, Berg G, Lindgren R. "Does physical exercise influence the frequency of postmenopausal hot flushes?" *Acta Obstetricia et Gynecologica Scandinavica* 1990;69(5): 409–12.

14. Christy CJ. "Vitamin E in menopause." *American Journal of Obstetrics and Gynecology* 1945: 50;84–87; McLaren HC. "Vitamin E in the menopause." *British Medical Journal* 1930ii:1378–81.; Finkler RS. "The effect of vitamin E in the menopause." *Journal of Clinical Endocrinology and Metabolism* 1249; 9: 89–94.

15. Smith C. "Non-hormonal control of vasomotor flushing in menopausal patients." *Chicago Medical School Quarterly* 1964;67:193–95.

16. Hudson T. *Woman's Encyclopedia of Natural Medicine* (Los Angeles: Keats Publishing) 1999, p. 146.

17. Gruenwald J. "Standardized Black Cohosh (Cimicifuga) extract Clinical Monograph." *Quarterly Review of Natural Medicine* 1998 Jun 30: 117–25.

18. Lloyd JU. *Origin and history of all the Pharmacopeial Vegetable Drugs, Chemicals and Preparations,* vol. 1. (Cincinnati: The Caxton Press)1921, p. 54.

19. Foster S. "Black cohosh: Cimicifuga racemosa; a literature review." *HerbalGram* 1999 Jan (45): 35–49.

20. McKenna DJ, Jones K, Humphrey S, Hughes K. "Black cohosh: efficacy, safety, and use in clinical and preclinical applications." *Alternative Therapies in Health and Medicine* 2001;7(3): 93–100.

21. Lehmann-Willenbrock E; Riedel HH. "Klinische und endokrinologische Untersuchungen zur Therapie ovarieller Ausfallserscheinungen nach Hysterektomie unter Belassung der Adnexe" (Clinical and endocrinologic studies of the treatment of ovarian insufficiency manifestations following hysterectomy with intact adnexa) [Article in German] *Zentralblatt Fur Gynakologie* 1988;110 (10): 611–18.

22. Liske E. "Therapeutic efficacy and safety of Cimicifuga racemosa for gynecologic disorders." *Advances in Therapy* 1998;15(1): 45–53.

23. Einer-Jensen N, Zhao J, Andersen KP, Kristoffersen K. "Cimicifuga and Melbrosia lack oestrogenic effects in mice and rats." *Maturitas* 1996;25(2):149–53.

24. Jarry H, Harnischfeger G, Duker E "[The endocrine effects of constituents of Cimicifuga racemosa. 2. In vitro binding of constituents to estrogen receptors]." [Article in German] *Planta Medica* 1985 Aug;(4):316–19.

25. Dixon-Shanies D, Shaikh N. "Growth inhibition of human breast cancer cells by herbs and phytoestrogens." *Oncology Reports* 1999;6(6): 1383–87.

26. Fugh-Berman A, Kronenberg F. "Red clover (Trifolium pratense) for menopausal women: current state of knowledge." Review. *Menopause* 2001;8(5): 333–37.

27. Zava DT, Dollbaum CM, Blen M. "Estrogen and progestin bioactivity of foods, herbs, and spices." *Proceedings of the Society for Experimental Biology and Medicine* 1998; 217(3): 369–78.

28. Wang W, Tanaka Y, Han Z, Higuchi CM. "Proliferative response of mammary glandular tissue to formononetin." *Nutrition and Cancer* 1995;23(2): 131–40.

29. Costello CH, Lynn EV. "Estrogenic substances from plants: I. Glycerrhiza." *Journal of the American Pharmaceutical Association.* 1950;39:177–80.

30. Kumagai A, Nishino K et al. "Effect of glycerrhizin on estrogen action." *Endocrinologia Japonica* 1967;14:34–38.

31. Hopkins MP et al. "Ginseng face cream and unexplained vaginal bleeding." *American Journal of Obstetrics and Gynecology* 1988;159(5):1121–22.

32. Punnonen R. "Oestrogen-like effect of ginseng." *British Medical Journal* 1980; 281: 1110.

33. Komesaroff PA, Black CV, Cable V, Sudhir K. "Effects of wild yam extract on menopausal symptoms, lipids and sex hormones in healthy menopausal women." *Climacteric* 2001; 4(2): 144–150.

34. Lindahl O. "Double blind study of a valerian preparation." *Pharmacology, Biochemistry, and Behavior* 1989;32(4): 1065–66.

35. Leatherwood PD, Chauffard F. "Aqueous extract of valerian reduces latency to fall asleep in man." *Planta Medica* 1985;(2):144–48.

36. Balderer G. "Effect of valerian on human sleep." *Psychopharmacology* 1985;87 (4):406–409.

37. Leatherwood PD et al. "Aqueous extract of valerian root improves sleep quality in man." *Pharmacology, Biochemistry, and Behavior* 1982;17(1): 65–71.

Chapter 5

1. Schwartz H. *Never Satisfied: A Cultural History of Diets, Fantasies and Fat* (New York: The Free Press, A Division of Macmillan, Inc., NY, Collier Macmillan Publishers) 1986, p. 5.

2. Chrisler JC, Ghiz L. "Faces of women and aging." *Women and Therapy* 1993; 14: 69.

3. Speroff, L, Glass RH, Kase NG. *Clinical Gynecologic Endocrinology and Infertility* (Baltimore, MD: Lippincott, Williams and Wilkins) 1999, p. 784.

4. Poehlman ET, Toth MJ, Gardner AW. "Changes in energy balance and body composition at menopause: A controlled longitudinal study." *Annals of Internal Medicine* 1995;123(9): 673–75.

5. Armellini F, Zamboni M, Mino A, Bissoli L, Micciolo R, Bosello O. "Postabsorptive resting metabolic rate and thermic effect of food in relation to body composition and adipose tissue distribution." *Metabolism* 2000;49(1): 6–10.

6. Toth MJ, Tchernof A, Sites CK, Poehlman ET. "Effect of menopausal status on body composition and abdominal fat distribution." *International Journal of Obesity and Related Metabolic Disorders* 2000;24(2): 226–31.

7. Wang Q, Hassager C, Ravn P, Wang S, Christiansen C. "Total and regional body-composition changes in early postmenopausal women: Age-related or menopause-related?" *American Journal of Clinical Nutrition* 1994;60(6):843–48.

8. Svendsen OL, Hassager C, Christiansen C. "Age- and menopause-associated variations in body composition and fat distribution in healthy women as measured by dual-energy X-ray absorptiometry." *Metabolism* 1995;44(3):369–73.

9. Toth MJ, Tchernof A, Sites CK, Poehlman ET. "Effect of Menopausal Status . . ."

10. Ijuin H, Douchi T, Oki T, Maruta K, Nagata Y. "The contribution of menopause to changes in body-fat distribution." *Journal of Obstetrics and Gynaecology Research* 1999;25(5): 367–72.

11. Kerner Furman F. *Facing the Mirror: Older Women and Beauty Shop Culture.* (New York: Routledge Press) 1997.

12. North America Menopause Society. "Effects of Menopause and Estrogen Replacement Therapy of Hormone Replacement Therapy in Women With Diabetes Mellitus: Consensus Opinion of the North America Menopause Society." *Menopause* 2000;7(2): 87–95.

13. Sites CK, Calles-Escandon J, Brochu M, Butterfield M, Ashikaga T, Poehlman ET. "Relation of regional fat distribution to insulin sensitivity in postmenopausal women." *Fertility and Sterility* 2000;73(1): 61–5.

14. Galvard H, Elmstahl S, Elmstahl B, Samuelsson SM, Robertsson E. "Differences in body composition between female geriatric hip fracture patients and healthy controls: Body fat is more important as explanatory factor for the fracture than body weight and lean body mass." *Aging* (Milano) 1996;8(4):282–86.

15. Douchi T, Yamamoto S, Kuwahata R, Oki T, Yamasaki H, Nagata Y. "Effect of non-weight-bearing body fat on bone mineral density before and after menopause." *Obstetrics and Gynecology* 2000;96(1): 13–17.

16. Heiss CJ, Sanborn CF, Nichols DL, Bonnick SL, Alford BB. "Associations of body fat distribution, circulating sex hormones, and bone density in postmenopausal women." *Journal of Clinical Endocrinology and Metabolism* 1995;80(5): 1591–96.

17. Van Pelt RE, Jones PP, Davy KP, Desouza CA, Tanaka H, Davy BM, Seals DR. "Regular exercise and the age-related decline in resting metabolic rate in women." *Journal of Clinical Endocrinology and Metabolism* 1997;82(10): 3208–12.

18. Withers RT, Smith DA, Tucker RC, Brinkman M, Clark DG. "Energy metabolism in sedentary and active 49- to 70-yr-old women." *Journal of Applied Physiology* 1998;84(4):1333–40.

19. Astrup A. "Physical activity and weight gain and fat distribution changes with menopause: Current evidence and research issues." *Medicine and Science in Sports and Exercise* 1999;31(11 Suppl): S564–67.

20. Murray M. *Encyclopedia of Nutritional Supplements* (Rocklin, CA: Prima Publishing) 1996, p. 317.

20a. Avenell A, Richmond PR, Lean ME, Reid DM. "Bone loss associated with a high fibre weight reduction diet in postmenopausal women." *European Journal of Clinical Nutrition* 1994;48(8):561–6.

21. Bahadori B, Wallner S, Schneider H, Wascher TC, Toplak H. "[Effect of chromium yeast and chromium picolinate on body composition of obese, non-diabetic patients during and after a formula diet]," in German. *Acta Medica Austriaca* 1997;24(5): 185–87.

22. Hoeger WW, Harris C, Long EM, Hopkins DR. "Four-week supplementation with a natural dietary compound produces favorable changes in body composition." *Advances in Therapy* 1998;5(5): 305–14.

23. Trent LK, Thieding-Cancel D. "Effects of chromium picolinate on body composition." *Journal of Sports Medicine and Physical Fitness* 1995;35(4): 273–80.

24. Cerulli J, Grabe DW, Gauthier I, Malone M, McGoldrick MD. "Chromium picolitate toxicity." *Annals of Pharmacotherapy* 1998;32(4): 428–31.

25. White LM, Gardner SF, Gurley BJ, Marx MA, Wang PL, Estes M., "Pharmacokinetics and cardiovascular effects of ma-huang (Ephedra sinica) in normotensive adults." *Journal of Clinical Pharmacology* 1997;37(2): 116–22.

26. Gambacciani M, Ciaponi M, Cappagli B, Piaggesi L, De Simone L, Orlandi R, Genazzani AR. "Body weight, body fat distribution, and hormonal replacement therapy in early postmenopausal women." *Journal of Clinical Endocrinology and Metabolism* 1997;82(2):414–17.

27. Chmouliovsky L, Habicht F, James RW, Lehmann T, Campana A, Golay A. "Beneficial effect of hormone replacement therapy on weight loss in obese menopausal women." *Maturitas* 1999;32(3): 147–53.

28. Van Seumeren I. "Weight gain and hormone replacement therapy: Are women's fears justified?" Review. *Maturitas* 2000;34 Suppl 1: S3–8.

29. Brincat MP. "Hormone replacement therapy and the skin." *Maturitas* 2000;35(2):107–17.

30. Brincat M, Versi E, Moniz CF, Magos A, de Trafford J, Studd JW. "Skin collagen changes in postmenopausal women receiving different regimens of estrogen therapy." *Obstetrics and Gynecology.* 1987;70(1): 123–27.

31. Oikarinen A. "Systemic estrogens have no conclusive beneficial effect on

human skin connective tissue." *Acta Obstetricia et Gynecologica Scandinavica* 2000;79(4): 250–54.

32. Katsambas AD, Katoulis AC. "Topical retinoids in the treatment of aging of the skin." Review. *Advances in Experimental Medicine and Biology Biol.* 1999;455: 477–82.

33. Pugliese PT. "The skin's antioxidant systems." *Dermatology Nursing* 1998;10(6): 401–16; quiz 417–18. Review.

34. Jones SA, McArdle F, Jack CI, Jackson MJ. "Effect of antioxidant supplementation on the adaptive response of human skin fibroblasts to UV-induced oxidative stress." *Redox Report: Communications in Free Radical Research* 1999;4(6): 291–99.

35. Pugliese PT. "The skin's antioxident systems."

36. Gilchrest BA. "Treatment of photodamage with topical tretinoin: An overview." *Journal of the American Academy of Dermatology* 1997;36(3 Pt 2): S27–36. Review.

37. Hetter GP. "An examination of the phenol-croton oil peel: Part IV. Face peel results with different concentrations of phenol and croton oil." *Plastic and Reconstructive Surgery.* 2000;105(3): 1061–83; discussion 1084–87.

38. Cassano N, Alessandrini G, Mastrolonardo M, Vena GA. "Peeling agents: Toxicological and allergological aspects." *Journal of the European Academy of Dermatology and Venereology* 1999;13(1): 14–23. Review.

39. Ross EV, Grossman MC, Duke D, Grevelink JM. "Long-term results after CO_2 laser skin resurfacing: A comparison of scanned and pulsed systems." *Journal of the American Academy of Dermatology* 1997;37(5 Pt 1): 709–18.

40. Rapaport MJ, Rapaport V. "Prolonged erythema after facial laser resurfacing or phenol peel secondary to corticosteroid addiction." *Dermatologic Surgery* 1999;25(10): 781–84; discussion: 785.

41. Tosti A, Camacho-Martinez F, Dawber R. "Management of androgenetic alopecia." *Journal of the European Academy of Dermatology and Venereology* 1999;12(3):205–14. Review.

42. Georgala S, Gourgiotou K, Kassouli S, Stratigos JD. "Hormonal status in postmenopausal androgenetic alopecia." *International Journal of Dermatology* 1992;31(12): 858–59.

43. Callan AW, Montalto J. "Female androgenetic alopecia: An update." *The Australasian Journal of Dermatology* 1995;36(2):51–55; quiz 56–57. Review

44. Tosti A et al. "Management of androgenetic alopecia."

45. York J, Nicholson T, Minors P, Duncan DF. "Stressful life events and loss of hair among adult women, a case-control study," *Psychological Reports* 1998;82(3 Pt 1): 1044–46.

46. Jacobs JP, Szpunar CA, Warner ML. "Use of topical minoxidil therapy for androgenetic alopecia in women." *International Journal of Dermatology* 1993;32(10): 758–62.

47. Schmidt JB. "Hormonal basis of male and female androgenic alopecia: Clinical relevance." *Skin Pharmacology* 1994;7(1–2):61–66.

48. Isaak JA. *Feminism and Contemporary Art: The Revolutionary Power of Women's Laughter* (London and New York: Routledge) 1996.

49. Teitjens Meyers D. *Miroir, Memoire, Mirage: Appearance, Aging, and Women,* quoted in Urban Walker M. (ed.) *Mother Time* (New York: Rowman & Littlefield Publishers, Inc.) 1999, p. 40.

50. Bobbie Brown, quoted in Vienne V. "Looking Better All the Time." *O, The Oprah Magazine* 2000;1(4): 300.

51. Vienne V. Ibid., p. 234.

52. Adcock, F. *Poems 1960–2000,* (Bloodaxe Books) 2000.

Chapter 6

1. CDC-Nat Center for Chronic Disease Prevention and Health Promotion, web page: www.ccd.gov/nccdphp/cvd/aboutcardio.htm.

2. American Heart Association (AHA's) "Heart and Stroke, an A-Z Guide." www.americanheart.org/HeartandStrokeAZ Guide/women.html.

3. Emilio R, Guiliani, Gersh, McGoon, Hayes, Hartzell, Schaff. *Mayo Clinic Practice of Cardiology* (Third Edition) (St. Louis, MO: Mosby Press) 1996, p. 1882.

4. Guiliani Ibid.

5. AHA "Heart and Stroke . . ."

6. Anand SS, Yusuf S, Vuksan V, Devanesen S, Teo KK, Montague PA, Kelemen L, Yi C, Lonn E, Gerstein H, Hegele RA, McQueen M. "Differences in risk factors, atherosclerosis, and cardiovascular disease between ethnic groups in Canada: The Study of Health Assessment and Risk in Ethnic groups (SHARE.)" *Lancet* 2000;356(9226): 279–84.

7. Whitty CJ, Brunner EJ, Shipley MJ, Hemingway H, Marmot MG. "Differences in biological risk factors for cardiovascular disease between three ethnic groups in the Whitehall II study." *Atherosclerosis* 1999;142(2): 279–86.

8. AHA "Heart and Stroke . . ."

9. Emilio et al. *Mayo Clinic Practice of Cardiology*, p. 1885.

10. AHA "Heart and Stroke . . ."

11. NIH. *Facts About Heart Disease and Women: Are You At Risk?* (pamphlet). National Heart, Lung, and Blood Institute, NIH, 1998.

12. NIH, Ibid.

13. Vasan RS, Larson MG, Leip EP, Evans JC, O'Donnell CJ, Kannel WB, Levy D. "Impact of high-normal blood pressure on the risk of cardiovascular disease." *New England Journal of Medicine* 2001;345(18): 1291–1297.

14. NIH. "The Sixth Report of the Joint National Committee on Detection, Evaluation, and Treatment of High Blood Pressure." National Heart, Lung and Blood Institute, NIH, 1997.

15. AHA Ibid.

16. Speroff, L, Glass RH, Kase NG. *Clinical Gynecologic Endocrinology and Infertility*, (Baltimore, MD: Lippincott, Williams and Wilkins) 1999, pp.781–82.

17. Speroff L. Ibid, p. 782.

18. Speroff L. Ibid, p. 799.

19. NIH. *Facts About Heart Disease and Women: Are you at Risk?* (pamphlet). National Heart, Lung, and Blood Institute, NIH, 1998.

20. Greenwood DC, Muir KR, Packham CJ Madeley RJ. "Coronary heart disease: A review of the role of psychosocial stress and social support." *Journal of Public Health Medicine* 1996;18(2): 221–31. Review.

21. Tennant C. "Life stress, social support and coronary heart disease." *Australian and New Zealand Journal of Psychiatry.* 1999;33(5): 636–41. Review.

22. Greenwood DC, Muir KR, Packham CJ Madeley RJ. "Coronary Heart Disease."

23. Seeman TE. "Health promoting effects of friends and family on health outcomes in older adults." *American Journal of Health Promotion* 2000;14(6): 362–70. Review.

24. Reuters Health Information, "Heart Information Network." (heartinfo.org) Reuters, Nov. 15, 2000.

25. Georgiades A, Sherwood A, Gullette EC. "Effects of exercise and weight loss on mental stress-induced cardiovascular responses in individuals with high blood pressure." *Hypertension* 2000;36(2): 171–76.

26. American Heart Association. "American Heart Association dietary recommendations dish out a more individualized approach" (news release). American Heart Association, Journal Report, Oct. 5, 2000.

27. Denke MA. "Individual responsiveness to a cholesterol-lowering diet in postmenopausal women with moderate hypercholesterolemia."*Archives of Internal Medicine* 1994;154(17): 1977–82.

28. Titan SM, Bingham S, Welch A, Luben R, Oakes S, Day N, Khaw KT. "Frequency of eating and concentrations of serum cholesterol in the Norfolk population of the European prospective investigation into cancer (EPIC-Norfolk): cross sectional study." *British Medical Journal* 2001;323(7324):1286–1288.

29. Liu S, Manson JE, Stampfer MJ, Rexrode KM, Hu FB, Rimm EB, Willett WC.

"Whole grain consumption and risk of ischemic stroke in women: A prospective study." *Journal of the American Medical Association* 2000;284(12):1534–40.

30. Liu S, Manson JE, Lee IM, Cole SR, Hennekens CH, Willett WC, Buring JE. "Fruit and vegetable intake and risk of cardiovascular disease: The Women's Health Study." *American Journal of Clinical Nutrition* 2000;72(4):922–28.

31. Romero AL, Romero JE, Galaviz S, Fernandez ML. "Cookies enriched with psyllium or oat bran lower plasma LDL cholesterol in normal and hypercholesterolemic men from Northern Mexico." *Journal of the American College of Nutrition* 1998;17(6): 601–608.

32. Gerhardt AL, Gallo NB. "Full-fat rice bran and oat bran similarly reduce hypercholesterolemia in humans." *Journal of Nutrition* 1998;128(5): 865–69.

33. Keenan JM et al. "Randomized, controlled, crossover trial of oat bran in hypercholesterolemic subjects." *Journal of Family Practice* 1991;33(6): 600–608.

34. Davidson MH et al. "The hypocholesterolemic effects of beta-glucan in oatmeal and oatbran. A dose-controlled study." *Journal of the American Medical Association* 1991;265(14): 833–39.

35. Anderson JW, Johnstone BM, Cook-Newell ME. "Meta-analysis of the effects of soy protein intake on serum lipids." *New England Journal of Medicine* 1995;333(5): 76–82.

36. De Kleijn MJ, van der Schouw YT, Wilson PW, Grobbee DE, Jacques PF. "Dietary intake of phytoestrogens is associated with a favorable metabolic cardiovascular risk profile in postmenopausal U.S. women: the Framingham Study." *Journal of Nutrition* 2002;132(2): 276–282.

37. Nestel PJ, Yamashita T, Sasahara T, Pomeroy S, Dart A, Komesaroff P, Owen A, Abbey M. "Soy isoflavones improve systemic arterial compliance but not plasma lipids in menopausal and perimenopausal women." *Arteriosclerosis and Thrombosis* 1997;17 (12): 3392–98.

38. Williams JK, Clarkson TB. "Dietary soy isoflavones inhibit in vivo constrictor responses of coronary arteries to collagen-induced platelet activation." *Coronary Artery Disease* 1998;9(11): 759–64.

39. Washburn S, Burke GL, Morgan T, Anthony M. "Effect of soy protein supplementation on serum lipoproteins, blood pressure, and menopausal symptoms in perimenopausal women." *Menopause* 1999;6(1): 7–13.

40. Jenkins DJ et al. "The effect on serum lipids and oxidized low-density lipoprotein of supplementing self-selected low-fat diets with soluble-fiber, soy, and vegetable protein foods." *Metabolism* 2000;49(1): 67–72.

41. Gronbaek M, Becker U, Johansen D, Gottschau A, Schnohr P, Hein HO, Jensen G, Sorensen TI. "Type of alcohol consumed and mortality from all causes, coronary heart disease, and cancer." *Annals of Internal Medicine* 2000;133(6):411–19.

42. Gronbaek M, Sorensen TI. "Alcohol consumption and risk of coronary heart disease. Studies suggest that wine has additional effect to that of ethanol." *British Medical Journal.* 1996;313(7053): 365.

43. Bell RA, Mayer-Davis EJ, Martin MA, D'Agostino RB Jr, Haffner SM. "Associations between alcohol consumption and insulin sensitivity and cardiovascular disease risk factors: the Insulin Resistance and Atherosclerosis Study." *Diabetes Care* 2000;23(11): 1630–36.

44. Constant J. "Alcohol, ischemic heart disease, and the French paradox." *Coronary Artery Disease* 1997;8(10): 645–49.

45. Wang Z, Huang Y, Zou J, Cao K, Xu Y, Wu JM. "Effects of red wine and wine polyphenol resveratrol on platelet aggregation in vivo and in vitro." *International Journal of Molecular Medicine* 2002;9(1): 77–79.

46. Gronbaek M et al. *Annals of Internal Medicine.*

47. Hudson, T. *Women's Encyclopedia of Natural Medicine* (Los Angeles: Keats) 1999, p. 117.

48. Theobald H, Bygren LO, Carstensen J, Engfeldt P. "A moderate intake of wine is associated with reduced total mortality and reduced mortality from cardiovascular disease." *Journal of Studies on Alcohol* 2000;61(5):652–56.

49. Constant J. "Alcohol, ischemic heart disease . . ."

50. Weinberger MH. "Salt intake and blood pressure in humans." *Boletin de la Asociacion Medica de Puerto Rico.* 1989;81(4): 152–54.

51. Castillo-Richmond A, Schneider RH, Alexander CN, Cook R, Myers HF, Nidich S, Haney C, Rainforth M, Salerno J. "Effects of stress reduction on carotid atherosclerosis in hypertensive African Americans." *Stroke* 2000;31(3): 568–73.

52. Calderon R Jr, Schneider RH, Alexander CN, Myers HF, Nidich SI, Haney C. "Stress, stress reduction and hypercholesterolemia in African Americans: A review." *Ethnicity and Disease* 1999 Autumn;9(3): 451–62. Review.

53. Weed S. *Menopausal Years the Wise Woman Way.* (Ithica NY: Ashtree Publishing) 1992, p. 150.

54. Corry DB, Tuck AM. "Obesity, Hypertension and Sympathetic Nervous System Activity." *Current Hypertension Reports.* 1999;1(2):119–26.

55. Hagberg JM, Brown MD. "Does exercise training play a role in the treatment of essential hypertension?" *Journal of Cardiovascular Risk* 1995;2(4):296–302. Review.

56. Westheim A, Simonsen K, Schamaun O, Qvigstad EK, Staff P, Teisberg P. "Effect of exercise training in patients with essential hypertension." *Acta Medica Scandinavica. Supplementum* 1986;714: 99–103.

57. Ornish D, Scherwitz LW, Billings JH, Brown SE, Gould KL, Merritt TA, Sparler S, Armstrong WT, Ports TA, Kirkeeide RL, Hogeboom C, Brand RJ. "Intensive lifestyle changes for reversal of coronary heart disease." *Journal of the American Medical Association.* 1998;280(23):2001–2007.

58. Ornish D. "Avoiding revascularization with lifestyle changes: The Multicenter Lifestyle Demonstration Project." *American Journal of Cardiology* 1998;82(10B):72T–76T. Review.

59. Blazicek P, Kopcova J, Bederova A, Babinska K. "Homocysteine levels in vegetarians versus omnivores." *Annals of Nutrition and Metabolism* 2000;44(3):135–38.

60. Murray M. *Encyclopedia of Nutritional Supplements* (Rocklin, CA: Prima Publishing) 1996, p. 104.

61. Jha P, Flather M, Lonn E, Farkouh M, Yusuf S. "The antioxidant vitamins and cardiovascular disease. A critical review of epidemiologic and clinical trial data." *Annals of Internal Medicine* 1995;123(11):860–72. Review.

62. Dagenais GR, Marchioli R, Yusuf S, Tognoni G. "Beta-carotene, vitamin C, and vitamin E and cardiovascular diseases." *Current Cardiology Reports.* 2000;2(4):293–99. Review.

63. Yochum LA, Folsom AR, Kushi LH. "Intake of antioxidant vitamins and risk of death from stroke in postmenopausal women." *American Journal of Clinical Nutrition* 2000 Aug;72(2):476–83.

64. The Coronary Drug Project Group. "Clofibrate and niacin in coronary heart disease." *Journal of the American Medical Association* 1975;231(4): 360–81.

65. Canner PL et al. "Fifteen year mortality in Coronary Drug Project patients: Long-term benefit with niacin." *Journal of the American College of Cardiology.* 1986;8: 1245–55.

66. Murray M. *Encyclopedia of Nutritional Supplements* (Rocklin, CA: Prima Publishing) 1996.

67. Malloy MJ, Kane JP, Kunitake ST, Tun P. "Complementarity of colestipol, niacin, and lovastatin in treatment of severe familial hypercholesterolemia." *Annals of Internal Medicine* 1987;107(5): 616–23.

68. Schectman G, Hiatt J. "Dose-response characteristics of cholesterol-lowering drug therapies: Implications for treatment." *Annals of Internal Medicine* 1996;125(12): 990–1000. Review.

69. Bierenbaum ML et al. "Reducing atherogenic risk in hyperlipidemic humans with flax seed supplementation: A preliminary report. "*Journal of the American College of Nutrition* 1993;12: 501–504.

70. Schmidt EB, Dyerberg J. "Omega-3 fatty acids: Current status in cardiovascular medicine." *Drugs* 1994;47: 405–24.

71. Kromhout D et al. "Inverse relation between fish oil consumption and 20-year mortality from coronary heart disease." *New England Journal of Medicine* 1985;312: 1205–1209.

72. Stark KD, Park EJ, Maines VA, Holub JB. "Effect of a fish-oil concentrate on serum lipids in postmenopausal women receiving and not receiving hormone replacement therapy in a placebo-controlled, double-blind trial." *American Journal of Clinical Nutrition* 2000 Aug;72(2): 389–94.

73. Nestel PJ. "Fish oil and cardiovascular disease: Lipids and arterial function. " *American Journal of Clinical Nutrition* 2000 Jan;71(1 Suppl): 228S–31S.

74. Nestel PJ, Pomeroy SE, Sasahara T, Yamashita T, Liang YL, Dart AM, Jennings GL, Abbey M, Cameron JD. "Arterial compliance in obese subjects is improved with dietary plant n-3 fatty acid from flaxseed oil despite increased LDL oxidizability. " *Arteriosclerosis and Thrombosis* 1997;17(6): 1163–70.

75. Cobias L et al. "Lipid, lipoprotein, and hemostatic effect of fish vs. fish oil w-3 fatty acids in mildly hyperlipidemic males." *American Journal of Clinical Nutrition* 1991;53:1210–16.

76. Nestel PJ, Pomeroy S, Kay S, Komesaroff P, Behrsing J, Cameron JD, West L. "Isoflavones from red clover improve systemic arterial compliance but not plasma lipids in menopausal women." *Journal of Clinical Endocrinology and Metabolism* 1999 Mar;84(3): 895–98.

77. Samman S et al. "The effect of supplementation with isoflavones on plasma lipids and oxidisability of LDLs in premenopausal women." *Atherosclerosis* 1999;147: 277–83.

78. Singh RB, Niaz MA, Ghosh S. "Hypolipidemic and antioxidant effects of Commiphora mukul as an adjunct to dietary therapy in patients with hypercholesterolemia." *Cardiovascular Drugs and Therapy* 1994;8(4): 659–64.

79. Dalvi SS et al. "Effect of gugulipid on bioavailability of diltiazem and propranolol." *Journal of the Association of Physicians of India* 1994;42(6):454–55.

80. Heber D, Yip I, Ashley JM, Elashoff DA, Elashoff RM, Go VL. "Cholesterol-lowering effects of a proprietary Chinese red-yeast-rice dietary supplement." *American Journal of Clinical Nutrition* 1999;69(2):231–36.

81. Sotiriou CG, Cheng JW. "Beneficial effects of statins in coronary artery disease—beyond lowering cholesterol." *Annals of Pharmocotherapy* 2000;34(12):1432–39.

82. Wong HN, Ming S, Phou HY, Black HR. "A comparison of Chinese traditional and Western medical approaches for the treatment of mild hypertension." *Yale Journal of Biology and Medicine* 1991;64(1): 79–87.

83. Racz-Kotilla E, Racz G, Solomon A. "The action of Taraxacum officinale extracts on the body weight and diuresis of laboratory animals." *Planta Medica* 1974;26: 212–17.

84. "Monograph: Crataegus oxycantha." *Alternative Medicine Review* 1998;3(2): 138–39.

85. Miller A. "Botanical Influences on Cardiovascular Disease." *Alternative Medicine Review* 1998;3(6):423–31.

86. Schussler M, Holzo J, Fricke U. "Myocardial effects of flavonoids from Cratagus species." *Arzneimittel-Forschung* 1995;45:842–45.

87. Weikl A, Assmus KD, Neukum-Schmidt A et al. "Crataegus Special Extract WS 1442. Assessment of objective effectiveness in patients with heart failure." *Fortschritte der Medizin.* [Article in German] *Monographie* 1996;114: 291–96.

88. Uchida S, Ikari N, Ohta H et al. "Inhibitory effect of condensed tannins on angiotensin converting enzyme." *Japanese Journal of Pharmacology* 1987;43:242–45.

89. Herrington DM. "The HERS trial results: Paradigms lost? Heart and Estrogen/Progestin Replacement Study." *Annals of Internal Medicine* 1999;131(6):463–66.

90. Wells G, Herrington DM. "The Heart and Estrogen/Progestin Replacement Study: What heave we learned and what questions remain?" *Drugs & Aging* 1999;15(6): 419–22.

91. Blakely, JA. "The Heart and Estrogen/Progestin Replacement Study revisited: Hormone replacement therapy produced net harm, consistent with the observational data." *Archives of Internal Medicine* 2000;160(19): 2897–900.

92. Heckbert SR, Kaplan RC, Weiss NS, Psaty BM, Lin D, Furberg CD, Starr JR, Anderson GD, LaCroix AZ. "Risk of recurrent coronary events in relation to use and recent initiation of postmenopausal hormone therapy." *Archives of Internal Medicine.* 2001;161(14): 1709–13.

93. Alexander KP, Newby LK, Hellkamp AS, Harrington RA, Peterson ED, Kopecky S, Langer A, O'Gara P, O'Connor CM, Daly RN, Califf RM, Khan S, Fuster V. "Initiation of hormone replacement therapy after acute myocardial infarction is associated with more cardiac events during follow-up." *Journal of the American College of Cardiology* 2001;38(1): 1–7.

Chapter 7

1. Makin M. "Osteoporosis and proximal femoral fractures in the female elderly of Jerusalem." *Clinical Orthopedics* 1987;(218): 19–23.

2. Ling X, Cummings SR et al. "Vertebral fractures in Beijing, China: The Beijing Osteoporosis Project." *Journal of Bone and Mineral Research* 2000;15(10): 2019–25.

3. Brown S. *Better Bones, Better Body* (Los Angeles: Keats Publishing) 2000, pp. 37–39.

4. Seeman E, Hopper JL, Young NR, Formica C, Goss P, Tsalamandris C. "Do genetic factors explain associations between muscle strength, lean mass, and bone density? A twin study." *American Journal of Physiology* 1996;270(2 Pt 1): E320–27.

5. Kellie SE, Brody JA. "Sex-specific and race-specific hip fracture rates." *American Journal of Public Health* 1990;80:326.

6. Ling X et al. "Vertebral fractures in Beijing, China: The Beijing Osteoporosis Project." *Journal of Bone and Mineral Research* 2000;15(10): 2019–25.

7. Yang RS, Wang SS, Liu TK. "Proximal femoral dimension in elderly Chinese women with hip fractures in Taiwan." *Osteoporosis International* 1999;10(2): 109–13.

8. Iga T, Dohmae Y et al. "Increase in the incidence of cervical and trochanteric fractures of the proximal femur in Niigata Prefecture, Japan." *Journal of Bone and Mineral Metabolism* 1999;17(3): 224–31.

9. Morrison NA, Qi JC, Tokita A, Kelly PJ, Crofts L, Nguyen TV, Sambrook PN, Eisman JA. "Prediction of bone density from vitamin D receptor alleles." *Nature* 1994;367: 284–87.

10. Morrison NA, Yeoman R, Kelly PJ, Eisman JA. "Contribution of trans-acting factor alleles to normal physiological variability: Vitamin D receptor gene polymorphism and circulating osteocalcin." *Proceedings of the U.S. National Academy of Science* 1992;89: 6665–69.

11. Cadarette SM, Jaglal SB, Krieger N, McIsaac WJ, Darlington GA, Tu JV. "Development and validation of the Osteoporosis Risk Assessment Instrument to facilitate selection of women for bone densitometry." *Canadian Medical Association Journal* 2000;162(9):1289–94.

12. Guthrie JR, Dennerstein L, Wark JD. "Risk factors for osteoporosis: A review." *Medscape Womens Health.* 2000;5(4): E1. Review.

13. Liel Y, Shany S, Smirnoff P, Schwartz B. "Estrogen increases 1,25 dihydroxyvitamin D receptors expression and bioresponse in the rat duodenal mucosa." *Endocrinology* 1999;140: 280–85.

14. Byrne IM et al. "Identification of a hormone-responsive promoter immediately upstream of exon 1c in the human vitamin D receptor gene." *Endocrinology* 2000; 141(8): 2829–36.

15. McKane WR, Khosla S, Burritt MF, Kao PC, Wilson DM, Ory SJ, Riggs BL. "Mechanism of renal calcium conservation with estrogen replacement therapy in women in early postmenopause—a clinical research center study." *Journal of Clinical Endocrinology and Metabolism* 1995;80:3458–64.

16. Gray K. "Estrogens, Progestins, and Bone." World Congress on Osteoporosis 2000, *Medscape Women's Health* (www.medscape.com/womenshealthhome).

17. Jilka RL, Takahashi K, Munshi M, Williams DC, Roberson PK, Manolagas SC. "Loss of estrogen upregulates osteoblastogenesis in the murine bone marrow. Evidence for autonomy from factors released during bone resorption." *Journal of Clinical Investigation* 1998;101: 1942–50.

18. Tomkinson A, Gevers EF, Wit JM, Reeve J, Noble BS. "The role of estrogen in the control of rat osteocyte apoptosis." *Journal of Bone and Mineral Research* 1998;13: 1243–50.

19. Cooper GS, Sandler DP. "Long-term effects of reproductive-age menstrual cycle patterns on peri- and postmenopausal fracture risk." *American Journal of Epidemiology* 1997;145(9): 804-809.

20. Myerson M, Gutin B, Warren MP, Wang J, Lichtman S, Pierson RN Jr. "Total body bone density in amenorrheic runners." *Obstetrics and Gynecology* 1992;79: 973–78.

21. Snead DB, Weltman A, Weltman JY, Evans WS, Veldhuis JD, Varma MM, Teates CD, Dowling EA, Rogol AD. "Reproductive hormones and bone mineral density in women runners." *Journal of Applied Physiology* 1992;72(6):2149–56.

22. Baker D, Roberts R, Towell T. "Factors predictive of bone mineral density in eating-disordered women: A longitudinal study." *International Journal of Eating Disorders* 2000;27(1): 29–35.

23. Newton JR, Freeman CP, Hannan WJ, Cowen S. "Osteoporosis and normal weight bulimia nervosa—which patients are at risk?" *Journal of Psychosomatic Research* 1993;37(3): 239–47.

24. Ren Y, Zhu G. [The effects of progestin on the bone metabolism in post-menopausal women] [in Chinese] *Chinese Journal of Obstetrics and Gynecology.* 1995;30 (3): 135–37.

25. Roux C, Kolta S, Chappard C, Morieux C, Dougados M, De Vernejoul MC. "Bone effects of dydrogesterone in ovariectomized rats: A biologic, histomorphometric, and densitometric study." *Bone* 1996;19(5):463–68.

26. Prior JC. "Progesterone as a bone-trophic hormone." *Endocrine Reviews* 1990;11 (2): 386–98. Review.

27. Adler RA. "Sex steroids and osteoporosis. The role of estrogens and androgens." *Clinical Laboratory Medicine* 2000 Sep;20(3): 549–58, vii.

28. Birge SJ, Whedon GD. In: McCally M, ed. *Hypodynamics and Hypogravics; The Physiology of Inactivity and Weightlessness* (New York, NY: Academic Press) 1968 pp., 267–70.

29. Wolman RL. "ABC of sports medicine. Osteoporosis and exercise." *British Medical Journal* 1994;309(6951): 400–403. Review.

30. Jaglal SB, Kreiger N, Darlington G. "Past and recent physical activity and risk of hip fracture." *American Journal of Epidemiology* 1993;138(2): 107–18.

31. Jakes RW, Khaw K, Day NE, Bingham S, Welch A, Oakes S, Luben R, Dalzell N, Reeve J, Wareham NJ. "Patterns of physical activity and ultrasound attenuation by heel bone among Norfolk cohort of European Prospective Investigation of Cancer (EPIC Norfolk): Population based study." *British Medical Journal* 2001;322(7279): 140–43.

32. Sabatier JP, Guaydier–Souquieres G, Benmalek A, Marcelli C. "Evolution of lumbar bone mineral content during adolescence and adulthood: A longitudinal study in 395 healthy females 10–24 years of age and 206 premenopausal women." *Osteoporosis International* 1999;9(6): 476–82.

33. Heaney RP. "Thinking straight about calcium." New England Journal of Medicine 1993;328: 503–505.

34. Reid IR, Ames RW, Evans MC, Gamble GD, Sharpe SJ. "Effect of calcium supplementation on bone loss in postmenopausal women." New England Journal of Medicine 1993;328(7): 460–64.

35. Nordin BE, Need AG, Steurer T, Morris HA, Chatterton BE, Horowitz M. "Nutrition, osteoporosis, and aging." Annals of the New York Academy of Science 1998;854: 336–51.

36. Rao DS. "Perspective on assessment of vitamin D nutrition." Journal of Clinical Densitometry 1999;2(4): 457–64.

37. Glerup H, Mikkelsen K, Poulsen L, Hass E, Overbeck S, Thomsen J, Charles P, Eriksen EF. "Commonly recommended daily intake of vitamin D is not sufficient if sunlight exposure is limited." Journal of Internal Medicine 2000;247(2):260–68.

38. Obstetrics and Gynecology News 34;23 December 1999.

39. Dequeker J, Westhovens R. "Low dose corticosteroid associated osteoporosis in rheumatoid arthritis and its prophylaxis and treatment: Bones of contention." Journal of Rheumatology 1995;22(6): 1013–19.

40. Sambrook PN. "Corticosteroid osteoporosis." Zeitschrift fur Rheumatologie 2000; 59 Suppl1: 45–47. Review.

41. Valimaki MJ, Tiihonen M, Laitinen K, Tahtela R, Karkkainen M, Lamberg-Allardt C, Makela P, Tunninen R. "Bone mineral density measured by dual-energy X-ray absorptiometry and novel markers of bone formation and resorption in patients on antiepileptic drugs." Journal of Bone and Mineral Research 1994;9(5): 631–37.

42. Cummings SR, Nevitt MC, Browner WS, Stone K, Fox KM, Ensrud KE, Cauley J, Black D, Vogt TM. "Risk Factors for Hip Fracture in White Women." New England Journal of Medicine 1995;332(12): 767–73.

43. Brambilla DJ, McKinlay SM. "A prospective study of factors affecting age at menopause." Journal of Clinical Epidemiology 1989;42(11): 1031–39.

44. Seeman E, Allen T. "Risk factors for osteoporosis." Australian and New Zealand Journal of Medicine 1989;19(1): 69–75.

45. Aloia JF, Vaswani AN, Yeh JK, Ross P, Ellis K, Cohn SH. "Determinants of bone mass in postmenopausal women." Archives of Internal Medicine 1983;143(9): 1700–704.

46. Krall EA, Dawson-Hughes B. "Smoking and bone loss among postmenopausal women." Journal of Bone and Mineral Research 1991;6(4): 331–38.

47. Hoper JL, Seeman AL. "The bone density of female twins discordant for tobacco use." New England Journal of Medicine 1994;330(6): 387–92.

48. Cure-Cure C, Cure-Ramirez P. "Multiparity decreases risk of fractures in postmenopausal women." American Journal of Obstetrics and Gynecology 2001;184: 580–83.

49. Ganry O, Baudoin C, Fardellone P. "Effect of alcohol intake on bone mineral density in elderly women: The EPIDOS Study." American Journal of Epidemiology 2000; 151(8): 773–80.

50. Massey LK, Whiting SJ. "Caffeine, urinary calcium, calcium metabolism and bone." Journal of Nutrition. 1993;123(9): 1611–14. Review.

51. Cummings SR et al. "Risk Factors for Hip Fracture."

52. Nordin BE, Need AG, Steurer T, Morris HA, Chatterton BE, Horowitz M. "Nutrition, osteoporosis, and aging." Annals of the New York Academy of Science 1998:854: 336–51.

53. Itoh R, Suyama Y, Oguma Y, Yokota F. "Dietary sodium, an independent determinant for urinary deoxypyridinoline in elderly women. A cross-sectional study on the effect of dietary factors on deoxypyridinoline excretion in 24-h urine specimens from 763 free-living healthy Japanese." European Journal of Clinical Nutrition 1999;53(11): 886–90.

54. Ho SC, Chen YM, Woo JL, Leung SS, Lam TH, Jankus ED. "Sodium is the lead-

ing dietary factor associated with urinary calcium excretion in Hong Kong Chinese adults." *Osteoporosis International* 2001;12: 723–31.

55. Munger RG, Cerhan JR, Chiu BC. "Prospective study of dietary protein intake and risk of hip fracture in postmenopausal women." *American Journal of Clinical Nutrition* 1999;69(1):147–52.

56. Hannan MT et al. "Effect of dietary protein on bone loss in elderly men and women: The Framingham Osteoporosis Study." *Journal of Bone and Mineral Research* 2000;15(12):2504–12.

57. Nordin et al. "Nutrition, osteoporosis"

58. Marsh AG, Sanchez TV, Midkelsen O, Keiser J, Mayor G. "Cortical bone density of adult lacto-ovo-vegetarian and omnivorous women." *Journal of the American Dietetics Association* 1980;76(2): 148–51.

59. Ho SC et al. *Medscape Women's Health* (Reuters Health) Jan 24, 2001.

60. Pennington J. et al. "Mineral content of food and total diets: The selected minerals in foods survey, 1982 to 1984." *Journal of the American Dietetics Association* 1986; 86: 876–91.

61. Wyshak G. In Jocelyn Selim. "Pop, Crackle, Snap." *Discover Magazine* 2000;21 (11): 28.

62. New SA, Robins SP, Campbell MK, Martin JC, Garton MJ, Bolton-Smith C, Grubb DA, Lee SJ, Reid DM. "Dietary influences on bone mass and bone metabolism: Further evidence of a positive link between fruit and vegetable consumption and bone health?" *American Journal of Clinical Nutrition* 2000;71(1): 142–51.

63. Tucker KL, Hannan MT, Chen H, Cupples LA, Wilson PW, Kiel DP. "Potassium, magnesium, and fruit and vegetable intakes are associated with greater bone mineral density in elderly men and women." *American Journal of Clinical Nutrition* 1999;69(4): 727–36.

64. Yamaguchi M, Kakuda H, Gao YH, Tsukamoto Y. "Prolonged intake of fermented soybean (natto) diets containing vitamin K2 (menaquinone-7) prevents bone loss in ovariectomized rats." *Journal of Bone and Mineral Metabolism* 2000;18(2): 71–76.

65. Feskanich D, Weber P, Willett WC, Rockett H, Booth SL, Colditz GA. "Vitamin K intake and hip fractures in women: A prospective study." *American Journal of Clinical Nutrition* 1999;69(1): 74–79.

66. Frost ML, Blake GM, Fogelman I. "Can the WHO criteria for diagnosing osteoporosis be applied to calcaneal quantitative ultrasound?" *Osteoporosis International* 2000;11(4): 321–30.

67. He YQ, Fan B, Hans D, Li J, Wu CY, Njeh CF, Zhao S, Lu Y, Tsuda-Futami E, Fuerst T, Genant HK. "Assessment of a new quantitative ultrasound calcaneus measurement: Precision and discrimination of hip fractures in elderly women compared with dual X-ray absorptiometry." *Osteoporosis International* 2000;11(4):354–60.

68. "Prevention: Who's at Risk" and "Osteoporosis: Bone Mass Measurement." National Osteoporosis Foundation website (www.nof.org).

69. Adachi JD. "The correlation of bone mineral density and biochemical markers to fracture risk." *Calcified Tissue International* 1996;59 Suppl 1: 16–19.

70. Table adapted from the World Health Organization Study Group. WHO Technical Report Series 843. World Health Organization, Geneva, Switzerland, 1994.

71. Dresner-Pollak R, Parker RA, Poku M, Thompson J, Seibel MJ, Greenspan SL. "Biochemical markers of bone turnover reflect femoral bone loss in elderly women." *Calcified Tissue International* 1996;59(5): 328–33.

72. Garnero P, Dargent-Molina P, Hans D, Schott AM, Breart G, Meunier PJ, Delmas PD. "Do markers of bone resorption add to bone mineral density and ultrasonographic heel measurement for the prediction of hip fracture in elderly women? The EPIDOS prospective study." *Osteoporosis International* 1998;8(6): 563–69.

73. Hedstrom M, Svensson J, Dalen N. "Biochemical bone markers and bone den-

sity in hip fracture patients: weak correlation in 106 women." *Acta Orthopaedica Scandinavica.* 2000,71(4): 409–13.

74. Feskanich D, Willet WC, Stampfer JM, Colditz GA. "Mild, dietary calcium, and bone fractures in women: A 12-year prospective study." *American Journal of Public Health* 1997;(6):992–97.

75. Chiu JF, Lan SJ, Yang CY, Wang PW, Yao WJ, Su LH, Hsieh CC. "Long-term vegetarian diet and bone mineral density in postmenopausal Taiwanese women." *Calcified Tissue International* 1997;60(3): 245–49.

76. Heaney RP. "Calcium, dairy products and osteoporosis." *Journal of the American College of Nutrition* 2000;19(2 Suppl): 83S–99S.

77. Heaney RP, McCarron DA, Dawson-Hughes B, Oparil S, Berga SL, Stern JS, Barr SI, Rosen CJ. "Dietary changes favorably affect bone remodeling in older adults." *Journal of the American Dietetics Association* 1999;99(10):1228–1233.

78. Adapted from Murray M. *Encyclopedia of Nutritional Supplements* (Rocklin, CA: Prima Publishing) 1996.

79. Horiuchi T et al. "Effect of soy protein on bone metabolism in postmenopausal Japanese women." *Osteoporosis International* 2000;11(8):721–24.

80. Somekawa U. "Soy intake related to menopausal symptoms, serum lipids, and bone mineral density in postmenopausal Japanese women." *Obstetrics and Gynecology* 2001;97(1): 109–15.

81. Kung AWC. *Journal of Clinical Endrocrinology and Metabolism* 2001;86: 5217–21.

82. Alekel DL et al. "Isoflavone-rich soy protein isolate attenuates bone loss in the lumbar spine of perimenopausal women." *American Journal of Clinical Nutrition* 2000;72(3): 844–52.

83. Bryant RJ, Cadogan J, Weaver CM. "The new dietary reference intakes for calcium: Implications for osteoporosis." *Journal of the American College of Nutrition* 1999;18(5 Suppl): 406S–412S.

84. Bourgoin BP, Evans DR, Cornett JR et al. "Lead content in 70 brands of dietary calcium supplement." *American Journal of Public Health* 1993; 83: 1155–60.

85. Recker RR. "Calcium absorption and achlorhydria." *New England Journal of Medicine* 1985;313(2): 70–73.

86. Murray M. *Encyclopedia of Nutritional Supplements* (Rocklin, CA: Prima Publishers) 1996, p. 152.

87. Heller HJ, Stewart A, Haynes S, Pak CY. "Pharmacokinetics of calcium absorption from two commercial calcium supplements." *Journal of Clinican Pharmacology* 1999;39(11): 1151–54.

88. Schieber MD, Rebar R. "Isoflavones and Postmenopausal Bone Health: A Viable Alternative to Estrogen Therapy?" *Menopause* 1999;6(3): 233–41.

89. Ohta H, Komukai S, Makita K, Masuzawa T, Nozawa S. "Effects of 1-year ipriflavone treatment on lumbar bone mineral density and bone metabolic markers in postmenopausal women with low bone mass." *Hormone Research* 1999;51(4): 178–83.

90. Halpner AD, Kellerman G, Ahlgrimm MJ, Arndt CL, Shaikh NA, Hargrave JJ, Tallas PG. "The effect of an ipriflavone-containing supplement on urinary N-linked telopeptide levels in postmenopusal women." *Journal of Women's Health and Gender Based Medicine* 2000;9(9): 995–98.

91. Arjmandi BH, Khalil DA, Hollis BW. "Ipriflavone a synthetic phytoestrogen, enhances intestinal calcium transport in vitro." *Calcified Tissue International* 2000;67 (3):225–29.

92. Arjmandi BH et al. "The synthetic phytoestrogen, ipriflavone, and estrogen prevent bone loss by different mechanisms." *Calcified Tissue International* 2000;66(1): 61–65.

93. Fujita T et al. "Comparison of antiresorptive activities of ipriflavone, an isoflavone derivative, and elcatonin, an eel carbocalcitonin." *Journal of Bone and Mineral Metabolism* 1999;17(4): 289–95.

94. Alexandersen P, Toussaint A, Christiansen C, Devogelaer JP, Roux C, Fechtenbaum J, Gennari C, Reginster JY. Ipriflavone Multicenter European Fracture Study. Ipriflavone in the treatment of postmenopausal osteoporosis: A randomized controlled trial." *Journal of the American Medical Association* 2001;285(11): 1482–88.

95. Oreffo RO, Kusec V, Virdi AS, Flanagan AM, Grano M, Zambonin-Zallone A, Triffitt JT. "Expression of estrogen receptor-alpha in cells of the osteoclastic lineage." *Histochemistry and Cell Biology* 1999;111(2): 125–33.

96. Robinson JA, Harris SA, Riggs BL, Spelsberg TC. "Estrogen regulation of human osteoblastic cell proliferation and differentiation." *Endocrinology* 1997;138(7): 2919–27.

97. Zaman G, Cheng MZ, Jessop HL, White R, Lanyon LE. "Mechanical strain activates estrogen response elements in bone cells." *Bone* 2000;27(2): 233–39.

98. Damien E, Price JS, Lanyon LE. "The estrogen receptor's involvement in osteoblasts' adaptive response to mechanical strain." *Journal of Bone and Mineral Research* 1998;13(8): 1275–82.

99. Wills M, Odegaard K, Persson U. "A cost-effectivenesss model of tibolone as treatment of the prevention of osteoporotic fractures in postmenopausal women in Sweden." 2002;21(2): 115–27.

100. Genant HK, Lucas J, Weiss S, Akin M, Emkey R, McNaney-Flint H, Downs R, Mortola J, Watts N, Yang HM, Banav N, Brennan JJ, Nolan JC. "Low-dose esterified estrogen therapy: Effects on bone, plasma estradiol concentrations, endometrium, and lipid levels. Estratab/Osteoporosis Study Group." *Archives of Internal Medicine* 1997; 157(22): 2609–15.

101. Prestwood KM, Kenny AM, Unson C, Kulldorff M. "The effect of low dose micronized 17ss-estradiol on bone turnover, sex hormone levels, and side effects in older women: A randomized, double blind, placebo-controlled study." *Journal of Clinical Endocrinology and Metabolism* 2000;85(12):4462–69.

102. Itoi H, Minakami H, Sato I. "Comparison of the long-term effects of oral estriol with the effects of conjugated estrogen, 1-alpha-hydroxyvitamin D3, and calcium lactate on vertebral bone loss in early menopausal women." *Maturitas* 1997;28(2): 11–17.

103. Lindsay R, Hart DM, MacLean A, et al. "Bone loss during oestiol therapy in postmenopausal women." *Maturitas* 1979;1: 279–85.

104. Head KA. "Estriol: safety and efficacy." *Alternative Medicine Review* 1998;3(2): 101–13. Review.

105. Riis BJ, Ise J, von Stein T, Bagger Y, Christiansen C. "Ibandronate: A comparison of oral daily dosing versus intermittent dosing in postmenopausal osteoporosis." *Journal of Bone and Mineral Research* 2001;16: 1871–78.

Chapter 8

1. Murray W. "Decreased libido in postmenopausal women." *Nurse Practitioner Forum* 2000;11(4):219–24.

2. Berman JR, Berman LA, Werbin TJ, Flaherty EE, Leahy NM, Goldstein I. "Clinical evaluation of female sexual function: Effects of age and estrogen status on subjective and physiologic sexual responses." *International Journal of Impotence Research* 1999;11 Suppl 1:S31–38.

3. Avis NE, Stellato R, Crawford S, Johannes C, Longcope C. "Is there an association between menopause status and sexual functioning?" *Menopause* 2000;7(5):297–309.

4. Avis NE, Stellato R, Crawford S, Johannes C, Longcope C. Ibid.

5. Mansfield PK, Koch PB. "Qualities midlife women desire in their sexual relationships and their changing sexual response." *Psychology of Women Quarterly* 1996;22: 285–303.

6. Mansfield PK, Koch PB. Ibid.

7. Kalogeraki A, Tamiolakis D, Relakis K, Karvelas K, Froudarakis G, Hassan E, Martavatzis N, Psaroudakis E. "Cigarette smoking and vaginal atrophy in post-menopausal women." *In Vivo* 1996;10(6): 597–600.

8. Brizzolara S, Killeen J, Severino R. "Vaginal pH and parabasal cells in post-menopausal women." *Obstetrics and Gynecology* 1999;94(5 Pt 1): 700–703.

9. Speroff L, Glass RH, Kase NG. *Clinical Gynecologic Endocrinology and Infertility* (Baltimore, MD: Lippincott, Williams and Wilkins) 1999, p. 623.

10. Burger HG, Dudley E, Cui J, Dennerstein L, Hopper JL. "A prospective longitu-dinal study of serum testosterone, dehydroepiandrosterone sulfate, and sex hormone-binding globulin levels through the menopause transition." *Journal of Clinical Endocrinology and Metabolism* 2000;85(8): 2832–38.

11. Davis SR, Burger HG. "Use of androgens in postmenopausal women." *Current Opinion in Obstetrics and Gynecology* 1997;9(3): 177–80.

12. Davis SR. "Androgen treatment in women." *Medical Journal of Australia* 1999; 170(11): 545–49.

13. Davis SR, Burger HG. "Use of androgens in postmenopausal women." *Current Opinions in Obstetrics and Gynecology* 1997;(3): 177–80.

14. Davis SR. "Androgen treatment in women." *Medical Journal of Australia* 1999:170(11): 545–49.

15. Gelfand MM, Wiita B. "Androgen and estrogen-androgen hormone replace-ment therapy: a review of the safety literature, 1941 to 1996." *Clinical Therapeutics* 1997;1993):383–404.

16. Slayden SM. "Risks of menopausal androgen supplementation." *Seminars in Reproductive Endocrinology* 1998;16(2):145–52.

17. Gelfand MM, Wiita B. "Androgen and estrogen-androgen . . ."

18. Sarrel PM. "Cardiovascular aspects of androgens in women." *Seminars in Repro-ductive Endocrinology* 1998;16: 121–28.

19. Worboys S, Kotsopoulus D, Teede H, McGrath B, Davis SR. "Evidence that par-enteral testosterone therapy may improve endothelium-dependent and -independent vasodilation in postmenopausal women already receiving estrogen." *Journal of Clinical Endocrinology and Metabolism* 2001;86(1): 158–61.

20. Barret-Connor E, Young R, Notelovitz M, Sullivan J, Wiita B, Yang HM, Nolan J. "A two-year double-blind comparison of estrogen-androgen and conjugated estrogens in surgically menopausal women. Effects of bone mineral density, symptoms and lipid profiles." *Journal of Reproductive Medicine* 1999;44(12): 1012–20.

21. Rosenberg MJ, Kind TD, Timmons MC. "Estrogen-androgen for hormone re-placement. A review." *Journal of Reproductive Medicine* 1997;42(7): 397–404.

22. Avis NE, Stellato R, Crawford S, Johannes C, Longcope C. Ibid.

23. Mansfield PK, Koch PB. "Qualities midlife women desire in their sexual relation-ships and their changing sexual response." *Psychology of Women Quarterly* 1998;22(2): 285–303.

24. Channon LD, Ballinger SE. "Some aspects of sexuality and vaginal symptoms during menopause and their relation to anxiety and depression." *British Journal of Medical Psychology* 1986;59 (Pt 2): 173–80.

25. Avis NE. Sexual function and aging in men and women: Community and population-based studies." *Journal of Gender Specific Medicine* 2000;3(2): 37–41.

26. Ganz PA, Rowland JH, Desmond K, Meyerowitz BE, Wyatt GE. "Life after breast cancer: Understanding women's health-related quality of life and sexual functioning." *Journal of Clinical Oncology* 1998;16(2): 501–14.

27. Davis AF. "Recent advances in female sexual dysfunction." *Current Psychiatry Reports* 2000;2(3): 211–14.

28. Shifren JL, Braunstein GD, Simon JA, Casson PR, Buster JE, Redmond GP,

Burki RE, Ginsburg ES, Rosen RC, Leiblum SR, Caramelli KE, Mazer NA. "Transdermal testosterone treatment in women with impaired sexual function after oophorectomy." *New England Journal of Medicine* 2000;343(10):682–88.

29. Melis GB, Ibba MT, Steri B, Kotsonis P, Matta V, Paoletti AM. ["Role of pH as a regulator of vaginal physiological environment"].[Article in Italian] *Minerva Ginecologica* 2000;52(4): 111–21.

30. Heimer G, Samsioe G. "Effects of vaginally delivered estrogens." Effects of vaginally delivered estrogens." *Acta Obstetricia et Gynecologica Scandinavica.* Supplement. 1996;163: 1–2.

31. Parsons CL, Schmidt JD. "Control of recurrent lower urinary tract infection in the postmenopausal woman." *Journal of Urology* 1982;128(6):1224–26.

32. Barentsen P, van de Weijer PH, Shram JH. "Continuous low dose estradiol released from a vaginal ring versus estriol vaginal cream for urogenital atrophy." *European Journal of Obstetrics, Gynecology, and Reproductive Biology.* 1999;71(1): 73–80.

33. Dugal R et al. "Comparison of usefulness of estradiol vaginal tablets and estriol vagitories for treatment of vaginal atrophy." *Acta Obstetricia et Gynecologica Scandinavica* 2000;79(4):293–97.

34. Heimer GM. "Estriol in the postmenopause." *Acta Obstetricia et Gynecologica Scandinavica* 1987;139: S1–S23.

35. WeiderPass E et al. "Low-potency oestrogen and risk of endometrial cancer: A case-control study." *Lancet* 1999;353(9167):1824–28.

36. Hustin J, Van der Eynde JP. "Cytological evaluation of the effect of various estrogens given in postmenopause." *Acta Cytologica* 1977;21:225–28.

37. Head KA. "Estriol: Safety and efficacy." *Alternative Medicine Review* 1998(2): 101–13. Review.

38. Losc G, Englev E, Oestradiol-releasing vaginal ring versus oestriol vaginal pessaries in the treatment of bothersome lower urinary tract symptoms." *British Journal of Gynecology* 2000;107(8): 1029–34.

39. Ishiko O et al. "Estriol, pelvic floor muscle exercises may combat postmenopausal stress incontinence." *Journal of Reproductive Medicine* 2001:46:213–20.

40. Choi YD, Rha KH, Choi HK. "In vitro and in vivo experimental effect of Korean red ginseng on erection." *Journal of Urology* 1999;162(4): 1508–11.

41. Zava DT, Dollbaum CM, Blen M. "Estrogen and progestin bioactivity of foods, herbs, and spices." *Proceedings of the Society for Experimental Biology and Medicine* 1998; 217(3):369–78.

42. Waynberg J, Brewer S. "Effects of Herbal vX on libido and sexual activity in premenopausal and postmenopausal women." *Advances in Therapy* 2000;17(5):255–62.

43. Cohen AJ, Bartlik B. "Ginkgo biloba for antidepressant-induced sexual dysfunction." *Journal of Sex and Marital Therapy* 1998;24(2): 139–43.

44. Sands R, Studd J. "Exogenous androgens in postmenopausal women," *American Journal of Medicine* 1995;16;98(1A): 76S–79S.

45. Kaplan SA, Reis RB, Kohn IJ, Ikeguchi EF, Laor E, Te AE, Martins AC. "Safety and efficacy of sildenafil in postmenopausal women with sexual dysfunction." *Urology* 1999;53(3): 481–86.

46. Basson R, McInnes R, Smith MD, Hodgson G, Spain T, Koppiker N. "Efficacy and safety of sildenafil in estrogenized women with sexual dysfunction associated with female sexual arousal disorder." *Obstetrics and Gynecology* 2000;95(4 Suppl 1): S54.

47. Rosenberg KP. "Sildenafil." *Journal of Sex and Marital Therapy* 1999;25(4): 271–79.

Chapter 9

1. Avis NE, McKinlay SM. "A longitudinal analysis of women's attitudes toward the menopause: Results from the Massachusetts Women's Health Study." *Maturitas* 1991:13(1): 65–79.

2. Avis NE, Brambilla D, McKinlay SM, Vass K. "A longitudinal analysis of the association between menopause and depression. Results from the Massachusetts Women's Health Study." *Annals of Epidemiology* 1994;4(3): 214–20.

3. Dennerstein L, Dudley E, Guthrie J, Barrett-Connor E. "Life satisfaction, symptoms, and the menopausal transition." *Medscape Women's Health* 2000:5(4): E4.

4. Weissman M and Klerman G. "Sex differences and the epidemiology of depression." *Archives of General Psychiatry* 1977;34: 98–111.

5. Sichel D and Driscoll J. *Women's Moods* (New York: Quill Publishers) 1999.

6. Sherwin, BB. "Hormones, mood, and cognitive functioning in postmenopausal women." *Obstetrics and Gynecology* 1996;87(2 Suppl): 20S–26S.

7. Goldman, H. *Review of General Psychiatry* (Norwalk, CT: Appleton & Lange) 1995, p. 77.

8. Sherwin B. "Hormones, mood, and cognitive functioning in postmenopausal women." *Obstetrics and Gynecology* 1996;87(2) (supplement): 20S.

9. Young E and Korszun A. "Psychoneuroendocrinology of depression." *Psychiatric Clinics of North America* 1998;21(2):309–23.

10. Woodward S, Freedman RR, "The thermoregulatory effects of menopausal hot flashes on sleep." *Sleep* 1994;17: 497.

11. Weed S. *The Menopausal Years The Wise Woman Way.* (Woodstock, NY: Ashtree Publishing) 1992, p. 71.

12. *The Diagnostic and Statistical Manual of Mental Disorders*, Fourth Edition. (Washington, D.C.: APA Press) 1994.

13. Yonkers KA. "The association between premenstrual disorder and other mood disorders." *Journal of Clinical Psychiatry* 1997;58(suppl 15): 19–25.

14. Sichel D and Watson J, *Women's Moods* (Quill Publishers) 1999, p. 107.

15. Childress AR, Burns D, "The basics of cognitive therapy." *Psychosomatics* 1981;22 (12):1017–27.

16. Milrod B et al. "Open trial of psychodynamic psychotherapy for panic disorder." *American Journal of Psychiatry* 2000;157(11): 1878–80.

17. Bateman AW, Fonagy P. "Effectiveness of psychotherapeutic treatment of personality disorder." *British Journal of Psychiatry* 2000;177: 138–43.

18. Bateman A, Fonagy P. "Effectiveness of partial hospitalization in the treatment of borderline personality disorder: A randomized controlled trial." *American Journal of Psychiatry* 1999;156(10): 1563–69.

19. McCarty MF. "High-dose pyridoxine as an 'anti-stress' strategy." *Medical Hypotheses* 2000;54(5): 803–807.

20. Wyatt KM et al. "Efficacy of vitamin B-6 in the treatment of premenstrual syndrome: Systematic review." *British Medical Journal* 1999;22;318(7195): 1375–81.

21. Coppen A, Bailey J. "Enhancement of the antidepressant action of fluoxetine by folic acid: A randomized, placebo-controlled trial." *Journal of Affective Disorders* 2000;60 (2): 121–30.

22. Bell IR, Edman JS, Morrow FD, et al. "Vitamin B1, B2 and B6 augmentation of tricyclic antidepressant treatment in geriatric depression with cognitive dysfunction" (Brief Communications). *Journal of the American College of Nutrition* 1992;11(2): 159–63.

23. Stoll AL et al. "Omega -3 fatty acids in bipolar disorder: A preliminary double-blind, placebo-controlled trial." *Archives of General Psychiatry* 1999;56: 407–12.

24. Perovic S, Muller WE. "Pharmacological profile of hypericum extract. Effect on serotonin uptake by postsynaptic receptors." *Arzneimittel-Forschung* 1995; 45: 1145–48.

25. Brenner R, Bjerkenstedt L, Edman GV. "Hypericum perforatum extract (St. John's wort) for depression." *Psychiatric Annals* 2002;32(1): 21–26.

26. Gaster B, Holroyd J. "St John's wort for depression: A systematic review." *Archives of Internal Medicine* 2000;160: 152–56.

27. Schrader E. "Equivalence of St. John's wort extract (Ze 117) and fluoxetine: a randomized, controlled study in mild-moderate depression." *International Clinical Psychopharmacology* 2000;15(2): 61–68.

28. Izzo AA, Ernst E. "Interactions between herbal medicines and prescribed drugs: a systematic review." *Drugs* 2001;61(15): 2162–2175.

29. Gorski JC, Hamman MA, Wang Z, et al. "The effects of St. John's wort on the efficacy of oral contraception." American Society for Clinical Pharmacology and Therapeutics Annual Meeting, March 24–27, 2002, Atlanta, GA; abstract MPI–80.

30. "Monograph: 5-Hydroxytryptophan." *Alternative Medicine Review* 1998; 3(3): 224–26.

31. Murray M. *5-HTP* (New York: Bantam Books) 1998.

32. "Piper methysticum (kava kava)." *Alternative Medicine Review* 1998;3(6): 458–60.

33. Mischoulon D. "The herbal anxiolytics kava and valerian for anxiety and insomnia." *Psychiatric Annals* 2002;32(1):55–60.

34. Pittler MG, Ernst E. "Efficacy of kava extract for treating anxiety: systematic review and meta-analysis." *Journal of Clinical Psychopharmacology* 2000;20(2):84–89.

35. Gaby A. "Kava-liver disease link questioned." *Healthnotes Newswire*, February 28, 2002.

36. "Piper methysticum (kava kava)" *Alternative Medicine Review*. Ibid.

37. Sherwin B. "Estrogen and Memory in Women." *Annals New York Academy of Sciences* 1994;743: 213–31.

38. Limouzin-Lamothe MA, Mairon N, Joyce CR, Le Gal M. "Quality of life after the menopause: Influence of hormonal replacement therapy." *American Journal of Obstetrics and Gynecology* 1994;170(2): 618–24.

39. Yonkers KA. "Antidepressants in the treatment of premenstrual dysphoric disorder." *Journal of Clinical Psychiatry* 1997;58(suppl 14): 4–10.

40. Steiner M, Romano SJ, Babcock S, Dillon J, Shuler C, Berger C, Carter D, Reid R, Stewart D, Steinberg S, Judge R. "The efficacy of fluoxetine in improving physical symptoms associated with premenstrual dysphoric disorder." *British Journal of Gynecology*. 2001;108(5): 462–68.

41. Dunner DL and Laird LK. "Comparative safety and tolerability of nefazodone." *Journal of Clinical Psychiatry* 2002;(63)(suppl 1): 33–38.

42. Caldwell BM, Watson UI. "An evaluation of psychologic effects of sex hormone administration in aged women. Results of therapy after six months." *Journal of Gerontology* 7:228–44.

43. Sherwin B. "Estrogen and Memory in Women." *Annals New York Academy of Sciences* 1994;753: 213–31.

44. LeBlanc ES et al. "Use of HRT may improve cognitive function in certain patients." *Journal of the American Medical Association* 2001;284: 1475–81;1489–99.

45. Fedor-Freybergh P. "The influence of estrogen on the well-being and mental performance in climacteric and postmenopausal women." *Acta Obstetricia et Gynecologica Scandinavica* 1977;64: 5–69.

46. Sichel D, Driscoll J. *Women's Moods* (New York: Quill Publishers) 1999, p. 281.

47. Ibid, p. 280.

48. Fauci AS, Braunwald E, Isselbacher KJ et al. *Principles of Internal Medicine* (New York: McGraw-Hill Publishers) 1998.

49. Henderson VW et al. "Estrogen replacement therapy in older women." *Archives of Neurology* 1994;51: 896–900.

50. Paganini-Hill et al. "Estrogen deficiency and risk of Alzheimer's disease in women." *American Journal of Epidemiology* 1994;140: 256–61.

51. Fillit H et al. "Observations in a preliminary open trial of estradiol therapy for senile dementia-Alzheimer's type." *Journal of Steroid Biochemistry* 1989;34: 521–25.

52. Drachman DA et al. "Estrogen replacement therapy does not reduce Alzheimer's risk." *Archives of Neurology* 2001;58:435–40.

53. Mulnard RA, Cotman CW, Kawas C et al. "Estrogen replacement therapy for treatment of mild to moderate Alzheimer disease: A randomized controlled trial." *Journal of the American Medical Association* 2000;283(8): 1007–15.

54. Yaffe K, Krueger K, Sarkar S, Grady D, Barrett-Connor E, Cox DA, Nickelsen T. "Cognitive function in postmenopausal women treated with raloxifene." *New England Journal of Medicine* 2001;344(16): 1207–13.

55. Kanowski S, Herrmann WM, Stephan K, Wierich W, Horr R. "Proof of efficacy of the ginkgo biloba special extract EGb 761 in outpatients suffering from mild to moderate primary degenerative dementia of the Alzheimer type or multi-infarct dementia." *Pharmacopsychiatry* 1996 Mar;29(2): 47–56.

56. Le Bars PL, Katz MM, Berman N, Itil TM, Freedman AM, Schatzberg AF. "A placebo-controlled, double-blind, randomized trial of an extract of Ginkgo biloba for dementia. North American EGb Study Group." *Journal of the American Medical Association* 1997;278(16): 1327–32.

57. Soholm B. "Clinical improvement of memory and other cognitive functions by Ginkgo biloba: Review of relevant literature." *Advances in Therapy* 1998;(1): 54–65.

58. Perry EK, Pickering AT, Wang WW, Houghton PJ, Perry NS. "Medicinal plants and Alzheimer's disease: From ethnobotany to phytotherapy." *Journal of Pharmacy and Pharmacology* 1999;51(5): 527–34.

59. Van Dongen MC, van Rossum E, Kessels AG, Sielhorst HJ, Knipschild PG. "The efficacy of ginkgo for elderly people with dementia and age-associated memory impairment: New results of a randomized clinical trial." *Journal of the American Geriatric Society* 2000;48(10): 1183–94.

60. Granger AS. "Ginkgo biloba precipitating epileptic seizures." *Age and Ageing*. 2001;30(6): 523–25.

61. Him H. "Isoflavones in soy may attenuate Alzheimer's disease in post-menopausal women." Presented to the 221st National Meeting of the American Chemical Society, Reuters Health, April 3, 2001. *Medscape Women's Health*.

62. Sheehy G. *The Silent Passage* (New York: Pocket Books) 1998, p. 267.

63. Weed S. *The Menopausal Years: The Wise Woman Way.* (Woodstock NY: Ashtree Publishing) 1992, p. 123.

Chapter 10

1. Spadola M. *Breasts.* (Berkeley, CA: Wildcat Canyon Press) 1998, p. 1.

2. Spadola M. ibid, pp. 1–2.

3. National Alliance of Breast Cancer Organizations, New York. 1(800) 719–9154.

4. Sources: National Cancer Institute "Cancer Facts" and the American Cancer Society.

5. Vogel VG. "Breast cancer prevention: A review of current evidence." *Cancer—A Cancer Journal for Clinicians* 2000;50(3): 156–70.

6. Austin S. co-author of *Breast Cancer: What you Should Know (But May Not Be Told) About Prevention, Diagnosis and Treatment)* (Rocklin, CA: Prima Publishing) 1994. p. 167.

7. Kuroishi T, Tominaga S. "[Epidemiology of breast cancer.]" Article in Japanese. *Gan To Kagaku Tyoho* 2001;28(2): 168–73.

8. Wakai K, Suzuki S, Ohno Y, Kawamura T, Tamakoshi A, Aoki R. "Epidemiology of breast cancer in Japan." *International Journal of Epidemiology* 1995;24(2): 285–91.

9. Baghurst PA, Rohan TE. "High-fiber diets and reduced risk of breast cancer." *International Journal of Cancer* 1994 Jan 15;56(2): 173–76.

10. De Stefani E, Correa P, Ronco A, Mendilaharsu M, Guidobono M, Deneo-

Pellegrini H. "Dietary fiber and risk of breast cancer: A case-control study in Uruguay." *Nutrition and Cancer* 1997;28(1): 14–19.

11. Freudenheim JL et al. "Premenopausal breast cancer risk and intake of vegetables, fruits, and related nutrients." *Journal of the National Cancer Institite* 1996;88(6): 340–48.

12. Ahmed MT, Loutfy N, El Shiekh E. "Residue levels of DDE and PCBs in the blood serum of women in the Port Said region of Egypt." *Journal of Hazardous Materials* 2002;89(1): 41–48.

13. Romieu I, Hernandez-Avila M, Lazcano-Ponce E, Weber JP, Dewailly E. "Breast cancer, lactation history, and serum organochlorines." *American Journal of Epidemiology* 2000;152 (4): 363–70.

14. Laden F, Hankinson SE, Wolff MS, Colditz GA, Willett WC, Speizer FE. "Plasma organochlorine levels and the risk of breast cancer; a follow-up in the Nurses' Health Study." *International Journal of Cancer* 2001;91(4)568–74.

15. Snedeker SM. "Pesticides and breast cancer risk: a review of DDT, DDE, and dieldrin." *Environmental Health Perspectives* 2001;109 Suppl 1: 35–47.

16. Duell EJ, Millikan RC, Savitz DA, Newman B, Smith JC, Schell MJ, Sandler DP. "A population-based case-control study of farming and breast cancer in North Carolina." *Epidemiology.* 2000;11(5): 523–31.

17. Hsieh CY, Santell RC, Haslam SZ, Helferich WG "Estrogenic effects of genestein on the growth of estrogen-receptor-positive human breast cancer (MCR-7) cells in vitro and in vivo." *Cancer Research* 1998;58(17):3833–38.

18. Barnes S. "The chemopreventive properties of soy isoflavonoids in animal models of breast cancer." *Breast Cancer Research and Treatment* 1997;46(2–3): 169–79.

19. Lamartiniere CA, Murrill WB, Manzolillo PA, Zhang JX, Barnes S, Zhang X, Wei H, Brown NM, "Genestein alters the ontogeny of mammary gland development and protects against chemically-induced mammary cancer in rats." *Proceedings of the Society for Experimental Biology and Medicine.* 199;217(3): 358–64.

20. Barnes S, ibid.

21. Murkies A, Dailais FS, Briganti EM, Burger HG, Healy DL, Wahlquist ML, Davis SR. "Phytoestrogens and breast cancer in postmenopausal women: a case control study." *Menopause* 2000;7(5): 283–85.

22. Rose DP, Connolly JM. "Regulation of tumor angiogenesis by dietary fatty acids and eicosanoids." *Nutrition and Cancer* 2000;37(2): 119–27. Review.

23. Rose DP, Connolly JM. "Omega-3 fatty acids as cancer chemopreventive agents" *Pharmacology and Therapeutics* 1999;83(3): 217–44. Review.

24. Nakagawa H, Yamamoto D, Kiyozuka Y, Tsuta K, Uemera Y, Hioki K, Tsutsui Y, Tsubura A. "Effects of genestein and synergistic action in combination with eicosapentanoic acid on the growth of breast cancer cells lines." *Journal of Cancer Research and Clinical Oncology* 2000;126(8): 448–54.

25. Schairer C, Lubin J, Triosi R, Sturgeon S, Brinton L, Hoover R. "Menopause estrogen and estrogen-progestin replacement therapy and breast cancer risk." *Journal of the American Medical Association* 2000;283:485–91.

26. Rockhill B, Willett WC, Hunter DJ, Manson JE, Hankinson SE, Colditz GA, "A prospective study of recreational physical activity and breast cancer risk." *Archives of Internal Medicine* 1999;159(19): 2290–96.

27. Latikka P, Pukkala E, Vihko V. "Relationship between the risk of breast cancer and physical activity. An epidemiological perspective." *Sports Medicine* 1998 Sep;26(3): 133–43.

28. McTiernan A, "Physical activity and the prevention of breast cancer." *Medscape Womens Health* 2000;5(5): E1.

29. Jansen MA, Muenz LR. "A retrospective study of personality variables associated with fibrocystic disease and breast cancer." *Journal of Psychosomatic Research* 1984;28(1): 35–42.

30. Lilja A, Smith G, Malmstrom P, Salford LG, Idvall I. "Psychological profile related to malignant tumours of different histopathology." *Psychooncology* 1998;7(5): 376–86.

31. Gilbar O. "The connection between the psychological condition of breast cancer patients and survival. A follow-up after eight years." *General Hospital Psychiatry* 1996; 18(4): 266–70.

32. Weihs KL, Enright TM, Simmens SJ, Reiss D. "Negative affectivity, restriction of emotions, and site of metastases predict mortality in recurrent breast cancer." *Journal of Psychosomatic Research.* 2000;49(1): 59–68.

33. Watson M, Haviland JS, Greer S, Davidson J, Bliss JM "Influence of psychological response on survival in breast cancer: A population-bascohort study." *Lancet* 1999; 354(9187): 1331–36.

34. Stanton AL, Danoff-Burg S, Cameron CL, Bishop M, Collins CA, Kirk SB, Sworowski LA, Twillman R. "Emotionally expressive coping predicts psychological and physical adjustment to breast cancer." *Journal of Consulting and Clinical Psychology* 2000; 68(5): 875–82.

35. National Cancer Institute, U.S. National Institutes of Health.

36. Persson K, Ek AC, Svensson PG. "Factors affecting women to practice breast self-examination." *Scandinavian Journal of Caring Sciences* 1997;11(4): 224–31.

37. Weed, S. *Breast Cancer? Breast Health!* (Woodstock, NY, Ash Tree Publishing) 1996, p. 57.

38. Weed S. Ibid.

39. Dooley WC, Veronesi U, O'Shaughnessy J, Ljung B-M, Arias R, "Detection of premalignant and malignant breast cells by ductal lavage." *Obstetrics and Gynecology* 2001;97: 2S.

40. Dooley WC, Ljung BM, Veronesi U, Cazzaniga M, et al. "Ductal lavage for detection of cellular atypia in women at high risk for breast cancer." *Journal of the National Cancer Institute* 2001;93(21):1624–1632.

41. Disaia et al. "Hormone replacement therapy in breast cancer survivors; A cohort study." *American Journal of Obstetrics and Gynecology* 1996; 174;1494–98.

42. Jacobson JS, Troxel AB, Evans J, Klaus L, Vahdat L, Kinne D, Lo KM, Moore A, Rosenman PJ, Kaufman EL, Neugut AI, Grann VR. "Randomized trial of black cohosh for the treatment of hot flashes among women with a history of breast cancer." *Journal of Clinical Oncology* 2001;19(10): 2739–45.

43. Einer-Jensen N, Zhao J, Andersen KP, Kristoffersen K. "Cimicifuga and Melbrosia lack oestrogenic effects in mice and rats." *Maturitas* 1996;25:149–53.

44. Liu J, Burdette JE, Xu H, Gu C, van Breemen RB, Bhat KP, Booth N, Constantinou AI, Pezzuto JM, Fong HH, Farnsworth NR, Bolton JL. "Evaluation of estrogenic activity of plant extracts for the potential treatment of menopausal symptoms." *Journal of Agricultural and Food Chemistry* 2001;49(5):2472–79.

45. Dixon-Shanies D, Shaikh N. "Growth inhibition of human breast cancer cells by herbs and phytoestrogens." *Oncology Reports* 1999;6(6): 1383–87.

46. Jarry H, Harnischfeger G, Duker E. [The endocrine effects of constituents of Cimicifuga racemosa. 2. In vitro binding of constituents to estrogen receptors] [article in German]. *Planta Medica* 1985;(4): 316–19.

47. Blumenthal M, Busse WR, Goldberg A, Gruenwald J, Hall T, Riggins CW, et al. Eds. Klein S, Rister RS. Trans. *The Complete German Commission E Monographs Therapeutic Guide to Herbal Medicines* (Austin, TX: American Botanical Council; Boston: Integrative Medicine Communications) 1998, p. 90.

48. Nesselhut T, Schellhas C, Deitrich R, Kuhn W. "Examination of the proliferative potential of phytopharmaceuticals with estrogen-mimicking action in breast carcinoma." *Archives of Gynecology and Obstetrics* 1993;817–18.

49. Zava DT, Dollbaum CM, Blen M. "Estrogen and progestin bioactivity of foods, herbs, and spices." *Proceedings of the Society for Expermental Biology and Medicine* 1998;217 (3):369–78.

50. Wang W, Tanaka Y, Han Z, Higuchi CM. "Proliferative response of mammary glandular tissue to formononetin." *Nutrition and Cancer* 1995;23(2):131–40.

51. Polkowski K, Mazurek AP. "Biological properties of genestein. A review of in vitro and in vivo data." *Acta Poloniae Pharmaceutica* 2000;57(2): 135–55.

52. Fotsis T, Pepper MS, Montesano R, Aktas E, Breit S, Schweigerer L, Rasku S, Wahala K, Adlercreutz H. "Phytoestrogens and inhibition of angiogenesis." *Bailliere's Clinical Endocrinology and Metabolism* 1998;12(4): 649–66. Review.

53. Fotsis T, Pepper MS, Montesano R, Aktas E, Breit S, Schweigerer L, Rasku S, Wahala K, Adlercreutz H. "Phytoestrogens and inhibition of angiogenesis, Ibid.

54. Fotsis T, Pepper MS, Aktas E, Breit S, Rasku S, Adlercreutz H, Wahala K, Montesano R, Schweigerer L. Flavonoids, dietary-derived inhibitors of cell proliferation and in vitro angiogenesis. *Cancer Research* 1997;57(14):2916–21.

55. Polkowski K, Mazurek AP. "Biological properties of genestein."

56. Polkowski K, Mazurek AP. Ibid.

57. Barnes S, Sfakianos J, Coward L, Kirk M. "Soy isoflavonoids and cancer prevention. Underlying biochemical and pharmacological issues." *Advances in Experimental Medicine and Biology* 1996;401: 87–100.

58. Santell RC, Kieu N, Helferich WG. "Genestein inhibits growth of estrogen-independent human breast cancer cells in culture but not in athymic mice." *Journal of Nutrition* 2000;130(7): 1665–69.

59. Barnes S. "The chemopreventive properties of soy isoflavonoids in animal models of breast cancer." *Breast Cancer Research and Treatment* 1997 Nov-Dec;46(2–3): 169–79.

60. Quella SK, Loprinzi CL, Barton DL, Knost JA et al. "Evaluation of soy phytoestrogens for the treatment of hot flashes in breast cancer survivors: A North Central Cancer Treatment Group Trial." *Journal of Clinical Oncology* 2000;18(5): 1068–74.

61. Barton DL, Loprinzi CL, Quella SK, Sloan JA, Veeder MH et al. "Prospective evaluation of vitamin E for hot flashes in breast cancer survivors." *Journal of Clinical Oncology* 1998;16(2): 495–500.

62. Warnecke G. "Psychosomatische Dysfunktionen im Weiblichen Klimakterium. Klinische Wirksamkeit und Vertraeglichkeit von Kava-Extrakt WS 1490." *Fortschritte der Medizin* 1991;109(4): 119–22.

63. Barton D, Loprinzi C, Wahner-Roedler D. "Hot flashes: Aetiology and management." *Drugs and Aging* 2001;18(8): 597–606.

Chapter 11

1. Colborn T, Dumanoski D, Peterson Myers J. *Our Stolen Future* (New York: Penguin) 1997, p. 48.

2. Duell EJ, Millikan RC, Savitz DA, Newman B, Smith JC, Schell MJ, Sandler DP. "A population-based case-control study of farming and breast cancer in North Carolina." *Epidemiology* 2000;11(5): 524–31.

3. Millikan R, DeVoto E, Duell EJ, Tse CK, Savitz DA, Beach J, Edmiston S, Jackson S, Newman B. "Dichlorodiphenyldichloroethene, polychlorinated biphenyls, and breast cancer among African-American and white women in North Carolina." *Cancer Epidemiology, Biomarkers and Prevention* 2000;9(11): 1233–40.

4. Romieu I, Hernandez-Avila M, Lazcano-Ponce E, Weber JP, Dewailly E. "Breast cancer, lactation history, and serum organochlorines." *American Journal of Epidemiology* 2000:15:152(4): 363–70.

5. Colborn T, Dumanoski D, Peterson Myers J. *Our Stolen Future,* p. 112.

6. Gore A. Foreword to *Our Stolen Future,* ibid., p.viii.

7. Whitten PL, Russell E, Naftolin F. "Influence of phytoestrogen diets on estradiol action in the rat uterus." *Steroids* 1994:59(7):443–9.

8. Medlock KL, Branham WS, Sheehan DM. "Effects of coumestrol and equol on

the developing reproductive tract of the rat." *Proceedings of the Society for Experimental Biology and Medicine* 1995;208(1): 679–71.

9. Gray K. "Estrogens, Progestins, and Bone." World Congress on Osteoporosis 2000, *Medscape Women's Health* (www.medscape.com/womenshealthhome).

10. *American College of Gynecology Educational Bulletin* 1998;May (no. 247).

11. Troisi RJ, Speizer FE, Willett WC, Trichopoulos D, Rosner B. "Menopause, post-menopausal estrogen preparations, and the risk of adult-onset asthma. A prospective cohort study." *American Journal of Respiratory and Critical Care Medicine* 1995;152(4 Pt 1): 1183–88.

12. Myers JR, Sherman CB. "Should supplemental estrogens be used as steroid-sparing agents in asthmatic women?" *Chest* 1994;106(1): 318–19.

13. Rodriguez C, Patel AV, Calle EE, Jacob EJ, Thun MJ. "Estrogen replacement therapy and ovarian cancer mortality in a large prospective study of US women." *Journal of the American Medical Association* 2001;285(11): 1460–65.

14. Garg PP, Kerlikowske K, Subak L, Grady D. "Hormone replacement therapy and the risk of epithelial ovarian carcinoma: A meta-analysis." *Obstetrics and Gynecology* 1998;92(3): 472–79.

15. Speroff L, Glass RH, Kase NG. *Clinical Gynecologic Endocrinology and Infertility,* (Baltimore MD: Lippincott, Williams and Wilkins) 1999, p. 624.

16. Genant HK, Lucas J, Weiss S, Akin M, Emkey R, McNaney-Flint H, Downs R, Mortola J, Watts N, Yang HM, Banav N, Brennan JJ, Nolan JC. "Low-Dose Esterified Estrogen Therapy: Effects on Bone, Plasma Estradiol Concentrations, Endometrium and Lipid Levels." *Archives of Internal Medicine* 1997;157:2609–15.

17. Longcompe C. "Estriol production and metabolism in normal women." *Journal of Steroid Biochemistry* 1984;20: 959–62.

18. Head KA. "Estriol: Safety and efficacy." *Alternative Medicine Review* 1998(2): 101–13. Review

19. Takahashi K, Okada M, Ozaki T, Kurioka H, Manabe A, Kanasaki H, Miyazaki K. "Safety and efficacy of oestriol for symptoms of natural or surgically induced menopause." *Human Reproduction* 2000;15(5): 1028–36.

20. Head KA. "Estriol . . ."

21. Arteaga E, Villaseca P, Rojas A, Arteaga A, Bianchi M. "[Comparison of the antioxidant effect of estriol and estradiol on low density lipoproteins in post-menopausal women]" [article in Spanish]. *Revista Medica de Chile* 1998;126(5): 481–87.

22. Nishibe A, Morimoto S, Hirota K, Yasuda O, Ikegami H, Yamamoto T, Fukuo K, Onishi T, Ogihara T. "Effect of estriol and bone density of lumbar vertebrae in elderly and postmenopausal women." [article in Japanese] *Nippon Ronen Igakkai Zashi* 1996;33(5): 353–59.

23. Itoi H, Minakami H, Iwasaki R, Sato I. "Comparison of the long-term effects of oral estriol with the effects of conjugated estrogen on serum lipid profile in early menopausal women." *Maturitas* 2000;31;36(3): 217–22.

24. Toy JL, Davies JA, McNicol GP. "The effects of long-term therapy with oestriol succinate on the haemostatic mechanism in postmenopausal women." *British Journal of Obstetrics and Gynecology* 1978;85: 363–66.

25. Tzingounis VA et al. "Estriol in the management of the menopause." *Journal of the American Medical Association* 1978;239: 1638–41.

26. Follingstad AH. "Estriol: The forgotten estrogen?" *Journal of the American Medical Association* 1978;239(1): 29–30.

27. Lemon HM. "Estriol prevention of mammary carcinoma induced by 7, 12-dimethylbenzanthracene and procarbazine." *Cancer Research* 1975; 35: 1341–53.

28. Follingstad AH. "Estriol: The forgotten estrogen."

29. Lippman M, Monaco M, Bolan, G. "Effects of estrone, estradiol and estriol on hormone-responsive human breast cancer in long-term tissue culture." *Cancer Research* 1977;17:1901–1907.

30. Wright J, Schliesman B, Robinson L. "Comparative measurements of serum estriol, estradiol, and estrone in non–pregnant, premenopausal women: A preliminary investigation." *Alternative Medicine Review* 1999;4(4): 266–70.

31. Nahata MC. "Licensing of medicine for children in the USA," *Pediatric and Perinatal Drug Therapy,* May, 1997, and Pfizer Inc., "The Value and Costs of Pharmaceuticals: Questions and Answers," 2000/2001, www.pfizer.com.

32. Warren MP, Shantha S. "Uses of progesterone in clinical practice." *International Journal of Fertility and Women's Medicine* 1999;44(2): 96–103.

33. Menopause Online, a division of Third Age. www.menopause-online.com/progestins.htm.

34. Speroff L, Glass RH, Kase NG. *Clinical Gynecologic Endocrinology and Infertility,* p. 623.

35. "HRT" Mayo Clinic Women's Healthsource, August 1999.

36. Hargrove J, Maxson, W et al. "Menopausal Hormone Replacement Therapy with Continuous Daily Oral Mictonized Estradiol and Progesterone." *Obstetrics and Gynecology* 1989;73(4): 606–12.

37. De Lignieres B. "Oral Micronized Progesterone." *Clinical Therapeutics* 1999; 21(1): 41–50.

38. Bolaji II, Mortimer G, Grimes H, Tallon DF, O'Dwyer E, Fottrell PF. "Clinical evaluation of near-continuous oral micronized progesterone therapy in estrogenized postmenopausal women." *Gynecological Endocrinology* 1996;10(1): 41–47.

39. Hargrove J, Maxson W et al. "Menopausal hormone replacement therapy."

40. O'Leary P, Feddema P, Chan K, Taranto M, Smith M, Evans S. "Salivary, but not serum or urinary levels of progesterone are elevated after topical application of progesterone cream to pre- and postmenopausal women." *Clinical Endocrinology* (Oxf) 2000;53(5): 615–20.

41. Carey BU, Carey AH, Patel S, Carter G, Studd JW. "A study to evaluate serum and urinary hormone levels following short and long term administration of two regimens of progesterone cream in postmenopausal women." BJOG: *An International Journal of Obstetrics and Gynecology* 2000;107(6): 722–26.

42. Burry KA, Patton PE, Hermsmeyer K "Percutaneous absorption of progesterone in postmenopausal women treated with transdermal estrogen." *American Journal of Obstetrics and Gynecology* 1999;180(6 Pt1): 1504–11.

43. Warren MP, Shantha S. "Uses of progesterone in clinical practice." *International Journal of Fertility and Women's Medicine* 1999;44(2): 96–103. Review

44. Komesaroff PA, Black CV, Cable V, Sudhir K. "Effects of wild yam extract on menopausal symptoms, lipids and sex hormones in healthy menopausal women." *Climacteric* 2001;4(2): 144–150.

45. Cicinelli E, de Ziegler D, Bulletti C, Matteo MG, Schonauer LM, Galantino P. "Direct transport of progesterone from vagina to uterus." *Obstetrics and Gynecology* 2000;95(3):403–406.

46. De Ziegler D, Ferriani R, Moraes LA, Bulletti C. "Vaginal progesterone in menopause: Crinone 4% in cyclical and constant combined regimens." *Human Reproduction* 2000;15 Suppl 1: 149–58.

47. Davis SR, Tran J. "Testosterone influences libido and well being in women." *Trends in Endocrinology and Metabolism* 2001;12(1):33–37.

48. Davis SR, McCloud P, Strauss BJ, Burger H. "Testosterone enhances estradiol's effect/s on postmenopausal bone density and sexuality." *Maturitas* 1995;21(3): 227–36.

49. Davis SR. "The therapeutic use of androgens in women." *Journal of Steroid Biochemistry and Molecular Biology* 1999;69(1–6): 177–84.

50. Burger HG, Dudley E, Cui J, Dennerstein L, Hopper JL. "A prospective longitudinal study of serum testosterone, dehydroepiandrosterone sulfate, and sex hormone-binding globulin levels through the menopause transition." *Journal of Clinical Endocrinology and Metabolism* 2000;85(8): 2832–38.

51. Burger HG, Dudley E, Cui J, Dennerstein L, Hopper JL. Ibid.

52. Stomati M, Monteleone P, Casarosa E et al. "Six-month oral dyhydroepiandros-terone supplementation in early and late postmenopause." *Gynecological Endocrinology* 2000;14(5): 342–63.

53. Villareal DT, Holloszy JO, Kohrt WM. "Effects of DHEA replacement on bone mineral density and body composition in elderly women and men." *Clinical Endocrinology* (Oxf) 2000;53(5): 561–68.

54. Curtis MG. "Selective Estrogen Receptor Modulators: A Controversial Approach for Managing Postmenopausal Health." *Journal of Women's Health* 1999;3(3): 323.

55. Curtis MG. Ibid.

56. Etingin O. M.D. "Estrogen vs. Raloxifene." *Women's Health Advisor, Cornell University Medical College,* "Estrogen vs. Raloxifene, Aug, 1998.

57. Matthews J, Celius T, Halgren R, Zacharewski T. "Differential estrogen receptor binding of estrogenic substances: a species comparison." *Journal of Steroid Biochemistry and Molecular Biology* 2000;74(4): 223–34.

58. Whitten PL, Patisaul HB. "Cross-Species and Interassay: Comparisons of Phytoestrogen Action." *Environmental Health Perspectives* 2001;109 Suppl 1: 5–20.

59. Tamir S, Eizenberg M, Somjen D, Stern N, Shelach R, Kaye A, Vaya J. "Estrogenic and antiproliferative properties of glabridin from licorice in human breast cancer cells." *Cancer Research* 2000;60(20): 5704–7099.

60. Cotroneo MS, Wang J, Eltoum IA, Lamartiniere CA. "Sex steroid receptor regulation by genestein in the prepubertal rat uterus." *Molecular and Cellular Endocrinology* 2001;173(1–2):135–145.

Chapter 12

1. SEER. *Cancer Statistics Review,* 1973–1994. National Cancer Institute, NIH publication No. 97–2789.

2. Shike M. "Body weight and colon cancer." *American Journal of Clinical Nutrition* 1996;63(3 Suppl): 442S–44S.

3. Slattery ML. "Diet, lifestyle, and colon cancer." *Seminars in Gastrointestinal Disease* 2000;11(3): 142–46.

4. Potter JD, Bostick RM, Grandits GA, Fosdick L, Elmer P, Wood J, Grambsch P, Louis TA. "Hormone replacement therapy is associated with lower risk of adenomatous polyps of the large bowel: The Minnesota Cancer Prevention Research Unit Case-Control Study" *Cancer Epidemiology Biomarkers and Prevention* 1996;5: 779–84.

5. Paganini-Hill A. "Morbidity and mortality changes with estrogen replacement therapy." In Lobo RA. (Ed.) *Treatment of the Perimenopausal Woman: Basic and Clinical Aspects.* Second Edition. (Philadelphia: Lippincott Williams & Wilkens) 1999.

6. Grodstein F, Newcomb PA, Stampfer MJ. "Postmenopausal hormone therapy and the risk of colorectal cancer: A review and meta-analysis." *American Journal of Medicine* 1999;106: 574–82.

7. Nanda et al. "HRT and the risk of colorectal cancer: A meta-analysis." *Obstetrics and Gynecology* 1999;93: 880–88.

8. Lointier et al. "The effects of steroid hormones on a human colon cancer line in vitro." *Anticancer Research* 1992,12: 1327–30.

9. Colditz GA, Cannuscio CC, Frazier A. "Physical activity and reduced risk of colon cancer: Implications for prevention." *Cancer Causes and Control* 1997;8(4): 649–67.

10. Augustsson K, Skog K, Jagerstad M, Steineck G. "Assessment of the human exposure to heterocyclic amines." *Carcinogenesis* 1997;18(10): 1931–35.

11. Layton DW, Bogen KT, Knize MG, Hatch FT, Johnson VM, Felton JS. "Cancer risk of heterocyclic amines in cooked foods: An analysis and implications for research." *Carcinogenesis* 1995;16(1): 39–52.

12. Michels KB, Giovannucci E, Joshipura KJ, Rosner BA, Stampfer MJ, Fuchs CS, Colditz GA, Speizer FE, Willett WC. "Prospective study of fruit and vegetable consumption and incidence of colon and rectal cancers." *Journal of the National Cancer Institute* 2000;92(21): 1740–52.

13. Voorrips LE, Goldbohm RA, van Poppel G, Sturmans F, Hermus RJ, van den Brandt PA. "Vegetable and fruit consumption and risks of colon and rectal cancer in a prospective cohort study: The Netherlands Cohort Study on Diet and Cancer." *American Journal of Epidemiology* 2000;1;152(11): 1081–92.

14. Zhou SB, Wang GJ, Zhu Y, Chen BQ. "Effect of dietary fatty acids on colon tumorigenesis induced by methyl nitrosourea in rats." *Biomedicine and Environmental Sciences* 2000;13(2):105–16.

15. Bujanda L. "The effects of alcohol consumption upon the gastrointestinal tract." *American Journal of Gastroenterology* 2000;95(12): 3374–82.

16. Kono S, Ahn YO. "Vegetables, cereals and colon cancer mortality: Long-term trend in Japan." *European Journal of Cancer Prevention* 2000;9(5):363–65.

17. Grasten SM, Juntunen KS, Poutanen KS, Gylling HK, Miettinen TA, Mykkanen HM. "Rye bread improves bowel function and decreases the concentrations of some compounds that are putative colon cancer risk markers in middle-aged women and men." *Journal of Nutrition* 2000;130(9): 2215–21.

18. Reddy BS, Hirose Y, Cohen LA, Simi B, Cooma I, Rao CV. "Preventive potential of wheat bran fractions against experimental colon carcinogenesis: Implications for human colon cancer prevention." *Cancer Research* 2000;60(17): 4792–97.

19. Nagao M, Sugimura T. "Carcinogenic factors in food with relevance to colon cancer development." *Mutation Research* 1993;290(1): 43–51.

20. p,p'-dichloro-diphenyldicholoroethylene and dichloro-diphenyl-trichloroanthane, respectively.

21. Soliman AS, Smith MA, Cooper SP, Ismail K, Khaled H, Ismail S, McPherson RS, Seifeldin IA, Bondy ML. "Serum organochlorine pesticide levels in patients with colorectal cancer in Egypt. *Archives of Environmental Health* 1997;52(6): 409–15.

22. Shike M. "Body weight and colon cancer." *American Journal of Clinical Nutrition* 1996;63(3 Suppl): 442S–44S.

23. Nadkar MY, Samant RS, Vaidya SS, Borges NE. "Relationship between osteoarthritis of knee and menopause." *Journal of the Association of Physicians of India* 1999;47(12)· 1161–63

24. Felson DT, Nevitt MC "The effects of estrogen on osteoarthritis." *Current Opinions in Rheumatogy* 1998;10(3): 269–72.

25. Wluka AE, Davis SR, Bailey M, Stuckey SL, Cicuttini FM. "Users of oestrogen replacement therapy have more knee cartilage than non-users." *Annals of Rheumatic Diseases* 2001;60(4): 332–36.

26. Maheu E, Dreiser RL, Guillou GB, Dewailly J. "Hand osteoarthritis patients' characteristics according to the existence of a hormone replacement therapy." *Osteoarthritis Cartilage* 2000;8 Suppl A: S33–37.

27. Hochberg MC. "What a Difference a Year Makes: Reflections on the ACR Recommendations for the Medical Management of Osteoarthritis." *Current Rheumatology Reports.* 2001;3(6): 473–78.

28. Reginster JY, Deroisy R, Rovati LC, Lee RL, Lejeune E, Bruyere O, Giacovelli G, Henrotin Y, Dacre JE, Gossett C. "Long-term effects of glucosamine sulphate on osteoarthritis progression: A randomised, placebo-controlled clinical trial." *Lancet* 2001; 357(9252): 251–56.

29. Hochberg MC. "What a Difference a Year Makes: Reflections on the ACR Recommendations for the Medical Management of Osteoarthritis." *Current Rheumatology Reports.* 2001;3(6): 473–78.

30. Johnson KA, Hulse DA, Hart RC, Kochevar D, Chu Q. "Effects of an orally administered mixture of chondroitin sulfate, glucosamine hydrochloride and manganese ascorbate on synovial fluid chondroitin sulfate 3B3 and 7D4 epitope in a

canine cruciate ligament transection model of osteoarthritis." *Osteoarthritis and Cartilage* 2001;9(1):14–21.

31. Von Wowern et al. "Osteoporosis: A risk factor in periodontal disease." *Journal of Periodontology* 1994;65(12): 1134–38.

32. Grodstein F, Colditz GA, Stampfer MJ "Post-menopausal hormone use and tooth loss: A prospective study." *Journal of the American Dental Association* 1996;127: 370–77.

33. Otomo-Corgel J. "Periodontal Disease in Midlife Women." *Menopause Management* 2000:9(2): 14–18.

34. Petti S, Cairella G, Tarsitani G. "Nutritional variables related to gingival health in adolescent girls." *Community Dentistry and Oral Epidemiology* 2000;28(6): 407–13.

35. Genco RJ, Ho AW, Grossi SG, Dunford RG, Tedesco LA. "Relationship of stress, distress and inadequate coping behaviors to periodontal disease." *Journal of Periodontology* 1999;70(7): 711–23.

36. Congdon NG, West KP Jr. "Nutrition and the eye." *Current Opinions in Ophthalmology* 1999;10(6): 464–73.

37. McDermott JH. "Antioxidant nutrients: Current dietary recommendations and research update. *Journal of the American Pharmacy Association* (Wash) 2000;40(6): 785–99.

38. Delcourt C, Cristol JP, Tessier F, Leger CL, Descomps B, Papoz L. "Age-related macular degeneration and antioxidant status in the POLA study. POLA Study Group. Pathologies Oculaires Liees a l'Age." *Archives of Ophthalmology* 1999;117(10): 1384–90.

39. Richer S. "Multicenter ophthalmic and nutritional age-related macular degeneration study—part 2: Antioxidant intervention and conclusions." *Journal of the American Optometric Association* 1996;67(1): 30–49.

40. Diamond BJ, Shiflett SC, Feiwel N, Matheis RJ, Noskin O, Richards JA, Schoenberger NE. "Ginkgo biloba extract: Mechanisms and clinical indications." *Archives of Physical Medicine and Rehabilitation* 2000;81(5):668–78.

41. Yannuzzi LA, et al. "Risk Factors for Neovascular Age-Related Macular Degeneration." *Archives of Opthalmology,*1992;110: 1701–1708.

42. Smith W, Mitchell P, Wang JJ. "Gender, oestrogen, hormone replacement and age-related macular degeneration: Results from the Blue Mountains Eye Study." *Australian and New Zealand Journal of Opthamology* 1997;25(Suppl 1): 513–15.

43. Hammond CB. "Therapeutic options for menopausal health: Combating aging and disease." Monograph. July 2000, vol 2, pp. 30–32.

44. Mares-Perlman JA, Lyle BJ, Klein R, Fisher AI, Brady WE, VandenLangenberg GM, Trabulsi JN, Palta M. "Vitamin supplement use and incident cataracts in a population-based study. *Archives of Ophthalmology.* 2000;118(11): 1556–63.

45. Metka M, Enzelsberger H, Knogler W, Schurz B, Aichmar H. "Opthalmic complaints as a climacteric symptom." *Maturitas* 1991;14: 3–8.

INDEX

trans fatty acids, 107
trazodone, 220
tricyclic antidepressants (TCAs), 218
Tri-/Bi-est, 263–65

ultrasound bone density tests, 148, 150, 151, 153
ultraviolet (UV) radiation, 88–89
unopposed estrogen, 26, 266
urinary issues, 13
urinary symptoms, remedies for, 186–87
urinary urgency, 183, 184, 187
uterine artery embolization, 42
uterine cancer, 26
uterine fibroids, 6, 16, 255
Utian, W. H., 26

vaginal dryness, 172–74, 173(fig.); remedies for, 185–86, 249–50
vaginal estrogen tablets, 186
vaginal infections, 12, 182–83
vaginal issues, 12
vaginal pH, 173–74
vaginal ring, estradiol-releasing, 186, 187
valerian, 73
vasomotor changes, 11, 18, 58; choosing the right remedy for you, 75–76; heart palpitations, 61–62; hot flashes and night sweats, 58–60; keeping up with your changing body, 76–77; non-hormonal remedies for vasomotor symptoms, 248–49; perimenopausal insomnia, 60–61; remedies for, 62–75, 64(table); vasomotor symptom relief and breast cancer, 245–48
venlafaxine, 219
viable eggs, 5, 5(fig.), 44
Viagra®, 190–91
Vienne, Veronique, 94
vitamin B6: for heart health, 116; for mental wellness, 212; for PMS symptoms, 53
vitamin C: for hot flashes, 67; for iron absorption, 50–51
vitamin D, for bone health, 19, 140–41, 160–61
vitamin E: for heart health, 116–17; for hot

flashes, 67; vitamin E oil for vaginal dryness, 185, 249
vitamins, minerals, and bone health, 144–45
vitex, 44, 54, 56, 70
von Bingen, Hildegard, 31

warfarin, 48
Weed, Susun, 201, 225, 241
weight: adolescent weight, 101, 103; bone density and, 133; exercise and, 85–86; heart disease and, 100–101; optimal weight plan, 112; thin women and menopause, 9–10; weight chart, 102(fig.); weight gain, 13–14;weight loss, 110–11; weight-loss approaches using supplements, 86–87; weight loss using HRT, 87–88
weight-bearing activity, for bone density, 137–38
Whole Lesbian Sex Book: A Passionate Guide for All of Us, The (Newman), 179
Whole Soy Cookbook, The (Greenberg), 64
wild yam creams, 70, 271–72
Wilson, Robert, 24–25, 26
Winfrey, Oprah, 34
Wolman, Roger, 163–64
Women's Encyclopedia of Natural Medicine (Hudson), 42
Women's Health Initiative (WHI) Study, 164–65, 255, 257
Women's Moods (Sichel and Driscoll), 194–95, 207–8
workplace, menopause in the, 29
World Congress on Osteoporosis 2000, 164, 165–66
World Health Organization (WHO), 148, 151
Wright, Jonathan, 263
wrinkles, 88
Wyshak, Grace, 144

xeno-estrogens, 254

yarrow, 46
your menopause is unique, 36